LIBRARY
EDUCATION CENTRE
PRINCESS ROYAL HOSPITAL

W 20 HoL £2

KT-148-498

Qualitative Research in Health Care

TELFORD
CB014261

Qualitative Research in Health Care

Edited by Immy Holloway

Open University Press

Open University Press
McGraw-Hill Education
McGraw-Hill House
Shoppenhangers Road
Maidenhead
Berkshire
England
SL6 2QL

email: enquiries@openup.co.uk
world wide web: www.openup.co.uk

and Two Penn Plaza, New York, NY 10121–2289, USA

First published 2005

Copyright © Immy Holloway 2005. Individual chapters © The Contributors 2005

All rights reserved. Except for the quotation of short passages for the purposes of criticism and review, no part of this publication may be reproduced, stored in a retrieval system, or transmitted, in any form, or by any means, electronic, mechanical, photocopying, recording or otherwise, without the prior permission of the publisher or a licence from the Copyright Licensing Agency Limited. Details of such licences (for reprographic reproduction) may be obtained from the Copyright Licensing Agency Ltd of 90 Tottenham Court Road, London, W1T 4LP.

A catalogue record of this book is available from the British Library

ISBN -13: 978 0335 21293 4 (pb) 978 0335 21294 1 (hb)
ISBN -10: 0 335 21293 X (pb) 0 335 21294 8 (hb)

Library of Congress Cataloging-in-Publication Data
CIP data applied for

Typeset by YHT Ltd, London
Printed in the Poland by OzGraf. S.A.
www.polskabook.pl

To my grandchildren, Hazel, Dochas and Chian.

Contents

Notes on contributors

Mark Avis is Reader in Social Contexts of Health at the University of Nottingham with a Master's degree in the Sociology of Health and Illness and a degree in philosophy. He is also a registered nurse, and has practised in both acute mental health and health care of the elderly settings. His research and publications have focused on patient and user experiences of care and, more recently, on the use of health- and social-care services by people from deprived communities, minority ethnic groups, or who are excluded because of mental health problems. He has taken the opportunity to apply his continued interest in philosophy to a critical analysis of the epistemological basis of qualitative techniques in health- and social-care research.

Dr Rosalind Bluff was a Midwifery Lecturer at the School of Nursing and Midwifery, in the University of Southampton and has recently retired. She is an experienced midwife and lecturer with a particular interest in qualitative research and the contribution it can make to the provision of quality midwifery care. She is co-editor of *Principles and Practice of Research in Midwifery* published by Bailliére Tindall in 2000; a second edition is in preparation.

Professor Dawn Freshwater PhD currently holds the position of Chair, Faculty of Regional Professional Studies at the Southwest (Bunbury) Campus of Edith Cowan University Australia. She is also Director of the Centre for Regional Development and Research and Professor in Primary Health Care and Mental Health at Bournemouth University in the United Kingdom. Professor Freshwater is the editor of the *Journal of Psychiatric and Mental Health Nursing*; the President of the International Association for Human Caring and a Director of the Florence Nightingale Foundation in the UK. She was awarded a Fellowship of the Royal College of Nursing in 2002 for her contribution to nursing. She has authored over 100 peer-reviewed papers and books and has co-edited texts relating to research, practice improvement, reflective practice and therapeutic nursing. In 2004 she published three books.

Professor Kathleen Galvin PhD is Chair in Health Research and currently Head of Research at IHCS, Bournemouth University. She has been involved in over 20 evaluation projects of services in health- and social-care sector. Professor Galvin's background is in nursing and her areas of interest and expertise comprise action research in a range of contexts, multiple methods in service evaluation, user involvement and perspectives, health promotion, nursing practice development and evaluation, and issues in doctoral education. Professor Galvin has an active role in the International Network for Doctoral Education in Nursing, and currently is an editorial board member of *Journal of Clinical Nursing* (Blackwell Publishing). She has published widely and her publications include several articles in the area of qualitative evaluation.

Professor Immy Holloway PhD was a medical sociologist who specialised in the area of qualitative research. Retired from full-time work a few years ago, she still works part-time in the Institute of Health and Community Studies, Bournemouth University and leads its Centre for Qualitative Research with Les Todres. Her interest lies in all areas of qualitative research, particularly in patient/client and professional perspectives on health and illness. Having written extensively in this field, she is the author and co-author of several books, some of which have been translated into languages other than English. Her most recent book is *Qualitative Research in Nursing*, 2nd edn, Oxford: Blackwell, which was written with Stephanie Wheeler.

Dr Ron Iphofen is Director of Postgraduate Research in the Faculty of Health, University of Wales, Bangor. He is recent past Vice Chair of the Social Research Association, led the updating of the Association's ethical guidelines and is currently engaged on a European Union project to establish professional standards in socio-economic research. He has contributed chapters to edited collections on public health and health research. His clinical work is in hypnotherapy. His textbook *Sociology in Practice for Health Professionals* was published by Macmillan in 1998. He has also been involved with developing an EU code of ethics and is publishing a website on ethical issues in cross-national research.

Professor Jenny Kitzinger PhD is Professor of Media and Communication Research at the Cardiff School of Journalism, Media and Cultural Studies, Cardiff University. She is co-editor of *Developing Focus Group Research: politics, theory and practice* (Sage, 1999). Her most recent book, *Framing Abuse: media influence and public understanding of sexual violence against children* was published by Pluto Press (2004). Besides writing and co-writing books, Professor Kitzinger has also published over 100 chapters and articles in well known journals.

Dr Debbie Kralik holds the position of Senior Research Fellow with the University of South Australia and the Royal District Nursing Service Research Unit. Committed to collaborative inquiry and as a strategy to foster ongoing dialogue with women, she has initiated, developed and evaluated correspondence (email and letter writing) as an effective mode for nursing inquiry. Her work was instrumental in the establishment of an internationally recognized chronic illness research programme. Understanding the experiences of transition when living with chronic illness will be the focus of the Post Doctoral Fellowship awarded by the Australian Research Council which commenced during 2003. Dr Kralik is editor of the *Journal of Advanced Nursing* and has published widely.

Dr John Aggergaard Larsen is a Research Fellow at the European Institute of Health and Medical Sciences at the University of Surrey. He has an MA in anthropology (Copenhagen) based on ethnographic fieldwork in China studying the cultural representation of an ethnic minority group. Dr Larsen's research interest concerns the socio-cultural shaping of experience and life trajectory, that is, ways in which individual experience and agency are influencing and influenced by social institutions and social/health interventions. He is currently facilitating an action research project supporting health-care practice development in south-east England and working on a research project exploring the experiences and employment opportunities of overseas-trained health-care professionals working in the UK.

Dr Frances Rapport holds the position of Julian Tudor Hart Senior Research Fellow at the University of Wales, Swansea. Her research interests are in the areas of reproductive technology and new qualitative methodologies. She has particular expertise in hermeneutic phenomenology and has explored women's motivation to donate eggs using phenomenological techniques. Dr Rapport is the editor of *New Qualitative Methodologies in Health and Social Care Research* (2004) London: Routledge and has written numerous research articles on research.

Dr Siobhan Sharkey has degrees in anthropology and qualifications in nursing. She entered mental health nursing, followed by posts in research and development and was a Royal College of Nursing Advisor in Mental Health. Currently she is working as a lecturer at the Highland Campus, University of Stirling, based in Inverness. Her research interests focus in particular on families and mental health. Her current research explores social networks of families and the importance of communities and context on well-being. She has published research on both risk and transitional care models in mental health. She has published widely in her areas of expertise.

Professor Andrew C. Sparkes PhD is Director of the Qualitative Research Unit in the School of Sport and Health Sciences, St Luke's Campus, University of Exeter, Devon, UK. His interdisciplinary research interests include: performing bodies, identities and selves; interrupted body projects and the narrative reconstruction of self; sporting auto/biographies; and the lives of marginalized individuals and groups. He is the author of a book *Telling Tales in Sport & Physical Activity: A Qualitative Journey*, Champaign, IL: Human Kinetics Press (2002) and has written a large number of articles on qualitative methodology and research in the field of health and illness.

Dr Clare Taylor is a Principal Lecturer in the School of Health and Social Sciences at Coventry University. She originally qualified as an occupational therapist. She subsequently embarked on a more academic path with an OU degree in Psychology and an MA in Sociological Research in Healthcare before completing her PhD. Her current areas of interest are evidence-based practice and researching the experiences of disabled occupational therapy students. Her publications include a number of research articles and chapters on evidence-based practice and education for occupational therapists and a book in 2000, *Evidence-based Practice for Occupational Therapists*, Oxford: Blackwell Science.

Professor Les Todres PhD is a clinical psychologist and Professor of Qualitative Research and Psychotherapy at the Institute of Health and Community Studies, Bournemouth University, UK. His previous occupational roles have included head of a student counselling service and director of a clinical psychology training programme. He has also worked within National Health Service clinics and GP practices. He has published in the areas of phenomenological psychology and integrative psychotherapy. In his current position, he co-founded and co-leads the Centre for Qualitative Research at Bournemouth University. He also provides clinical supervision to psychological therapists at the Intensive Psychological Therapies Service in Poole, Dorset.

Dr Stephen Wallace has worked in a variety of academic and clinical settings during his career. He maintains an abiding interest in knowledge-making of all kinds and introduced the formal teaching of qualitative methods to psychology students at Deakin University in Australia. During his period as Reader in Clinical Governance at Bournemouth University he became interested in the crisis of postmodern scholarship, especially as it related to researching the health and welfare arena. He has published a great number of articles in international journals.

Foreword

Why should a separate qualitative text be necessary for graduate students in health care disciplines? This is an interesting question. Are not qualitative research methods texts basically the same, regardless of one's discipline? Do the guidelines for conducting focus groups, or the rules for grounded theory, change according to context or participants? What is so special about *health care*?

If one believes that qualitative research focuses on the *person*, rather than, for instance, the person's *scores* obtained on a structured instrument; on the *person* as a member of a family, or as an employee, a student or whatever, rather than a *subject* within a population; on the person who is *ill*, rather than on the *illness*, then probably qualitative methods need to be used. These methods may need to be adapted *if* those adaptations ease access to the participant and make the patients' participation possible despite the illness. But there is another caveat – these adaptations should only be attempted *if* they ease the process of qualitative inquiry without altering the nature of the method. Making these decisions is not a task for the student, but for the expert.

When illness strikes (and I note that common metaphor contains the essence of suddenness and force) people become overwhelmed with change. They struggle to comprehend what is happening to their bodies. Patients learn that everyday taken-for-granted functions are no longer easy or possible, and they may be overwhelmed with pain and sleeplessness. Therapies, which are supposed to *help*, may also cause astonishing and unwelcome side effects. Relationships with loved ones will be drastically altered. Facing loss of employment, disability, and even death, people who are ill find themselves drastically altered. In this bewildering and unwanted state, the participation in a student's research becomes a challenge, another task, and burden – but sometimes, a therapy – for the patient-participant. The researcher, willing or not, becomes a part of the professional team interacting with the patient. Data collection is transformed into something that involves asking about intimate, embarrassing and terrifying aspects of this changed life that the participant sometimes does not want to think about, let alone discuss.

The context of health care, the place that data are collected, is also unique. Whether a clinic, a hospital, or care provided in the home, sickness and its trappings, its syringes and stethoscopes, uniforms and rules, bandages and wheelchairs, dramatically define the setting. Researchers must learn to negotiate the hierarchy of personnel in the hospital, learn their place and priority, learn to be interrupted and learn to make the most of a golden moment in which data can actually be collected without disruption. Students of research methods have to come to grips with the sights, sounds and smells of hospitals, as well as attending to their research. In hospitals, behaviour that would be bizarre 'outside' becomes everyday. If the student is to observe, the smells of sickness must be overcome, and the groans and moans of agony tolerated. Tears become ordinary; laughter valued. Visitors, people so confident outside, become tentative and compliant within. Rules, both written and unwritten, mask normal behaviour and new forms of behaviours become ordinary.

It is in this context that our students must learn to do qualitative inquiry. They are observers standing still in the rush of life-saving business. Their task, if they have one, is not to get in the way. Their interviews inquire into suffering; they record graphic descriptions of pain, and responses to failed therapy. Their research makes explicit the aspects of experience that the caregivers find difficult to hear.

Therefore, qualitative research in health care is learned in the most difficult of all contexts. Our students have to learn how to attend to the individual without disclosing their identity. In very distressing situations, they have to focus on the participant and not on their own feelings. They must learn discretion, and to be trustworthy. And when the stakes are high, they must learn to minimally disturb their participants, their therapies, and their precious time with their families. Opportunities to collect data must not be wasted: they must be expert and efficient and excellent in their researching. Thus, the significance of this book.

In answer to the questions posed in the first paragraph, a specialist text in qualitative research *is* needed for the health care disciplines. Sometimes methods have to be altered to fit the context, the participant's needs, or the ongoing action. But such changes should be done cautiously, with full awareness of the ramifications these changes will have on the final product.

Qualitative research is fast becoming the mainstream research method in health care programmes within the social science disciplines, such as nursing, occupational therapy, rehabilitation and counselling. With this exponential rise in demand, qualitative inquiry has become out of step—we have many introductory texts, but relatively few that will assist the more advanced student, those actually doing research. The pragmatic approach and the major methods detailed in this book will ease the process of doing research and fill a very large gap.

Finally, the text will make a contribution in a very important way. Health care professionals are now making demands for evidence (and I use that term in its broadest sense) with an unprecedented intensity. This book will prepare health care practitioners to develop this knowledge and to become experts in qualitative inquiry, thus contributing to filling this critical need.

Janice M. Morse
Professor and Scientific Director of the International Institute for
Qualitative Methodology
University of Alberta
Canada

Introduction

Qualitative research has become very popular in Britain over the last two or three decades particularly in the health-care field. This type of research answers questions that are equally valid but quite different from those of quantitative research. A number of books have been published in the area of qualitative inquiry in health care, many American, most exclusively for nurses and an occasional text for the medical profession or the professions allied to medicine. This book is aimed at health professionals in general, be they academics in the health-care field, professionals in clinical practice, or students who are undertaking postgraduate degrees in the area of health studies such as MA/MSc, and those who are beginning a PhD, a professional or a taught doctorate. The writers hope that their chapters address some of the needs of mature students or professionals and academics with some experience of research rather than as novice researchers. The book should not be seen as an 'unproblematic toolkit' or a prescription how to use qualitative research but might help researchers in the choice of data collection procedures and to make decisions about specific qualitative approaches. The techniques and procedures of collection and analysis are discussed in relation to specific approaches.

Health-care research is becoming ever more interprofessional and multidisciplinary, parallel to the growth in collaboration between different professions, and most of us have been involved in research with people from other disciplines and professions. The writers are academics and/or practitioners from a variety of health professions, belonging to different disciplines and specialities in the health arena. The studies described are useful examples not only for the specific setting or discipline in which they were carried out, but also for those in other fields of health care and education. The text is intended in particular to help health professionals – such as clinical psychologists, nurses, doctors and professions allied to medicine (for instance, physiotherapists and occupational therapists) and academics in this field (not merely researchers but also educators) – carry out qualitative research. This type of inquiry might extend their understanding of clients and improve clinical practice on the basis of evidence from patients and colleagues.

I realize that the contributions vary widely, some are easily readable and others more demanding, but – apart from minor revisions – I have not changed the style or content of individual contributors. The variations reflect the character of qualitative research, which includes a number of approaches that differ a great deal. The chapters on data collection methods are relatively straightforward (though data collection itself is not); researchers at the start of their research often like to be introduced slowly. I have also added a discussion about the status of method to help create awareness that researchers need to reflect on the choice of approach which, after all, depends on the research question as well as on the ideology and personality of the researcher. Some approaches such as document analysis and conversation analysis are not described as they are used less often in health-care research (though, of course, they can be of use, especially document analysis).

The chapters on the specific approaches also differ: there is the philosophical density of phenomenology, the systematic approach of grounded theory, the practical/critical slant of action and evaluation research and the seductive quality of narrative approaches. The contributors gave examples of the approach discussed in their chapter. A section on feminist research is included, as a feminist stance is becoming increasingly popular among health academics and professionals.

Most of these chapters attempt to show that qualitative research is 'scientific' – albeit social science – and can produce 'evidence' for evidence-based practice, though a different type of evidence from that which is generated by quantitative inquiry. Indeed the two main methodologies (I hesitate to use the word 'paradigms') answer different types of research questions; they are not in opposition to each other but both useful for different purposes. As the references are extensive, researchers will be able to search further for literature about a particular approach or procedure. I do hope that this book contains something useful for those carrying out qualitative inquiry.

Perhaps I should admit that I left out several issues that could have been discussed. I do not apologize for leaving out a section on the use of computer analysis in qualitative research. Although computers may be useful, they are more effective when researchers carry out studies with very large samples, and this is not usual in qualitative research. This book might also have included a discussion of triangulation between qualitative and quantitative methods. For health researchers the use of both methods together can be useful as they may complement each other. Most *qualitative* health researchers, however, have a particular view of the world and about the questions they want to ask. These researchers are most often focused on the social world and the experiences of people, and therefore generally, though not always, triangulate within qualitative methods.

I would like to thank the contributors to this book – all experts in their field. They have tried to keep to the deadlines in spite of having busy working lives. My thanks is also due to the many reviewers of these chapters, in particular Liz Norton, Sabi Redwood, Jan Walker, Les Todres and Nigel Rapport.

PART 1
Starting out

Why qualitative research in the health professions?

Many potential researchers wish to investigate a problem or major issue in clinical practice or education for practice that cannot be answered by quantitative research. There are some major reasons why they choose qualitative research.

- Qualitative research can be an important tool in understanding the emotions, perceptions and actions of people who suffer from a medical condition.
- The meanings that health professionals give to their work will only be uncovered if researchers observe their interaction with clients and ask them about their experience. This also applies to students destined for the health-care field.
- Qualitative research is person-centred; hence researchers consider the participants in the research as whole human beings not as a collection of physical parts.
- The reasons for particular types of behaviour can only be understood when it is observed and people are asked about it. Therefore health or education policies can be developed through this type of research; policies for changing health behaviour can only be effective if the reasons for this behaviour are clearly understood.

Research questions in health care and education for the health professions arise from issues, puzzles or problems that potential researchers encountered in the field. They are answered within a specific philosophical, ethical and political context and can only be solved within this framework.

Generally qualitative researchers start without a hypothesis, although they cannot avoid 'hunches' or making certain assumptions. This is particularly so for health professionals who have been in the clinical field for many years and have much experience. This can be 'sensitizing' them to certain important issues in the field that they might investigate. They must try, however, to uncover them and remain flexible and open minded and become, at least to some extent, 'strangers' in a familiar setting so that they do not miss the unexpected or unusual. The data from the research have primacy, not the researcher's preconceptions, nor the literature connected to their area of inquiry.

To undertake qualitative research, researchers in the health-care arena have to understand its principles and underlying *epistemology*. In Chapter 1, in the introduction to qualitative research, **Mark Avis** develops the ideas and philosophical background of qualitative inquiry. He discusses its nature, but claims that there is a lack of consensus about its defining characteristics, its procedures and evaluation. It is often defined by its difference and reaction to positivist forms of inquiry but Avis also suggests that researchers in the quantitative tradition do not agree on its principles. Neither qualitative nor quantitative research can be seen as a methodological monolith.

Without engaging in the 'paradigm wars', this chapter states as the main purpose of qualitative research the understanding of social behaviour and thought through people's own accounts and observations of their interaction with others, and stresses the researcher's involvement with the participants.

Ethical behaviour is the prime consideration of a researcher in the field of health care and does not stop when Ethics Committees have reviewed a proposal. Ensuring that research is carried out ethically requires careful consideration. In Chapter 2, **Ron Iphofen** clarifies that ethical issues in research are similar whatever the approach, although differences do exist. The key issues where qualitative health research differs are linked to:

- The issue of informed consent: participants cannot always be fully informed at the beginning of the research because it is exploratory in nature and is guided by the ideas of the participants.

- People's vulnerability in times of illness: participants may not be fully aware of their actions and words during the in-depth interviews and observations.

- The anonymity of the participants: this might be threatened by the detailed description of the research process and participants as well as the excerpts from interview and observation data.

- Power relationships: the health professional is in a powerful position and patients (or students) may feel obliged to participate. Their autonomy may be threatened.

A variety of issues are discussed in the chapter, many of which researchers might not have considered. Iphofen explores these and other problems. Although they are complex and cannot always be solved, he draws the researcher's attention to them. He uncovers the conflicting responsibilities and obligations of researchers who are both health professionals and researchers, focusing on and explaining not only the principles of ethical behaviour but also stating the guidelines for ethical action from the standpoint of a sociologist and clinical therapist.

1

MARK AVIS
Is there an epistemology for qualitative research?

Introduction: what is qualitative research?

Qualitative research is not easy to define in a way that would be acceptable to everyone who does qualitative research. At one end of the spectrum, qualitative research may be regarded as the use of techniques of data production and analysis that relate to textual or non-numerical data. At the other, qualitative research entails the explicit employment of distinctive methodological and epistemological theories, such as grounded theory, phenomenology or ethnography, to investigate people's understanding of their lives and social context. It has been noted that there is little consensus among qualitative researchers regarding the defining characteristics of qualitative research (Silverman 2001). Although its development is largely associated with the disciplines of anthropology and sociology (Denzin and Lincoln 1994), during the last fifty years qualitative methods have become established in a range of other academic disciplines such as education, social policy, human geography, social psychology, history, organizational studies, and health sciences. As a result, qualitative research has evolved in different ways as it accommodates the theoretical and methodological assumptions of the host discipline. In consequence, almost every aspect of qualitative research, what it is, what it is for, how it is done, and how it is to be judged, is the subject of controversy.

One of the central difficulties is that most characterizations of qualitative inquiry tend to rely on and respond to what it is not. Qualitative researchers often describe their methods in ways that demonstrate how they differ from quantitative methods. This seems understandable, even useful, until it becomes apparent that there is no agreed definition of quantitative methods. It is often assumed that quantitative methods are based on, among other things, objective measurement, hypothesis testing, law-like generalization, reproducible designs, and the pursuit of factual knowledge. These principles are often brought together under the label of *positivism*. The problem with positivism as a methodological label is that it is both imprecise and anachronistic (Avis 1997). Most quantitative researchers would not consider themselves to be positivists. Even among quantitative researchers there is often little common understanding of what the term 'quantitative research' means. These ambiguities tend to create a circular argument; qualitative methods are defined as not quantitative, and quantitative methods are defined as not qualitative.

In part, these puzzles about the nature of qualitative research arise from writers taking a prescriptive view of epistemology. That is, by starting from assumptions about the nature of knowledge, writers deduce what methodological requirements must be met if researchers want a particular type of research activity to lead to knowledge. I will start from a more practical point of view; observing that the purpose of a research project is to generate credible evidence to answer a question that is open to empirical inquiry. Particular kinds of research questions will lend themselves to the use of particular types of research method. In writing about their projects, researchers offer a rationale for their choice of research methods, provide assurance that their methods generate credible evidence, and argue that the evidence generated provides a valid answer to the research question. An analysis of the arguments that researchers use to convince their audiences that their research practices are justified and their findings credible may highlight similarities between qualitative and quantitative research rather than differences.

What characterizes qualitative research?

Qualitative researchers usually start with research questions that ask how we can acquire an understanding of social behaviour by exploring people's subjective accounts of social life. The importance of investigating the interaction between the social and individual is acknowledged rather well by Popay (1992: 100); she states that qualitative inquiry 'explores the meanings people attach to their experiences and identifies and describes the social structures and processes that shape these meanings'. Other qualitative researchers have emphasized the importance of providing a 'thick description' of social behaviour (Geertz 1973), an account of social action that helps us unravel the implicit rules and conventions that make social behaviour meaningful. Another way that qualitative researchers have talked about their enterprise has been to capture social events from the perspective of the people being studied, or to provide an insider's view of social life. Bryman has referred to it as 'seeing through the eyes of the people you are studying' (Bryman 1988: 61). None of these characterizations of qualitative research questions are entirely satisfactory; there are technical differences between exploring meanings and describing perspectives, and between providing an explanation and achieving understanding. However, for the moment, I suggest that the research questions that drive qualitative research concern the need to provide an understanding of social behaviour by exploring people's accounts of social life. Accepting a research objective that gives precedence to obtaining an 'insider's view', brings with it certain methodological commitments. It is these commitments that are used to justify the methods necessary to produce credible evidence about the 'insider's view'. I will outline four methodological commitments that provide a basic characterization of qualitative research methods.

First, qualitative research gives priority to obtaining and analyzing *textual data*.

In simple terms, qualitative research predominantly uses methods of inquiry that produce text rather than numbers. Textual data could include transcripts of interviews or conversations, free text comments on a questionnaire, diary entries, observation notes, case histories, or entries in medical and nursing records. In some cases, qualitative data can also include pictorial and video evidence. The importance of textual data is that they allow people to express their thoughts and beliefs in their own words and on their own terms. An emphasis on text allows qualitative researchers to accept the importance of unexpected and unanticipated information. This is not to say that measurement of relevant information is not of interest to qualitative researchers. A commitment to narrative detail does not imply that qualitative data cannot or should not be summarized in quantitative form, but there is a responsibility to analyze and present textual data in a way that preserves their narrative and social character. This commitment is often demonstrated in qualitative researchers' use of direct quotations to illustrate their findings.

Second, qualitative research relies on *extensive interaction* with the people being studied. In order to explore the meanings that people attach to their experiences, or to view the social world through the eyes of the participants in the research, it is necessary for the researcher to interact with them over an extended period and in a fairly unconstrained manner. Therefore, precedence is usually given to research methods that allow open, often unstructured, interactions with the people being studied. Qualitative researchers refer to this period of interaction with individuals and groups as *fieldwork*. The typical methods used during fieldwork are participant observation, and unstructured or semi-structured interview techniques. An important consequence of this commitment to an interactive approach is that qualitative researchers recognize that the people being studied are not simply passive subjects but active contributors to the research project. It is an approach that one qualitative researcher has described as learning from people rather than studying them (Spradley 1979). Once it is recognized that data are produced through interaction, then the metaphor of collection becomes difficult to sustain. Although this point applies equally to all research methods, qualitative researchers find it hard to maintain the fiction, and often prefer to use terms such as data generation or production, which acknowledge that data arise out of the interaction between researchers and participants.

Third, qualitative research usually involves a *flexible plan of inquiry*. Since qualitative researchers aim to interact with people in an open and unconstrained manner, it is important that they can respond constructively to the ideas expressed by the participants. Consequently, qualitative researchers usually employ a plan of inquiry that evolves as the research study progresses. As a result, qualitative researchers rarely have a rigidly predefined protocol for sampling, data collection and analysis. Instead, they will start with a broad research question and, after negotiating access to people who have relevant experiences to offer, they go on to develop their plan for sampling, data generation and analysis as the study progresses. Qualitative researchers in the field are highly sensitive to unanticipated factors or puzzling features in the way people interact or talk about their lives that they consider will have a bearing on the research question. Becker (1998: 153) provides an entertaining account of the way that, during his seminal study of student doctors, he spent days trying to unravel what one of the students had meant when he called a patient a 'crock'.

This flexible plan of inquiry is highly characteristic of qualitative research as it allows researchers to develop hunches and hypotheses as the study progresses. These new hypotheses or 'working propositions' will be tested as the study progresses by expanding the sample, using new methods, or employing extra analytical techniques. As Michael Agar (1986: 12) puts it:

> Such work requires an intensive personal involvement, an abandonment of traditional scientific control, an improvisational style to meet situations not of the researcher's making, and an ability to learn from a long series of mistakes.

Recognition that it is the researcher who is the research instrument, and that the plan of inquiry should be developed as the study progresses means that qualitative researchers cannot rely on standardized procedures to deal with concerns such as bias and reproducibility. In view of this, the importance of 'learning from a long series of mistakes' is an essential aspect of qualitative research. It requires qualitative researchers to reflect constantly and critically on the decisions they make during the course of a study. They need to reflect on their own role in the social process of producing data (Mason 2002). This practice is usually referred to as *reflexivity*, and is regarded as an intrinsic feature of qualitative research (see also Chapter 15). Similarly, since qualitative researchers cannot rely on the reproducibility of their techniques to establish the credibility of evidence, they rely instead on the idea of *transparency*. Qualitative researchers attempt to demonstrate transparency in their decision-making through reflexivity, and by leaving what has been referred to as an *audit trail*, a record of the researchers' design decisions, as the study progresses, about gaining access, selection of field role, choice of participants, ethical considerations, and analytical methods. Transparency is an attempt to demonstrate the credibility of qualitative research evidence by allowing the reader to 'see through' the researchers' decision-making and their analytical approach to the data. As a result of their improvisational, flexible plan of inquiry qualitative researchers rely on reflexivity and transparency as a means to provide assurance about the credibility of the evidence.

Finally, the emphasis on trying to understand people's experiences and their interpretation of the social world entails *naturalism* in study methods. Methodological naturalism holds that research techniques should be familiar to people being studied, respect their beliefs, have similarities with normal social interaction, and leave people undisturbed as far as is possible. Hence, highly structured or manipulated social settings like the experiment or formal interview are avoided. A commitment to naturalism is not to overlook the fact that any form of investigation is likely to influence participants' behaviour. On the contrary, the use of highly interactive methods and the emphasis on reflexivity will entail recognition that the research study itself is a social process. Researchers cannot detach themselves from the evidence they are generating. Naturalism forces on researchers a recognition that research activity is itself a social process and, as such, open to interpretation.

Another way in which the application of sociological theory becomes an essential element in qualitative inquiry concerns how its findings can be applied to other settings. The focus on providing a contextual understanding of particular social processes from individuals' points of view means that qualitative researchers are less concerned to produce findings that can be generalized to a wider population. This does not mean that the findings of qualitative studies cannot be applied to a broader range of settings than those of the specific study. However, the application of qualitative research findings to other situations will not depend upon sampling theory, but in the way that the results can be made to fit with general social theory (Dingwall 1992). Application of the findings of a qualitative study to other groups and other contexts is contingent upon arguments to show that the findings are credible in the light of existing theory, and that they are consistent with social theories that have wider application. For this reason, we need to be very careful about approaches to qualitative inquiry that reduce it to a series of techniques devoid of theoretical context. The danger in stripping out substantive social and anthropological theory is that qualitative research findings can be reduced to anecdotal and banal descriptions (Lambert and McKevitt 2002). In my view, any research method that is conducted without an adequate theoretical context will lead to a form of mindless empiricism that offers very little explanation of the topic under investigation.

Theory and qualitative research

The need for the use of social theory in the development of empirical research studies raises further problems for qualitative research. A flexible plan of inquiry means that qualitative researchers use social theory in various ways to develop their lines of inquiry, their hypotheses and hunches to be followed up during the course of fieldwork. It must be recognized that all evidence generated during the course of an empirical inquiry is the result of the explicit or implicit deployment of particular theories that researchers considered useful in framing the research question and guiding the conduct of the inquiry. Qualitative researchers must face, head on, the problem that evidence cannot be dissociated from the theories that were used to guide its generation.

In essence, a theory is simply an explanatory story that helps people make sense of their experience. In our culture, we generally favour the explanatory stories that science offers, but that is largely pragmatic. Scientific theories are useful in helping us make sense of our experience. Without taking a view on what a scientific theory should involve, we can see that explanation and understanding are closely related. We understand something when an explanatory story helps us make sense of it; the story provides us with a credible account of why it occurred. An important legacy of empiricism reminds us that the credibility of a theory depends on its ability to explain the evidence of our senses. However, it is not quite as straightforward as this. Critics of empiricism have pointed out there is no clear demarcation between the evidence of the senses and theory (Quine 1953). What we think we hear, see, smell, taste and touch depends upon interpretation. We use theory all the time in making sense of our empirical evidence. In fact, the evidence of our senses would tell us very little about the world if we did not use theory to help us interpret those sensory stimuli. Empirical researchers acknowledge, in some cases reluctantly, that all evidence is dependent upon theory.

Worse still, we must also face up to the recognition that the credibility of a theory depends on its ability to make sense of the evidence, while also accepting that evidence cannot be divorced from the theory involved in its generation. This observation seems to give rise to a circularity about evidence and theory that denies the possibility of stepping outside the circle to resolve the problem. The temptation is to look for an epistemological point of view that could allow the researcher to step off the merry-go-round of theory and evidence by finding some fixed, objective ground on which to make a judgement, while others have embraced the impossibility of ever getting off.

In keeping with a pragmatic approach, I observe that all empirical evidence must be treated with extreme caution. Any evidence generated in the course of a research project cannot be separated from the theoretical standpoint of the researcher; this observation serves to reinforce the need for *critical reflexivity*. Quantitative researchers can address concerns about the interconnectedness of theory and evidence during the design stages of the project; they can be explicit about the hypotheses to be employed and tested. The use of emergent designs arising from an interactive and flexible approach to inquiry means that qualitative researchers must reflect on the connections between their hypotheses and the evidence generated as the study progresses. This third principle combines both reflexivity and transparency in that it requires a *critical reflection on the relationship between theory and the evidence* obtained as a result of the decisions taken by the researchers. It is the clarity and cogency of the researchers' consideration of the ways in which their theoretical assumptions informed the emergent research design that matters in addressing the credibility of qualitative research evidence.

Credibility of qualitative evidence

The four methodological commitments I have identified are not meant to set out the necessary or sufficient conditions for the conduct of qualitative inquiry. On the contrary, in some cases a qualitative investigation can involve little more than that the analysis of textual data arising from open-ended questionnaire items. However, in order to meet the broader objective of trying to explain social behaviour using the perspective of the people involved, qualitative research will usually also require an in-depth, interactive, and naturalistic approach to the inquiry.

Up until now I have identified four methodological commitments in the conduct of qualitative research about which there is some degree of consensus: narrative data, extensive interaction with research participants, a flexible plan of inquiry, and a naturalistic focus on social processes. The interactive, emergent, and idiosyncratic nature of qualitative design makes it impossible for qualitative researchers to demonstrate the same degree of reliability and detachment as quantitative researchers. As a result, qualitative researchers depend upon alternative principles to provide assurance of the credibility of qualitative evidence. I have suggested that these are reflexivity, transparency, and critical examination of evidence in the light of relevant theory. These principles are significant because they are an essential element of the argument that researchers put forward to assure audiences of the credibility of their evidence. The role of these three principles in establishing the credibility of evidence from qualitative inquiry would seem, on the face of it, to have something in common with principles of elimination of bias, reproducibility, and objectivity in the justification of quantitative evidence.

Epistemology and qualitative methodology

As noted earlier, one of the great difficulties that anyone faces in trying to provide an intelligible account of qualitative research is to acknowledge the depth of the disagreements that exist between qualitative researchers. It is likely that many qualitative researchers would regard my characterization of the nature of qualitative research as dependent upon a trivial account of four methodological commitments. Critics might argue that an account of qualitative research methods must start with epistemological considerations regarding the nature of social reality, how it can be known, and whether the social world can be treated in the same way as the physical world. They would argue that it is essential to take a view on what can be known and by what means; these considerations will tell us how different forms of research should be conducted and how one form of research should be distinguished from another. I will refer to these qualitative researchers as 'separatists', since they maintain that qualitative research depend on a collection of beliefs about the nature of social phenomena, and how they can be known, that sets them apart from quantitative researchers. I will examine the extent of this epistemological separation between qualitative and quantitative research methods by considering a central aspect of their argument, whether we should treat social reality as constructed rather than found.

Social construction

We have noted that qualitative research is based on an investigation of social phenomena that gives precedence to the perspective of the people being studied. This approach to inquiry encourages researchers to view social reality as *constructed* out of different social perspectives. A simple version of this social constructionist point of view recognizes that all social facts, even those as apparently objective as a medical diagnosis, are not simply discovered but created through the application of social norms, and that these norms may differ from one social group to another. As Dingwall (1992: 165) points out:

> This point is important in understanding the boundaries between social and natural scientific studies in medicine. There are no diseases in nature, merely relationships between organisms [...]. Diseases are produced by the conceptual schemes imposed on the natural world by human beings, which value some states of the body and disvalue others. This is not to say that biological changes may not impose themselves on us, but rather that the significance of those changes depends upon their location in human society. The normal

physiology of ageing is relevant in very different ways to an East African herdsman who sees it as a mark of advancing status, power and sexual attractiveness and to a Californian actress who sees it as the beginning of her decline as a social being.

People make implicit classifications of the social world they experience. However, the reality of a social concept such as 'disease' depends upon a particular way of classifying our experience, and that differences in classification will reflect the beliefs and values of particular social group. Furthermore, the underlying reasons for the classification are not always readily apparent to the person or social group making the classification. The idea of disease is so deeply ingrained in our way of thinking about the world that we can overlook the point that it does not pick out an objective feature of the natural world but a classification that relates to our social norms. Becker's (1998) protracted attempts to get medical students to define the concept of a 'crock' to him illustrates the difficulty that people have in explaining their ways of classifying their experience. In fact, Becker (1998: 157) was eventually only able to understand the significance of the concept of a 'crock' through the use of social theory to explain implicit values in the medical practice that the medical students were learning:

> Like their teachers, students hoped to perform medical miracles, and heal the sick, if not actually raise the dead. They knew that wasn't easy to do, and that they wouldn't always be successful, but one of the real payoffs of medical practice for them was to 'do something' and watch a sick person get well. But you can't perform a medical miracle on someone who was never sick in the first place. Since crocks, in the student view, weren't 'really sick', they were useless as the raw material of medical miracles.

We can see that the conventions people use for classifying their social experiences reflect the implicit shared beliefs and interests of various social groups. It also illustrates the point that different social groups may experience the same event very differently depending upon their shared norms and beliefs. The 'social world' is itself a product of various social conventions for classifying social actions and events. Perhaps the first sociological text explicitly to consider the application of this point was the book *The Social Construction of Reality* by Berger and Luckmann (1966) which drew attention to the way in which the experience of social reality is multi-layered and constructed through processes of social interaction.

A central aspect of the epistemological debate about the distinctiveness of qualitative research concerns investigators' responses to the recognition that social reality is constructed, and what implications it has for a social research methodology. Separatists maintain that a recognition that social reality is constructed rather than found, means giving up the notion that there is an objective social reality out there to be discovered through the application of a scientific, quantitative methodology (Schutz 1972; Lincoln and Guba 2000). An epistemology that can recognize and deal with the insider's view, and constructed social realities will be radically different from an epistemology that supports scientific knowledge based on an assumption that there is an objective reality that can be studied using standardized observational techniques. By rejecting the idea that there is a social reality that exists independently of inquiry, and against which the results of an inquiry can be tested for truth, separatists challenge positivist scientific episte- mology as a means to deliver knowledge about the social world. Indeed, some versions of constructivism have turned the tables on science by pointing out that science itself is simply another constructed social reality that reflects the norms and interests of a particular social group: scientists. It is argued, therefore, that quali- tative research operates within a different paradigm of inquiry, one that allows recognition of its ontological and epistemological commitments and particular forms of research practice (Lincoln and Guba 2000). Consequently, qualitative research must be based on fundamentally different epistemology from scientific inquiry.

This is a well-rehearsed argument; the lines are familiar but the plot is not so well understood. The argument relies heavily on the device of identifying positi- vism with quantitative research methods and scientific knowledge. However, positivism is a red herring; neither empiricists such as Quine (1953) nor realists like Searle (1995) or Bhaskar (1998) have any time for this largely discredited epistemology. Once we strip out the vestiges of positivism, and its residual influ- ence on scientific practice, such as its hostility to theory and its emphasis on observation, then we are less likely to be taken in by the distinction between what is found and what is constructed. Modern-day realists (Bhaskar 1998) are quite able to accept that reality is both constructed and found. Searle (1995) finds no dif- ficulty in accepting that social facts depend upon convention and social interaction to make them so. The conventions and social rules that allow cultures to recognize and acknowledge social facts such as marriage, class, and alienation are inter- subjective events based on observable social processes that can be studied. Simi- larly, Hacking (1999) recognizes that many social concepts, such as 'mental disease', 'child abuse', or 'teenage pregnancy', are social inventions in the sense that their identification and introduction into social discourse reflects the interests of particular social groups. However, he argues that the events that they describe are real; they are features of a social reality that exist independently of the terms we use to describe them. The social processes and the interests of the groups that maintain the currency of socially constructed terms such as 'child abuse' or 'teenage pregnancy' are available for study. Becker's (1998) explanation of med- ical students' use of the term 'crock' depended upon his obtaining an insider's view of social phenomena to show how their use of the term reflected their interests. However, the students were using the term 'crock' to describe a feature of medical practice that was also observable by Becker, it picked up an aspect of social reality that Becker could recognize and discuss independently of the concept. It should be recognized that the existence of multiple social perspectives does not equate to multiple social realities. The metaphor of different perspectives only really makes sense when we have a common set of coordinates on which to plot them. After all, multiple points of views are all perspectives on something.

The epistemological distinctions made between qualitative and quantitative methods appear to rest on the use of positivism as an exaggerated version of the epistemology of science and a rather overdrawn comparison between social and physical reality. In avoiding some of the more extreme claims of constructivists that all observable reality is socially constructed (Searle 1995), we can acknowledge that social reality is both socially constructed and that there are social events and processes that can be observed by researchers using a range of techniques. Observing socially constructed phenomena may be more complex than looking at physical phenomena, requiring an extended range of research techniques and careful reflexive scrutiny of the relation between observation and theory. However, this does not provide a reason to abandon a commitment to an intersubjectively observable social reality or consider that qualitative research is based on a different epistemology to quantitative research. We should avoid making the same kind of error as the positivists who, during the last century, also took a prescriptive view of epistemology. An alternative approach to epistemological questions regarding qualitative research is to be non-dogmatic and grounded in practice. If we start from the way in which researchers work and examine the logic of their approach, we can then consider whether there are important epistemological distinctions that need to be drawn between qualitative and quantitative research.

A common logic for research?

I started from the point of view that research is a method for generating robust evidence in response to a question open to an empirical answer. An effective empirical inquiry will produce reliable and credible evidence that could form the basis of a knowledge claim or an answer to a practical problem. Therefore, the value of research activity depends upon the ability of the researcher to substantiate a number of claims about the suitability of the research question for a research design, the credibility of the research evidence, the validity of their interpretation of the evidence in the light of theory. The research process is, in effect, a series of logical arguments advanced to support these claims (Avis 1995). Once we set aside the dogma that positivist science provides a ready set of rules and procedures for dealing with these arguments, then we must acknowledge that we have to evaluate the strength of the arguments that researchers put forward to substantiate their claims on their own merits.

The key concept that underpins the strength of the arguments, and therefore the logic of empirical inquiry, is validity. Many research textbooks suggest that validity concerns whether a measure measures what it is supposed to measure. Validity is not a procedural matter; it refers to the quality and strength of the arguments that researchers put forward to substantiate claims about the reliability of their evidence and the credibility of their conclusions. Therefore, validity is more properly an evaluative concept in considering the arguments researchers put forward to justify their claims, although following established procedures is sometimes an important element in providing a justification for researchers' claims.

IBRARY
DUCATION CENTRE
RINCESS ROYAL HOSPITAL

Validity and qualitative research

However, once again, we find that qualitative researchers are deeply divided about the application of the concept of validity to qualitative research findings. Some writers reject the application of validity to qualitative research on the grounds that the concept belongs to the quantitative research paradigm and has no place in qualitative investigations (Smith and Heshusius 1986) or suggest alternative criteria (Guba 1981). An alternative is to accept the application of validity to qualitative research by treating it as an evaluative concept that applies to all empirical evidence (LeCompte and Goetz 1982).

Underlying these differences is a re-emergence of disagreements about the nature of the relationship between research evidence and social reality. Some who reject the application of validity to qualitative research also reject the idea that there is an objective social reality. They argue that every social group constructs its own view of the world, its own social reality. Guba and Lincoln (1986: 236) suggest that validity

> is nothing more than an assessment of the degree of isomorphism between the study findings and the real world [it] cannot have any meaning as a criterion in a paradigm that rejects realist ontology. If realities are only assumed to exist in mentally constructed form, what sense could it make to look for isomorphisms?

If research evidence is simply another social perspective, and there are multiple social realities each with its own internal logic, there can be no criterion that could allow us to decide whether one perspective is more valid than another. The emphasis can only be on the internal consistency of accounts of a social perspective. Guba (1981) and Lincoln and Guba (1985) have presented a number of criteria, consistent with the qualitative paradigm, that allow us to judge whether a research evidence is an authentic representation of a particular social perspective. The main criterion that has been offered as a qualitative equivalent of validity is *credibility*. Credibility has a more restricted meaning than validity; credibility is used to express research participants' endorsement of research evidence as an authentic statement of their perspective. This seems a very limited ambition; it appears to reduce qualitative investigations to little more than descriptions of a social perspective that participants recognize as their own.

If the emphasis in qualitative inquiry is on providing the thickest possible description of the insider's view, or capturing the 'lived-experience' of the participant, this seems to ignore the use of social theory to provide explanations of social phenomena based on an understanding of the insider's view. The distinctiveness of qualitative research is to explain social processes from the perspective of those participating in the study; that is more than an attempt to provide a description of a social perspective that is corroborated by participants. Indeed, if we acknowledge that theory influences all aspects of qualitative inquiry then we cannot judge the authenticity of a qualitative account through internal consistency alone. The value of validity is that it allows us to examine the researchers' use of general social theory to explain particular social perspectives. In their classic paper, LeCompte and Goetz (1982) present an application of the concept of validity to qualitative research. They provide a comprehensive list of the ways that qualitative researchers use validity to argue that their evidence can provide an explanatory account of social reality based on investigation of the subjective point of view. Validity has a central role in justifying claims that research evidence and social theory can be combined to explain, rather than describe, the content of various social perspectives.

Conclusion

It would be misleading to treat qualitative research as a unified body of research practice or as unambiguously opposed to quantitative research. It is clear that the conduct of qualitative research differs in a number of important respects from the highly standardized methods used in quantitative studies. The text based, interactive, flexible, and naturalistic methods used by qualitative researchers arise from their concern to explain social phenomena from the point of view of the people in the study. The principles of reflexivity, transparency and critical examination of the evidence in the light of theory are used during the processes of data generation to reflect on the credibility of the evidence. However, although the techniques of qualitative inquiry differ markedly from those of quantitative research methods, this should not lead us to conclude that there are no underlying similarities in the logic of inquiry.

I have avoided giving a definition of qualitative research, partly because there is no formulation of the characteristics of qualitative research that would be acceptable to all, and partly because I see no point in assuming from the outset that qualitative research should be separated from any other form of research without considering the underlying logic of inquiry. Instead, I have placed an emphasis on methodological commitments that arise from the particular kind of research question that qualitative researchers are concerned about.

An epistemological claim that research evidence arising from a particular inquiry can be used as a basis for knowledge depends upon the researchers' arguments to convince their audiences that their evidence is credible and supports their inferences. In doing this, researchers will offer several lines of reasoning to justify their research question; draw attention to the reliability of their evidence; and provide a defence of their interpretation of the evidence. Audiences will evaluate these arguments by examining their validity. They will look for flaws in the construction of the research question, defects in the transparency of data production and handling, errors in the critical evaluation of the evidence in the light of the theoretical assumptions of the researchers. Although quantitative researchers have more formalized procedures for presenting assurances that their evidence fulfils these principles, that does not imply that the text-based, interactive, flexible and naturalistic methods of qualitative research are irrational or any less rigorous. As Mason (2002) points out, a commitment to flexibility and naturalism does not entail an ad hoc, casual and unplanned approach to inquiry. She argues that qualitative research can be *strategic* without relying on rigid, highly structured plans, or on a toolkit of well-rehearsed techniques and procedures. Qualitative researchers have developed research techniques that allow them to provide a reasoned defence of their approach, and assurances about the reliability of their evidence while recognizing that their use of interactive and flexible techniques means that they cannot be neutral or detached from the evidence they are generating.

In answer to the question posed by the chapter, it should be clear that I do not think that there is any need to outline an epistemology for qualitative research that is distinctive or separates it from other forms of inquiry. Although there are substantial differences in technique between qualitative and quantitative methods, these can be explained by the nature of the research questions that qualitative researchers ask. The main argument used to separate qualitative and quantitative research is that social reality is constructed rather than found; therefore, the methods used to investigate social phenomena from the point of view of the research participants must be based on an epistemology that can accommodate multiple and constructed realities. Quantitative research methods, based on positivist epistemology, cannot make this accommodation. Qualitative methods must, therefore, be based on a separate paradigm of inquiry. This prescriptive argument misses the point on several counts. An empiricist epistemology indicates that the perspective of the human observer is both the starting point and the arbiter of knowledge claims, but reality has turned out to be far more complex than it appears to our senses. As a result, epistemology has taught us to be cautious in our claims. Epistemology is not a sermonizing discipline that tells people what to do if they want their research evidence to enter the kingdom of knowledge.

Researchers are, by and large, pragmatic people who recognize that their practices have to be trustworthy and reliable so that the evidence they produce will be believed. Research practice is justified by its success in providing credible evidence to resolve practical problems or provide a coherent answer to questions of theory. The validity of a claim that research evidence has answered these questions will be assessed against the credibility of the evidence and the plausibility of the claim that the evidence is supporting. Empirical research does not depend upon a particular epistemology to justify its methods. A prescriptive approach to epistemology must yield, in the end, to what works. In the words of Hilary Putnam (1974: 240), concluding that Popper's attempt to prescribe the principle of falsification as a solution to the problem of induction, does not describe how scientists actually work: 'practice is primary'.

References

Agar, M. (1986) *Speaking of Ethnography*. Newbury Park, CA: Sage.

Avis, M. (1995) Valid arguments? A consideration of the concept of validity in establishing the credibility of research findings, *Journal of Advanced Nursing*, 22: 1203–1209.

Avis, M. (1997) Letting sleeping dogmas lie: an examination of positivism in the nursing research literature, *Social Sciences in Health*, 3: 52–63.

Becker, H. (1998) *Tricks of the Trade: How to Think about Your Research While You're Doing It*. Chicago: The University of Chicago Press.

Berger, P. and Luckmann, T. (1966) *The Social Construction of Reality*. London: Penguin.

Bhaskar, R. (1998) *The Possibility of Naturalism*, 3rd edn. London: Routledge.

Bryman, A. (1988) *Quantity and Quality in Social Research*. London: Unwin Hyman.

Denzin, N.K. and Lincoln, Y.S. (1994) Introduction: entering the field of qualitative research. In Denzin, N.K. and Lincoln, Y.S. (eds) *The Handbook of Qualitative Research*. London: Sage, 1–18.

Dingwall, R. (1992) 'Don't mind him – he's from Barcelona': qualitative methods in health studies. In Daly, J., McDonald, I. and Willis, E. (eds), *Researching Health Care: Designs, Dilemmas and Disciplines*. London: Routledge, 161–175.

Geertz, C. (1973) *The Interpretation of Cultures*. New York: Basic Books.

Guba, E. (1981) Criteria for assessing the trustworthiness of naturalistic inquiries, *Educational Communication and Technology Journal*, 29: 75–92.

Guba, E. and Lincoln, Y. (1986) *Fourth Generation Evaluation*. Thousand Oaks: Sage.

Hacking, I. (1999) *The Social Construction of What?* Cambridge, MA: Harvard University Press.

Lambert, H. and McKevitt, C. (2002) Anthropology in health research: from qualitative research to multi-disciplinarity, *British Medical Journal*, 325: 210–213.

LeCompte, M. and Goetz, J. (1982) Problems of reliability and validity in ethnographic research, *Review of Educational Research*, 52: 31–60.

Lincoln, Y. and Guba, E. (1985) *Naturalistic Inquiry*. Newbury Park, CA: Sage.

Lincoln, Y. and Guba, E. (2000) Paradigmatic controversies, contradictions, and emerging confluences. In Denzin, N.K. and Lincoln, Y.S. (eds) *The Handbook of Qualitative Research*, 2nd edn. London: Sage, 163–188.

Mason, J. (2002) *Qualitative Researching*, 2nd edn. London: Sage.

Popay, J. (1992) 'My health is alright, but I'm just tired all the time': women's experience of ill health. In Roberts, H. (ed.) *Women's Health Matters*. London: Routledge, 99–120.

Putnam, H. (1974) The 'corroboration' of theories. In Schilpp, P. (ed.) *The Philosophy of Karl Popper*. La Salle: Open Court, 221–240.

Quine, W. (1953) *From a Logical Point of View*. Cambridge, MA: Harvard University Press.

Schutz, A. (1972) *The Phenomenology of the Social World*. London: Heinemann.

Searle, J. (1995) *The Construction of Social Reality*. London: Penguin.

Silverman, D. (2001) *Interpreting Qualitative Data: Methods for Analysing Talk, Text and Interaction*, 2nd edn. London: Sage.

Smith, J. and Heshusius, L. (1986) Closing down the conversation: the end of the quantitative–qualitative debate among educational inquirers, *Educational Researcher*, 15: 4–12.

Spradley, J. (1979) *The Ethnographic Interview*. New York: Holt, Rinehart & Winston.

2

RON IPHOFEN
Ethical issues in qualitative health research

Introduction: the problem of ethical research

Being an ethical researcher is difficult whatever one's profession or discipline. The newspaper headline-grabbing issues appear to be mainly in the field of genetic modification and the use of human embryos. But whenever research has an effect upon the lives of humans ethical problems will emerge. This chapter aims to lay out the fundamental problems associated with behaving ethically as a researcher, to outline some particular difficulties confronting qualitative research in health and to offer practical advice both on gaining permission to conduct such research and in ensuring that the research is conducted ethically. Qualitative inquiry in health care does not focus on biomedical matters but is social research in a health-care context.

Moral philosophy

This is not the place to raise the many theoretical and conceptual difficulties that philosophers have examined over many centuries in trying to understand 'good' behaviour. It is likely that health practitioners will have received tuition in ethics during their initial training. There is an extensive literature in the field and the competent health researcher would be well advised to spend a little time studying it. (See, for example: Thompson 2000; La Follette 2002.) It is enough for our purposes here to establish that ethics are concerned with behaving 'properly' and making the right choices.

The branch of ethics that concerns health research is primarily normative ethics – it is about the way one *ought* to behave as a researcher. Those normative principles have been established over time from considering moral choices at an abstract level in ethical theorizing, from the codes of behaviour established by professional institutions and from the observation in practice of what happens when research is done for the 'wrong' reasons or in questionable ways as well as observing the benefits from doing research the 'right' way. Thus theorizing about ethics can never be divorced from the application of principles in practice (La

Follette 2002: 8). The central point about normative ethics is that it entails value judgements and how one chooses to behave, as a researcher can never be proven to be right or wrong by appealing to empirical facts. The role of normative ethics is not to recommend any particular course of action but to set out possibilities, help to assess values and assist in the making of informed, thoughtful choices (Thompson 2000: 30–32).

The autonomous professional and the good scientist

A major problem facing modern professionals lies in the many lines of account-ability they have to deal with. Health workers in particular face clinical account-ability to their professional institution and their colleagues, to the service organization which employs them, and, of course, to the patient and public. They are also likely to be expected to fulfil obligations to their profession (such as keeping their knowledge and skills up to date) and to their employing organization (such as in keeping accurate case notes and comprehensive administrative records).

It is not easy to prioritize ethical issues, since they all present dilemmas – difficult choices. It might seem simple to advocate a fundamental treatment principle such as 'first do no harm'. Those working in the field of public health know that such a principle is sometimes difficult to apply in practice – the law requiring a notification of infectious diseases undoubtedly restricts the liberty of any person with such a disease. Vaccination carries a risk to each individual vaccinated, but the interests of public heath require the balancing of such a risk against the reduced risk of infection to the rest of society. So sometimes indivi-duals, in the interests of protecting or doing some good for the rest of a community or society, may have been exposed to some risk.

There is a clear link between professional and research ethics. Ethical dilem-mas in research merely compound these issues since health professionals *as researchers* add many more lines of accountability to those they already serve. As health researchers they raise obligations to other researchers in their field, to patients again who now also become 'research subjects', to science in general in terms of the advancement of human knowledge and to society in terms of human benefit. (For a discussion on the dilemmas of professional accountability in formal organizations see Bovens (1998).)

Behaving ethically in conducting qualitative health research is like moving through a moral maze. The next section will draw out the fundamental elements in this maze and help highlight the central choices that must be made to engage in ethical research. These principles are moral dilemmas common to all forms of inquiry, not just qualitative research.

Beauchamp and Childress (2001) outline four basic principles on which health researchers base their actions, and although they apply them to the bio-medical field, they are equally important in social research.

- Respect for autonomy: respecting the independent decision-making of autonomous participants.

- Non-maleficence: avoiding harm based on balancing benefits against risks and costs.
- Beneficence: providing benefits and balancing these against risks and costs.
- Justice: distributing benefits and risks fairly.

Issues arising from these principles will be further discussed throughout this chapter.

Consequently being a good health researcher means:

(a) not doing (too much) harm;

(b) doing (some) good.

However, these terms are by no means clear. What is understood by the terms 'harm' and 'good'?

By (b) is meant a range of actions with the scientific intent of improving human knowledge about health and illness: describing, understanding and explaining. Good research also produces benefits in the form of improved health policy and advice on best practice, drawn from systematically produced evidence.

By (a) is meant that, as a consequence of doing (b), one is necessarily intervening in people's normal daily routines and activities. Just that intervention alone might be seen as disturbing. People may not like being observed or being asked questions about their thoughts, attitudes and actions. Sometimes that intervention changes people's lives in unforeseen ways and, sometimes, such change might be a deliberate part of the scientific process. We might ask people to do things differently to see if the difference produces an improvement in their lives or the lives of those with whom they associate.

The choices one makes as a researcher are about getting the right balance between (a) and (b). That is, if the goals of science (b) are not valued relatively highly, if they are not considered worth doing, then no interventions in the lives of human beings (a) can ever be justified.

Things do get more complex, however, if some people think science worth doing (b) even if others don't – especially if it means too much interference in people's lives (a). Whether science then gets done depends on the relative power of those supporting research set against the power of those opposing it as well as on available resources. To illustrate with a typical scenario: college and university students used to be the most frequently studied category of individuals. Lecturers often used them as 'research subjects' and could justify their actions on the grounds that the students would also be learning about research while they were experiencing being the subjects of research. Students had little choice in the matter and could feel obliged to participate in the research whatever their wishes.

Of course, those opposing research will not always be the participants in research. There are plenty of groups in society that hold moral objections to some of the topics studied by researchers and/or to some of the methods they use. Thus, for example, some religious organizations once objected to the study of homosexuality on the grounds that it was a moral perversion and should simply be condemned. In some respects they felt that researching it led to condoning such behaviour. Similarly some people hold that no studies should be covert or deceive the participants being studied on the grounds that deception is wrong – whatever the purpose – even if the research advances human knowledge.

Whether such research ever gets done, then, depends on the relative power and the resources of those supporting it against those opposing it. Research on genetically modified (GM) food crops offers a useful example. Ecologically oriented groups in the 'green' or organic food movement hold that such studies are potentially a fundamental threat to the environment. Scientists working in the GM field, many Western governments, large corporations and investors (and perhaps some who make donations to political parties) currently support such work and so it continues to be conducted – subject only to damage from occasional 'guerrilla' tactics from the more ardent ecologically-conscious groups.

Equivalent examples in the qualitative research field are harder to find since it is often more difficult to see the consequences for society of such research actions or interventions. At least we can say that if both the *observers* (researchers and other interested groups) and the *observed* (people being studied) agree that the intervention should be allowed in the interests of scientific advance then some part of our first set of moral dilemmas is on the way to being solved.

But agreeing to research, in principle, must then be qualified by further fundamental ethical decisions. Whether the proposed research actually goes ahead will then be dependent upon questions in three further areas:

- What precisely is the research being done for?
- Who does it?
- How do researchers propose doing it?

These might be represented as concerns of purpose, profession and practice. Each of these questions poses a further series of potential ethical dilemmas that may conflict with each other. These will now be examined in turn.

The purpose of research

The general discourse about ethical research behaviour was developed in the post-Second World War trials of Nazi war crimes (The Nuremburg Code 1947). The behaviour of Nazi medical scientists was judged to be unethical and led to the establishment of a general agreement that the ends of research can never justify the means. Thus, merely wanting to understand more about how human beings 'work' is unlikely to be a sustainable justification for research activity. The ethical judgement involved here has to do with whether or not research with no immediately evident added value constitutes responsible research activity, when research resources are being competed for in terms of all the other resources needed for health services, and when the pressure for relevance is high and when time and energy are also in short supply.

That there may be some form of human/communal/societal benefit does act as an overarching principle in carrying out research.

Many people will participate in research if they believe it benefits their group, community and/or society. It might be impossible to estimate a value to society accurately assessed separately from the interests of the researcher. Although the researcher is not best placed to make a judgement that balances the costs against the benefits to participants – what researcher could not see some general benefit to the work in which they have invested a great deal of energy? Thus, for example, if feminist researchers engage in research to fulfil an emancipatory or empowering project for women this is likely to have an effect upon how they do that work and the outcomes of their research. Gillies and Aldred (2002: 38) advocate '... locating research in terms of its objectives and outcomes, by fully articulating the motivating political intentions'.

Recently governments in the so-called advanced societies have willingly financed health research that has subsequently made significant contributions to public health policy and, in many cases, to service practice. Opportunities to contribute to policy and practice from research look set to continue to grow. It is vital, then, that the contributions made by researchers are sensible, apt, valued, and ethical problems satisfactorily resolved. Again this raises issues of the sustained responsibility of individual researchers if such an opportunity is not to be squandered. In the same way, since research knowledge/information does constitute a marketable product, outputs are subject to quality assessment, estimates of worth and value for money. Researchers in independent research agencies, for example, are acutely aware of how delays occasioned by ethical review or legal challenges prompted by ethical compromise can jeopardize the 'added-value' of research knowledge. All researchers have to face dilemmas of knowledge production such as: Who (agency or group) is financing the research and under what conditions? Why are they funding the work and what do they seek to gain from it?

Whatever the health researcher's sector of activity (public, private, academic) there is little doubt that the research product has become an assessed determinant of career progress. For academics in the UK a Research Assessment Exercise (RAE) attempts to quantify this. For the private sector it has more to do with how well business accounts are managed. In public service the research product is primarily aimed at enhancing evidence-based practice. When research success determines individual career enhancement ethical review cannot solely lie in the hands of the researchers engaged in the project – given their personal investment in successful research products, some form of independent ethical review is seen as essential.

Consequently qualitative health researchers must demonstrate to themselves and to others that the research they propose will offer benefits to scientific understanding, to policy and to practice that makes the resources spent engaged in the study worthwhile.

Profession

Given the preceding argument it seems essential qualitative health researchers exert adequate controls over research in the field. Scandals in such research are unlikely ever to be as traumatic as those involving child organ retention. But such scandals do illustrate the taint on all research activity that is a consequence of ethically unregulated behaviour. The research field can be contaminated by many factors that include researchers posing as clinicians or the over-evaluation of routine patient–professional interactions. Unethical behaviour in clinical and other areas diminishes trust in the act of research and in the actions of other health researchers. Also important are the rules given by Beauchamp and Childress (2001) based on ethical principles:

- Veracity: telling the truth and informing participants in terms that they can understand.
- Privacy: this needs to be respected and is closely linked to confidentiality.
- Confidentiality: essential in a professional and in a research relationship (this will be discussed later).
- Fidelity: professional loyalty – a complex concept raising other difficulties that cannot be discussed fully in the space available here.

One professional device for enhancing ethical awareness is expert mentorship – the sharing of experiences and solutions to problems. Expert researchers can aid novices in their ethical decision-making by offering mentorship and advice in response to specific issues. When confronting a difficult ethical dilemma it is a good idea to ask colleagues how they would deal with it, or have dealt with similar problems in the past. A more systematic maintenance of ethical standards would recommend that researchers should be required to attend training courses in ethical decision-making. At the very least this could offer a way of ensuring that they have read and considered the available professional guidelines. In fact, the status and application of ethical guidelines has been a recurring concern within professional research associations. The issue is one of whether or not such codes can be applied, creating effective sanctions against researchers who behave un-ethically and do not follow rules and guidelines.

More recently increased consideration has been given to the safety of field researchers. An awareness of the risks (physical and emotional) to field researchers is both an ethical and a practical managerial concern to do with danger on the job. Dangers in qualitative research may arise from interviewing or observing in potentially threatening locations such as hospital A&E units, or from the discussion of unanticipated or sensitive topics in interviewing in residential care homes (Lee-Treweek and Linkogle 2000). There is now awareness that consideration for the safety of 'subjects' should be matched by a consideration for those doing the 'subjecting' (see Craig *et al.* 2001). The whole issue of calling participants 'subjects' is, of course, problematic (see later in this chapter).

Qualitative health researchers should recognize the particular ethical implications in the nature of the research they do and its ethical consequences for all participants (researchers and researched). Finding an experienced mentor and the sharing of concerns with others working in the same field is vital to seeking a balanced professional response to ethical dilemmas.

Practice

The experimental ideal in positivist approaches to research requires full control of all intervening variables and the ability validly and reliably to observe and measure the consequences of the research intervention. Qualitative research necessarily sacrifices such control desires in favour of accessing the authentic and natural behaviours and attitudes of those being studied. This means methodologically seeking not to deprive participants of their power to act as they would, even if they were not being studied.

Fortunately, this is consistent with the ethical purpose of seeking not to take away the power of the people we study, to preserve their autonomy and to behave as democratically as possible in the conduct of the research. But it would be dishonest to imply that qualitative researchers need no power to direct the research. They will choose to adopt methods or practices that are intended to help seek answers to the set research questions and, therefore, entail some form of intervention into and direction of the lives of the people being studied.

So questions do have to be asked about precisely what methods the researchers propose using:

1. Might such methods result in unacceptable forms of intervention in the lives of those being studied?
2. Should a competent professional engage in research which compromises methodological principles to prevent potential harm coming to research participants if that harm is estimated to be slight?
3. Who is qualified to make the judgement that harm might be minimal?

Concern for the rights and well being of research participants lies at the root of ethical review, such as that carried out by Research Ethics Committees. People who are vulnerable are of prime concern for both researchers and reviewers; the very young and the very old, together with those with learning difficulties are seen to be worthy of special attention. Vulnerability is linked to the problem of routinely socially excluded participants, and one might ask whether or not the potential for social exclusion in research was an ethical or methodological concern (or both).

When methods are compared there does seem to be a view among some observers that there are inherently unethical procedures. Covert observation is seen by some as particularly problematic since it necessarily implies deception – yet to let people know they were being observed might result in an alteration of their behaviour. Even conventional randomized controlled trials depend upon the subtle coercion of 'captive' subjects – i.e. patients. It is difficult to ensure that patients do not feel pressured into participation. In qualitative research it may be impossible to maintain a neat distinction between covert and overt research. Settings are more complex and changeable than may be anticipated (Murphy and Dingwall 2001: 342).

Advances in information technology have implications for research ethics – even in qualitative research. Enhanced data archiving makes possible the recording, retaining and re-analyzing of data. This has, in turn, encouraged researchers to retain data longer than was previously thought necessary – thereby enhancing the dangers of leaking confidentiality and anonymity. Similarly enhanced data management ('fusion', matching and transfer) captures the popular imagination more than all the other concerns: 'What do they know about me? Who else could gain access to that information?' (Mauthner *et al.* 1998).

In practice, the particular skills required of the qualitative researcher include balancing the control necessary for systematic and rigorous observation against allowing the attitudes and behaviour of interest to occur naturally. In this instance what is required for qualitative theoretical perspectives neatly meets ethical requirements – don't interfere too much! It is the practical difficulty of doing that that creates the problem.

The individual researcher's responsibility

These issues will be clarified as we look at specific dilemmas. But it is vital here to stress a few central principles. These are all linked to the idea that, in qualitative research in particular, whatever formal ethical review has been gone through. Whatever the professional codes that apply, the ultimate arbiter of the 'correct' moral decision has to be individual researchers themselves, and their thinking should be based on fundamental ethical principles.

1. Given the need to prioritize research goals in different ways at different times, in the progress of the research only the researchers in practice know the detail about what is going on and where the research is taking them. They will be the first to notice if harm is being done or if there is a potential for harm to be done as the research progresses. In this sense qualitative health research, in particular, is a 'coalface' activity. Often the individual researcher is directly involved with the respondent or individual or group under study – either in observing them, asking questions or participating in their daily lives in some way. Ethical choices and moral dilemmas may arise at any point during the research process and to attempt to pass the problem on to a supervisor, manager, or any other agency, is to evade it. In any case, it is not always possible in the course of the research. The 'coalface' researcher has an insight into the effects of the research process that may not be available to anyone else.

2. There is no simple 'decision-tree' that one can follow to help in making ethical research decisions. This is because moral views are not factual in the way that clinical decisions can be based upon available evidence. Moral views are judgements that change over and through time. What was acceptable behaviour in any one community or society many years ago may not be acceptable

now. This means that there is rarely ever one correct solution to many ethical problems. No ethical code or set of guidelines could be devised to produce the best of all possible outcomes for all stakeholders. Trade-offs are always required. This is not to say that the balance of harm and benefit is always a *zero sum* transaction (that one person's gain has to be another person's loss). Rather the *potential* for harm must always be considered and balanced against the *potential* for benefit. As indicated above the problem is getting the right balance of harm and benefit. The researcher's problem is to estimate whether that balance of harm and benefit is being achieved. Participants in a qualitative research project might, for example, initially be flattered to be asked lots of questions about themselves. But as the questioning persists it might become more of a burden than they had anticipated – and this might present a particular problem in health research with someone who may already be burdened by an illness, pain or disability.

3.   In fact, that judgement of the balance of harm and benefit frequently has to be taken in a dynamic situation. Once again this may be a particular feature of a central assumption of qualitative research – that life cannot be treated as a static phenomenon. People's experience of health and illness is an ongoing social process and it continues to be so even while they are being researched. What may have seemed straightforward and morally uncomplicated at the outset may turn out to be fraught with difficulty once the project is underway. The availability of detailed formal ethical guidelines and the apparently systematic process of ethical review that precedes most health research imply a rather static view of the research act. Qualitative research is better characterized by '... fluidity and inductive uncertainty' (Mauthner *et al.* 2002: 2). Unanticipated harm (and benefit of course) can emerge during a study when the only ethical decision-taker available is the researcher. Only the researcher can assess whether a particular set of questions is disturbing the respondent to such an extent that they cannot justifiably continue to ask them.

4.   Finally, the health professional researcher who also has professional responsibilities as a clinician and/or carer has to decide if they are first and foremost a health worker or a researcher. If the latter, the limiting of harm to the individual patient becomes the primary requirement – whatever the potential gains to society from their research. For the health researcher who is also a clinician there may be a problem of conflicting principles within each of the professional codes to which they are supposed to adhere. The potential for divided loyalties has to be addressed so that all involved in the research are clear as to the researchers' value hierarchy (see Bell and Nutt 2002).

Indeed, this last principle is one which is carefully watched for by those responsible for the ethical review of health research. It is seen to be of primary importance that patients, clients and those in the care of the health services are not harmed by the research and that their individual treatment is not affected in a negative way.

Typical problems

'Principles guide our perceptions of how to conduct ethical research ... specific circumstances and contexts inform our decisions' (Mauthner *et al.* 2002: 6).

All of the above principles and the issues discussed next are typically faced by all researchers, but qualitative research usually implies a different form of relationship with the research participant which leads to added complexities. This relationship can be summarized under the concept of 'trust' and tends to be of a more humanistic nature than research that produces quantitative data (Miles and Huberman 1994: 292). Quantitative data analysis is at one remove from the human nature of the person from whom it was generated. Qualitative data are methodologically required to remain close to the values, meaning, intentions, aspirations and goals of the participant. In that sense it is more personal.

Defining 'the subject'

Some contemporary qualitative researchers are uncomfortable with referring to the groups or individuals they study as 'subjects'. They regard this as an ethical concern in that the term suggests the kind of objectification of people one finds in more experimental or quantitative forms of research. This is more than a semantic concern and it is worth considering whether the people being studied are referred to as *participants, respondents* or *subjects* according to the precise nature of their engagement with the research project (Birch and Miller 2002).

Accessing participants and negotiating the research relationship

Who should be approached is largely a problem of choosing the most appropriate sample from the population and so is predominantly a methodological issue. In qualitative research the sample is usually chosen for convenience and/or purposively. But *how* people are accessed for research purposes remains both a practical and an ethical problem. It is hard to separate issues associated with accessing participants in the first place, re-accessing them as part of a continuing study, and remaining unimpeded in that access from gatekeepers who may seek to control what participants contribute to the study. Attempts to conduct qualitative research on residents in older people's care homes offer telling examples of such difficulties. Older people might not fully understand what is required of them and the sustained nature of that commitment, those caring for them might be sensitive to the older people's comments and, as a consequence, being able to interview them alone and without the participants' concern for what their carers might think they are saying influencing the honesty with which they participate raise myriad ethical concerns (Fisk and Wigley 2000).

Awareness of the balance of power between researcher and researched is vital. This may be even less clear in qualitative research studies (Murphy and Dingwall 2001: 344). Allowing a researcher into one's life for study may in itself imply a loss of power. The focus of the relationship is determined by the researcher's criteria, not by the other participants – otherwise the relationship would not exist. By their

interpretation and re-presentation of the participants' lives, resear
necessarily maintaining or challenging those people's location in the souiu
archy (Becker 1967).

To some extent exploitation of the research participant is inevitable. People,
opportunities, situations and meaningful spaces are all exploited to derive the 'rich,
deep data' that are sought in qualitative research (Birch and Miller 2002). The
establishment of rapport is an accomplished research skill, and even friendship can
be faked as part of the management of consent and the encouraging of continued
participation. In fact, researchers may expose themselves to unwanted personal
consequences if they disclose too much about themselves as a rapport-generating
strategy (Duncombe and Jessop 2002: 118–119). However, while there is a sense
in which friendship is necessarily implied in the establishment of rapport and the
development of trust, it is important to remember that the relationship is one of
'formal informality'. In all likelihood the relationship would not have existed
without the need for one party to secure a research goal. There is a danger in the
qualitative researcher seeking to avoid exploiting the partipant to such an extent
that no research goals are accomplished – a waste of everybody's time!

The negotiation of the research relationship particularly needs addressing by
health researchers who are also practitioners. Disclosure of their practitioner status
to participants is likely to have methodological consequences. Participants may say
and do different things for researchers they know to have other professional
obligations. Health and care workers conducting research might be perceived as
having more power in the research relationship than if they had not been practitioners. Ensuring participants have, and perceive themselves to have, adequate
power to determine their role in the research is ethically necessary to the implementation of all the following considerations.

Protecting participants: vulnerability and marginalization

Researchers have a duty to protect all participants in a study from any harmful
consequences that may arise out of their participation. This is even more the case
when those groups or individuals are less able to protect themselves. Children are
seen as particularly vulnerable, while older people may be both vulnerable and
marginalized. Children may lack the sophistication to perceive when a study is not
in their interests or when disclosure is damaging to them (Alderson 1995). Older
people may be excluded from most studies due to their lessened economic and
political importance. The ethical health researcher has to guard against all these
'disprivileging' possibilities.

It is unsurprising that increased awareness of the ethical problems associated
with the study of marginal and/or vulnerable groups or individuals should come
from feminist researchers. Gender biases in research arise from the assumption of
homogeneity in participants, and this can lead to the dominance of masculine
perspectives. Feminist research has succeeded in highlighting and making public
the traditionally private worlds of females, families and households (Cotterill
1992). That, in itself, is not without ethical concern – how those worlds are made
public and the consequences for the people in the study may then lie outside of

their control. Barron (1999) shows how intellectually disabled women are doubly disadvantaged research participants both in their status loss from cognitive impairment and from their gender. A self-appointed alliance with such groups may mask the superior position of the researcher.

More recently researchers have become concerned about the potential for harm to groups or individuals who may be typically excluded from studies as a consequence of their socio-cultural location. Such exclusion might mean that their interests are inadequately represented in a study and the researcher's (necessarily) limited perspective on the world cannot guarantee the inclusion of all groups. Typically this relates to lesser-abled individuals routinely being missed by all types of social survey – individuals with learning disability may be excluded from street interviews, those with vision impairments missed by postal questionnaires and so on. While *whom* to include is primarily a methodological problem, ethical concerns arise when routine exclusion perpetuates or exacerbates an individual's or a group's lowered status in society.

The key to how participants are ethically accessed and then protected lies in attending to the concerns noted under the five following sub-headings.

Seeking informed consent

To avoid harming participants in a study it is essential to gain their agreed consent to taking part. If they are to be able to consent, they need to know fully what their participation entails. They will need information, but here the ethical concern may conflict with a methodological one: how much information should they be given and in what form?

Too much information could act as a disincentive to participation by implying an excessive commitment of time or an inhibiting amount of emotional invest-ment. Or it may be too 'leading' in revealing too much about the researcher's interests. Too little information, however, could be construed as deceptive and result in participants' early withdrawal from the study when they find out more about it.

Even more difficult with qualitative research is that while the participant might not fully know what they are agreeing to, the researchers may know only a little more since the research can be allowed, or even encouraged, to move in directions that only become appropriate when the research is under way. This means that consent has to be ongoing and information-giving conceived as dynamically integrated into the life of the project (see, for example, Miller and Bell 2002).

Ethical review committees, particularly in health research, often insist upon formal consent being achieved before the commencement of a project. This is clearly impossible if change is an inherent part of the qualitative research process, in such cases the methodological limitations on gaining fully informed consent would have to be made clear at the outset. Indeed formal consent can be hard to achieve with some categories of groups and individuals who perceive themselves as vulnerable and/or marginalized. Reading and/or signing a formal consent form could appear to be establishing a more apparently official relationship than they had bargained for. The research relationship in such cases is inevitably tentative and gradualist.

Increasingly research ethics committees seek proof of consent in a written, signed and, in some cases, witnessed form. Clearly this could alienate some potential participants and, while it may protect the researcher against any future charge of not giving adequate information, it is by no means legally binding and would not even guarantee the respondent's continued participation in a project. The giving of oral consent on the telephone or in a face-to-face situation does appear more natural and consequently more consistent with the ethos of qualitative enquiry so, to ensure that as much information as necessary/possible can be demonstrated to have been given, researchers have taken to audio-tape recording the consenting process.

Eliciting 'data' and knowledge production

The source material for qualitative research is unlikely to be anonymous data. It is more usually people's accounts, stories, imagery, considered response and, in that sense at least, is primarily owned by them. Their agreement to participation in the research entails 'gifting' that experience to the researcher as data. It is likely in the first instance to be their re-presentation of a personal experience and has, therefore, a precious, human quality. If participants talk about the experience of pain in their illness or disease for example, they will be disclosing an intimacy – something that reveals a quality associated with the nature of their existence as a human being.

But then, as a necessary part of the process, the researcher manipulates these data in some way by coding, classifying, re-interpreting them and, ultimately, by disseminating them in a form accessible to interested others. The researcher's ethical responsibility is then associated with how that shared gift is cared for (how the data continue to be treated as 'precious' as they are analyzed and reproduced as knowledge), and how the person who shared the data is cared for as a consequence of those data being delivered – albeit in a different form – to a larger audience.

Part of the problem here is that one of the researcher's tasks is to select sufficient elements from the data to permit the description, understanding, explanation and so on that are part of the purposes of the research – the production of new knowledge. Conventionally this is known as data reduction, and is inevitable since the full richness of the person's unique and individual original experience can never be captured. Nor can it be fully reproduced. Another of the researcher's tasks is to help convey that experience authentically and in a way that might be useful for purposes of explanation, policy-making or practice. So there is always something of the researchers themselves that must be included in the re-presentation since they were party to the mediated reproduction of the experience. Researchers have to maintain a reflexive position, gauge how much of what emerges is dependent on or independent of them and consistently hold themselves accountable for the knowledge produced (Holland 1999).

There are added data protection problems associated with the secondary analysis of qualitative data collected for some other purpose. It is essential that the archiving principles adopted are declared and understood by both participants and researchers. These policies can be found at the major archive sites:

http://www.qualidata.essex.ac.uk

http://www.dipex.org.uk

Ensuring anonymity and confidentiality

The researcher can only strive to protect their respondent's identity and hold the information given in confidence. If persons choose to reveal their participation in a study there is little the researcher can do about it. If they wish their identity to be disclosed as part of the research report the researcher then has some dilemmas – what effect this might have on other subjects of their research (knowing the identity of one participant might help identify others who desire continued anonymity); and whether the personalization of reported data in any way affects its theoretical value.

Confidentiality is more than a matter of obeying the law on data protection. The information given by those being researched is introduced into a more public domain by virtue of its disclosure to the researcher. The researcher has to make clear to the participants precisely what the sharing of confidences – the researcher's data in qualitative research – might imply for them. There may be regret that so much has been disclosed and a need to address the emotional consequences of that. If criminal activity is disclosed the researcher has to choose between obedience to the law and a breach of the confidentiality originally promised. The researcher's moral integrity only remains intact if this is clearly understood by the participant prior to the commencement of the research. Yet making that clear may have methodological consequences in producing a tendency to minimal disclosure by the respondent as a safety precaution.

Developing and maintaining rapport and involvement

Being there, being interested, listening and hearing would seem to be a *sine qua non* of qualitative research. Participants usually have a way of knowing – as we all do as 'ordinary' human beings – if this is being accomplished authentically. More than that, there is an inherently long-term expectation of involvement between researcher and researched that is implied in any relationship of trust (Duncombe and Jessop 2002). Honest and immediate responses to potential breaches of trust have to be made. This can be as apparently trivial as requiring more time and energy investment of the participant than was originally implied. And this can happen in qualitative research when repeat visits are deemed necessary to enhance validity or as a check on the reliability of data gathered.

By consenting to participation, the people involved have already to some degree allowed the researcher into their lives. The degree to which that involvement is to be continued or deepened has to be continuously negotiated. Thus a participant who agreed originally only to receive a final report might be expected or expect to read, review, critically comment on and/or contribute to that report. The precise nature of the mutual expectations of researcher and researched will have to be continuously clarified for methodological as well as for ethical reasons.

There may be a limit to the degree to which participants can remain truly involved which depends upon the conceptual level or the detailed technical language adopted within research reports. The researcher comes from a professional and disciplinary tradition that the participants may not share. To ensure participants' continued understanding of how their contribution extends theoretical knowledge it might be necessary to 'translate' the research products for their benefit. There is clearly a danger of either demeaning the participants or of limiting the nature of their contribution by the inaccessibility of the terminology.

Here, again, the potential for conflict between researcher and health practitioner roles can emerge. 'Being listened to' is something patients often plead for. Ironically, more time may be spent with a patient as a participant within the context of a research project than in routine therapeutic engagements. While the health professional researcher may cope with that personally, a problem of appropriate disengagement from a research relationship that has therapeutic implications can arise. Preparations for that disengagement could be made both with research patients and service colleagues.

Facilitating participants' withdrawal from the research

The ultimate test of the enhanced power of research participants lies in their knowing that they have the ability to withdraw from the study at any point. No matter how inconvenient this may be to the researchers, they have only fulfilled their ethical obligations if they not only permit such withdrawal when it is sought, but facilitate it in terms of ensuring no harm comes to individuals as a consequence of their withdrawal from the study. This may mean going out of one's way to ensure they receive the same health-care treatment they would have done had they not joined the study in the first place.

Legal concerns and review procedures

Knowing the law

Ethically responsible qualitative health researchers have a duty to the people in their study, to society, to the funders of their research and to their profession, to remain aware of their legal obligations. Obedience to the law then becomes an individual moral choice. The ethical way to behave is to be informed of the law and then to decide whether or not the law should be obeyed. The law is not always moral since the law is established by the state, and it may not always suit the agencies of any particular state to act ethically. Hopefully this should be less the case with developing internationalism in legal matters and effective non-governmental agencies keeping a watch on the actions of states (such as the Red Cross, the Red Crescent, Oxfam, Amnesty International).

The major UK legislation that could affect consent, participation, and the protection of research participants' interests includes the Data Protection Act (1998), the Human Rights Act (1998), the law on Intellectual Property Rights, Freedom of Information and, of course, the full panoply of criminal law. For example, the Human Rights Act came into force in October 2000 and incorporates into UK law rights and freedoms guaranteed by the European Convention on Human Rights. Strictly it applies to action by public authorities, so it should not directly affect research conducted by private and independent research organizations – unless such work is being carried out on behalf of a Government department. Further information can be gained directly from the Human Rights Unit on: http://www.homeoffice.gov.uk/hract/.

The UK Medical Research Council has a thorough and comprehensive guidance document – Personal Information in Medical Research – which offers advice of use to all researchers working with personal data of any kind. This document can be found on: http://www.mrc.ac.uk/ethics_a.html.

In recent years a uniform procedure for ethical review of research proposals concerned with human health has been established. The Central Office for Research Ethics Committees (COREC) coordinates the development of operational systems for Local and Multi-Centre Research Ethics Committees (LRECs and MRECs) on behalf of the National Health Service (NHS) and the Department of Health (DoH) in England. It maintains an overview of the operation of the research ethics system in England, and alerts the DoH and other responsible authorities if the need arises for them to review policy and operational guidance relating to Research Ethics Committees. It also manages a national training programme for Research Ethics Committee members and administrators in England. It liaises with similar bodies having responsibilities for other regions within the UK. COREC can be contacted via the following website address: www.corec.org.uk.

There is a standardized form that must be completed by all applicants proposing research on NHS patients and/or staff and recommended standard procedures for seeking informed consent and producing patient information about the research. Examples of consent forms and patient information letters can be found in most introductory research texts (see, for example, Holloway and Wheeler (2002: 59–60)) but they must be written following COREC's guidelines.

The DoH have also established a Research Governance Framework for Health and Social Care that defines the broad principles of good research governance and attempts to ensure that health- and social-care research is conducted to high scientific and ethical standards. Research governance is concerned with proper accountability throughout the research process and the establishment of a framework is a formalized, administrative procedure intended to reduce unacceptable variations in research practice across health and social care. It is also intended to enhance the contribution of research to the partnership between services and science since it documents standards, details the responsibilities of the key people involved in research, outlines delivery systems and describes local and national monitoring systems. This can be found at: http://www.doh.gov.uk/research/rd3/nhsrandd/researchgovernance.htm.

This system only strictly covers access for research purposes to patients and staff in DoH and NHS institutions. The boundaries of the framework for social-care research are still far from clear; there is ambiguity about whether it should include research involving statutory social services, all social-care-related research, or non-clinical health services research. In fact, there is no equivalent national system covering the general public so researchers not operating within an institutionalized framework are still in a position to police their own ethical decisions. If people choose to participate without being accessed as patients or employees of the

NHS, they are free to do so. The researcher's problem then only pertains to how the formal organization of the NHS chooses to relate to them if they sidestep institutional review. Few modern researchers operate independently and systems of governance based on the NHS model are growing up elsewhere. Thus university-based researchers will increasingly be expected to submit proposals to institutional review boards (IRBs) – a system that has been in place in North America for some years.

Some of the problems that researchers face from these committees have already been hinted at. Qualitative researchers have experienced difficulties in the past because many members of LRECs and MRECs know little about such research and often critically scrutinize research designs and methodologies as they are seen to affect research ethics. They justify asking methodological questions on the grounds that an intervention in people's lives is unwarranted if a research design is flawed and unlikely to meet its intended objectives. The most common reasons for proposals in the social-care field being refused ethics committee approval seem to be criticisms of the proposed methodology. In addition, encounters between social researchers and LRECs often reveal a lack of consensus between the LRECs covering different geographical areas. There is also seen to be an emphasis on protecting staff and institutions against the potential threat of litigation rather than promoting the rights of research participants.

To help committees make informed judgements about qualitative health research projects, the Medical Sociology Group of the British Sociological Association agreed a short guidance document in 1996 on the criteria for the evaluation of qualitative research. (This has been reproduced in many sources – most recently as Appendix 1 in Alderson (2001).)

It is vital to encourage discussion and debate about the promotion and conduct of high quality ethical research since the development of formal governance and accountability structures is likely to increase. Janet Lewis, former Research Director of the Joseph Rowntree Foundation has proposed that the bodies that fund social-care research should be responsible for ensuring that proposed research designs are ethical. Thus she is suggesting that funding agencies should be more concerned about the judgement of ethical standards. Those involved in social-care research have been concerned to establish an ethical framework and accountability system that is not dominated by biomedical researchers who are less likely to understand the special concerns of qualitative health research. For further information see the Social Services Research Group website http://www.ssrg.org.uk.

Professional codes and ethical guidelines

There is only so much room in a chapter such as this to consider the full range of ethical dilemmas a researcher has to face. There are many other useful sources of ethical advice and guidance from the major relevant professional research associations:

• Social Research Association – http://www.the-sra.org.uk

- British Sociological Association – http://www.britsoc.org.uk/about/ethic.htm
- British Psychological Society – http://www.bps.org.uk/about/rules5.cfm

Growing international concern for the conduct of ethical research has led to a European Commission-funded project on the maintenance of research standards. Information about this can be found at: http://www.respectproject.org/main/index.php.

Such sources also suggest ways of seeking mentorship from individual researchers who have faced ethical dilemmas in the past and from internet discussion groups. However, Murphy and Dingwall (2001: 340) counsel caution in the application of codes in that they may not be adequately method-specific. Their generalized prescriptions may unnecessarily constrain valuable qualitative research or blunt researchers to the particular sensitivities of those currently under study. General principles may have to be operationalized in different ways that are directly linked to the methods and topics of study.

Miles and Huberman (1994: 288–297), Murphy and Dingwall (2001) and Holloway and Wheeler (2002) offer succinct discussions of qualitative research linked to the broader ethical dilemmas and with useful further reading suggestions.

Conclusion

The consideration of ethical dilemmas in qualitative health research is an exercise in professional integrity. Behaving responsibly as a researcher, health worker, and individual human being requires the sustained consideration of the ethical implications of one's activities – not to engage in such considerations is, in itself, unethical. The principle of researcher reflexivity has ethical as well as methodological import. The knowledge produced as a consequence of research cannot be seen as somehow detached from the many purposes for which the research was carried out, from the multiple professional loyalties to which the researcher is tied and from the precise ways in which the researchers engaged with the people they were studying.

While only the individual researchers are adequately placed during the conduct of a research project to make such judgements and to attend to their consequences for good health research, given their vested interests in research outcomes, some form of independent ethical review continues to be vital. Attempts to enhance the power of research participants suggests also the need for their inclusion in the judgement of ethical conduct – they may choose to disengage from, criticize, or seek redress for any grievance perceived as consequent on the research. Ethical qualitative research in health then becomes a mutual accomplishment of all these stakeholders: researcher, participants, funders and reviewers.

References

Alderson, P. (1995) *Listening to Children: Ethics and Social Research.* Barkingside: Barnardos.

Alderson, P. (2001) *On Doing Qualitative Research linked to Ethical Healthcare*. London: Wellcome Trust.

Barron, K. (1999) Ethics in qualitative social research on marginalized groups, *Scandinavian Journal of Disability Research*, 1 (1): 38–49.

Beauchamp, T.L. and Childress, J.F. (2001) *Principles of Biomedical Ethics*, 5th edn. New York: Oxford University Press.

Becker, H. (1967) Whose side are we on? *Social Problems*, 14 (Winter): 239–248.

Bell, L. and Nutt, L. (2002) Divided loyalties, divided expectations: Research ethics, professional and occupational responsibilities. In Mauthner, M., Birch, M., Jessop, J. and Miller, T. (eds) *Ethics in Qualitative Research*. London: Sage, 70–90.

Birch, M. and Miller, T. (2002) Encouraging participation: ethics and responsibilities. In Mauthner, M., Birch, M., Jessop, J. and Miller, T. (eds) *Ethics in Qualitative Research*. London: Sage, 91–106.

Bovens, M. (1998) *The Quest for Responsibility: Accountability and Citizenship in Complex Organisations*. Cambridge: Cambridge University Press.

Cotterill, P. (1992) Interviewing women: issues of friendship, vulnerability and power, *Women's Studies International Forum*, 15 (5/6): 593–606.

Craig, G., Corden, A. and Thornton, P. (2001) *A Code of Safety for Social Researchers*. London: SRA [http://www.the-sra.org.uk/Stay%20Safe.htm]

Duncombe, J. and Jessop, J. (2002) 'Doing rapport' and the ethics of 'faking friendship'. In Mauthner, M., Birch, M., Jessop, J. and Miller, T. (eds) *Ethics in Qualitative Research*. London: Sage, 107–122.

Fisk, M. and Wigley, V. (2000) Accessing and interviewing the oldest old in care homes, *Quality in Ageing – Policy, Practice and Research*, 1 (1): 27–33.

Gillies, V. and Aldred, P. (2002) The ethics of intention: research as a political tool. In Mauthner, M., Birch, M., Jessop, J. and Miller, T. (eds) *Ethics in Qualitative Research*. London: Sage, 32–52.

Holland, R. (1999) Reflexivity, *Human Relations*, 52 (4): 463–484.

Holloway, I. and Wheeler, S. (2002) *Qualitative Research in Nursing*, 2nd edn. Oxford: Blackwell.

La Follette, H. (ed.) (2002) *Ethics in Practice: An Anthology*. Oxford: Blackwell.

Lee-Treweek, G. and Linkogle, S. (2000) *Danger in the Field: Risk and Ethics in Social Research*. London: Routledge.

Mauthner, M., Birch, M., Jessop, J. and Miller, T. (eds) (2002) *Ethics in Qualitative Research*. London: Sage.

Mauthner, N.S., Parry, O. and Backett-Milburn, K. (1998) The data are out there, or are they? Implications for archiving and revisiting qualitative data, *Sociology*, 32 (4): 733–745.

Miles, M. and Huberman, A.M. (1994) *Qualitative Data Analysis*, 2nd edn. London: Sage.

Miller, T. and Bell, L. (2002) Consenting to what? Issues of access, gatekeeping and 'informed' consent. In Mauthner, M., Birch, M., Jessop, J. and Miller, T. (eds) *Ethics in Qualitative Research*. London: Sage, 53–69.

Murphy, E. and Dingwall, R. (2001) The Ethics of Ethnography. In Atkinson, P., Coffey, A., Delamont, S., Lofland, J. and Lofland, L. (eds) *Handbook of Ethnography*. London: Sage, 339–351.

The Nuremberg Code (1947) in *Doctors of Infamy: the Story of the Nazi Medical Crimes*. Mitscherlich, A. and Mielke, F. New York: Schuman (1949: xxiii–xxv).

Thompson, M. (2000) *Ethics (Teach Yourself series)*. London: Hodder Headline.

PART 2
Collecting data

Data sources in qualitative research

The most common types of data sources in qualitative inquiry are interviewing and observation. Increasingly, documentary sources such as diaries, letters and other documents from the field – for instance the clinical area, the doctor's surgery or the setting where students are being taught – are also used to generate data. In this book the focus is on interviewing and observation as these are still the most commonly used procedures that health professionals carry out, because they are more immediate, convey the thoughts, feelings and behaviour of people – and are more easily accessible.

The most popular data sources are in-depth, unstructured interviews with an *aide-mémoire* and one or two key questions that become progressively more focused throughout the process of the research. Semi-structured interviews with an interview guide, and, more recently, focus groups, are also used to generate data. There are many advantages to interviewing patients and clients, but it can also be problematic. One of the main characteristics of the qualitative interviews is the element of control that participants have over its direction and content (in contrast to structured interviews). Focus group interviews are group interviews and depend on the dynamic of the group – be they patients, students or health professionals – and generate interesting data, not only through the verbalization of experience and thought of the participants but also through their interaction during the interviews.

In their observations researchers watch action and interaction that take place in the health-care setting. These settings may be macro or micro, for example, a community, a culture, or a ward, an Accident and Emergency Department. Problems are inherent in this type of participant observation as the researchers themselves may influence the setting. Participant observation differs from structured observation in the sense that the framework is allowed to evolve during immersion in the setting, rather than being determined by the researcher.

The qualitative interview is 'a conversation with a purpose'. **Clare Taylor** explains about the nature of questioning and the reasons for carrying out interviews in Chapter 3. The interviewer needs special listening skills and should create an atmosphere of trust and respect so that the interview is conducive to exploring the experience of the participants without giving them a sense of lack of control or intimidation. The researcher therefore needs flexibility and sensitivity. As well as describing the characteristics of the qualitative interview and the advantages of interviewing, Taylor also exposes its problems. She describes differences between interviews in the main research approaches, and gives a number of examples from different health-care settings.

In Chapter 4, **Jenny Kitzinger** describes *focus group research* as an alternative to other data collection procedures and, in particular to one-to-one interviews. The nature and elements of focus groups are discussed, and advice is given about the situations and settings in which they might find useful and effective. Kitzinger compares focus group research to other qualitative and quantitative data collection techniques and demonstrates how they can be combined at times, depending on the type of research question. In the course of the chapter, potential problems and advantages of group research are also explored.

Observation, in particular participant observation, where the researcher is a participant in the setting is seen by many as the qualitative method *par excellence*. Unfortunately not all researchers have time to engage and immerse themselves in the setting they wish to explore. In Chapter 5, **Stephen Wallace** shows how 'naturally occurring data' are generated through observation by a skilled observer, especially in the clinical setting. These observations might help the health researcher understand social action and interaction, which has, of course, many implications for practice. Wallace discusses the underlying assumptions and dimensions of this type of data collection, while also revealing its difficulties such as, for instance, the influences of the researcher on the setting. Through observation of both explicit and 'tacit' aspects of culture are revealed.

3

M. CLARE TAYLOR
Interviewing

Interviewing is rather like a marriage: everybody knows what it is, an awful lot of people do it, and yet behind each closed front door there is a world of secrets.

Oakley 1981: 31

Introduction

This chapter will endeavour to explore and articulate some of the secrets behind the closed door of the qualitative research interview. Interviews are probably the most commonly utilized data collection method within qualitative research. They are frequently categorized as structured, semi-structured, in-depth or unstructured. However, structured interviews, while possibly asking open questions and generating some qualitative data (words), tend to rely on a rigid, unchanging format and are most commonly a tool for surveys and thus should be viewed as a quantitative data collection tool and, therefore, beyond the scope of this discussion. The term 'unstructured' can also provoke debate. Mason (2002) argues that no research interview can be entirely devoid of structure, even if that structure is the use of a single open question to prompt thought and discussion. The majority of qualitative research interviews will, therefore, be semi/lightly structured (Leicester and Lovell 1997), loosely structured or in-depth in format and aim.

Burgess (1984: 102) defines qualitative research interviews as 'conversations with a purpose', while Robson (2002) stresses the flexibility and adaptability of in-depth interviews. These definitions sum up the essence of qualitative research interviewing. The aim of the interview, as with any qualitative research data collection tool, is to explore the 'insider perspective'. To capture, in the participants' own words, their thoughts, perceptions, feelings and experiences. Thus, while interviews can be carried out in a number of formats (face-to-face, over the telephone or via the Internet), the tone of the interview is generally informal and conversational. It is a two-way process where researcher and participant engage in a dialogue to explore the topic at hand.

The informal and conversational tone of the qualitative research interview is highlighted by the nature of the questioning. The researcher will have an interview guide rather than a formal interview script. This guide will outline the themes, topics or scenarios to be explored within the interview and may include phrases to prompt the discussion. However, these will form a loose guide to the conversation, to allow the participants to explore things that are pertinent to them, rather than discuss aspects that may reinforce the researcher's preconceptions. The aim is to understand the world from the participant's perspective. This can provide a challenge for the health-care practitioner–researcher. As Britten (1995: 311) points out, for the practitioner 'the clinical task is to fit that problem into an appropriate medical category ... in a qualitative research interview the aim is to discover the interviewee's own framework of meanings'. While most health-care practitioners are skilled at the clinical information gathering interview, the skills of the qualitative research interview must be differentiated and developed.

Why interview?

Having acknowledged that interviews are the most commonly used data collection technique within qualitative research, the researcher might be tempted to choose to interview without critically exploring the reasoning behind this choice. Researchers must ask themselves the following questions:

- Does interviewing fit my philosophy of research and epistemological stance?
- Does interviewing fit my research aims and question?
  - Will interviews gather the best data to address these aims and questions?
- Do I have the skills for qualitative interviewing?
- What will the interview experience be like?

From the philosophical and epistemological perspective, qualitative interviews are appropriate for the researcher who seeks to access the participants' understanding of the world and their experiences. Qualitative interviews give participants the opportunity to describe experiences in detail and to give their perspectives and interpretations of these experiences. The interviewer has the opportunity to discuss and explore with the participants and to probe more deeply into their accounts. The researcher acknowledges that the process of interviewing will vary from participant to participant and that the process will be influenced by what each participant might say. The interview will, therefore, not be a uniform, standardized, replicable process. Each interview will be unique; it will describe, in the informants' own words, their account of the experience, their beliefs and their attitudes. This uniqueness is important for the researcher, who acknowledges the individuality, humanity and uniqueness of each individual and whose aim in research is to capture that unique and subjective account. However, an interview can only describe events, beliefs and attitudes. The research must take on trust the veracity of any descriptions of actions and behaviours. Interviews are opportunities for the participants to construct or reconstruct their daily lives and experiences. These constructions and reconstructions will be influenced by the participant's ability to articulate, reflect on and recall experiences and the accompanying emotions.

The philosophical and epistemological rationale for qualitative interviewing is succinctly conveyed in the following quotation:

> To understand other persons' constructions of reality we would do well to ask them (rather than assume we know merely by observing their overt behaviour) and to ask them in such a way that they can tell us in their terms (rather than those imposed rigidly and *a priori* by ourselves) and in a depth which addresses the rich context that is the substance of their meanings (rather than through isolated segments squeezed into a few lines of paper) (Jones 1985: 46).

If the aim of the qualitative interview is to learn 'what is important in the mind of informants: their meanings, perspectives, and definitions; how they view, categorize, and experience the world' (Taylor and Bogdan 1984: 88) researchers will not be aiming to test hypotheses within their research but addressing research questions. The types of research questions for which qualitative interviewing might be the most suitable data collection tool will focus on how participants understand and construct meanings about the experiences of their daily lives, exploring the 'meanings people hold for their everyday activities' (Marshall and Rossman 1989: 81). They also uncover how people view and explain their own behaviour and experience their environments (Taylor and Bogdan 1984; Jones 1985; Laliberte-Rudman and Moll 2001). These are the *how* and *why* questions rather than focus on the *what* or cause and effect hypotheses. To illustrate this with an example: to address the question 'what is the most effective way of organizing interventions when someone has a CVA?' (cardio-vascular accident). Randomized controlled trials (RCTs) (for instance, Evans *et al.* 2002) and systematic reviews (Stroke Unit Trialists' Collaboration 2004) have given very clear and strong statistical evidence for the value of Stroke Units in increasing survival post-CVA. However, these studies give no indication of how or why Stroke Units are so effective. Qualitative studies are needed to address these problems; qualitative studies using interviews have begun to explore these questions, for instance in the interview studies by Maclean *et al.* which explored perceptions, attitudes and beliefs about motivation for rehabilitation, following a stroke from the patients' (2000) and from the professionals' perspective (2002).

Interviews give the researcher the opportunity to discuss and explore past events. They can also be useful ways of exploring sensitive experiences or topics, which might not be accessible through more structured questionnaire methods. However, they will not give the researcher access to how the participants actually behave in real life. As Taylor and Bogdan (1984: 83) warn:

> Through interviewing, the skilful researcher can usually learn how informants view themselves and their world, sometimes obtain an accurate account of past events and current activities, and almost never predict exactly how an informant will act in a new situation.

LIBRARY
EDUCATION CENTRE
PRINCESS ROYAL HOSPITAL

Interviews can, however, be used as one data collection strategy in combination with others (e.g. observation) to gain greater depth of understanding of the phenomenon. This strategy of triangulation, using more than one data collection technique, can enhance the rigour and trustworthiness of any study (Lincoln and Guba 1985). Therapists' accounts of their clinical reasoning, explored within interviews, could be enhanced by observations of the therapists' interactions and interventions within the actual clinical encounters (Fleming 1991a; Fleming 1991b; Mattingly and Fleming 1994).

The skills of the qualitative interviewer

Before the interviewer can begin to address the in-depth, or 'meaty', aspects of the phenomenon under investigation, they must first establish a relationship with the participant that will facilitate the interview process and that ensures an atmosphere of trust, acceptance and mutual respect. The researcher must also be sensitive to issues around power and control and prepared to surrender control to participants so that they can tell their own story in their own way and according to their own agenda. As well as skills of communication, both verbal and non-verbal, the researchers must also be skilled in reflexivity, in order to be aware of their own impact on the interview environment.

The ways participants respond to questions may be influenced by perceptions of the role and status of the interviewer. Participants may respond differently to someone they perceive as of higher status (e.g. a doctor) in contrast to their response to a novice researcher or student. This is clearly illustrated in the discussion by Richards and Emslie (2000) of the different perceptions and responses of their interview participants based upon the status of the interviewer. Richards is a GP, while Emslie is a sociologist. They reflect on the similarities and differences that appeared to be associated with their status as doctor or sociologist. While informants to both interviewers found the interaction therapeutic and they disclosed sensitive and confidential information, the responses to the 'doctor' were often more deferential, especially with working-class participants. Middle-class persons tended to align themselves and assume commonalities with the 'doctor'. The sociologist described herself as a 'researcher' when introducing herself, and the assumption was often that she was a student, one participant described her as 'the girl from the University' (Richards and Emslie 2000: 74). In contrast to the 'doctor's' participants, the comments about health care and doctors to the sociologist were often less favourable. This paper clearly illustrates the potential influence of status, as well as highlighting issues of class, age and gender, which will be explored in more depth later in this chapter. These factors are important aspects of the context of the interview and must not be ignored; they should provide rich material for the reflexive researcher to explore when presenting the research findings.

The impact of power and authority has been particularly pertinent for in my own research studies (Taylor 1990, 1999, 2001). These studies have involved interviewing my own students, who might have perceived me as an 'expert' and as an authority figure. They might have felt that there was a 'right answer' and that they should attempt to give either the right answer or the answer they thought that I was expecting. However, responses were the opposite of those I might have expected. The following response to my question exploring the concept of 'empowerment' within the therapeutic encounter reassured me, that I was not being given the 'right' answer, and that my status as a lecturer was not having a detrimental impact on the interview process:

> It's very much one of those words, like holistic, which says everything, but how much does it really mean . . . it is a word that I put in my essay the other day . . . I come across it when I am revising . . . 'cos we feel we should be more professional, because at the end of the day it's all common-sense stuff (participant 4, year 3: Taylor 2001: 249).

Moll and Cook (1997) found that the occupational therapists in their study exploring occupational therapists' beliefs about the therapeutic value of activity within mental health settings, felt that the researchers were intimidating because the therapist perceived the interviewers to be 'experts'. They became reluctant to respond to the researchers' questions about their beliefs about the efficacy of their practice.

Differences in cultural background can also present a challenge to the researcher as Currer (1986) found in her study of the mental health of Pathan women in the UK. For her the challenges were not only linguistic but also practical. Many of her participants were unable to speak English with any degree of fluency, which necessitated the use of an interpreter, adding another dynamic to the interview relationship. The interview process was further complicated because many of the participants were not happy for their interviews to be tape-recorded, thus necessitating comprehensive note-taking while she carried out the interview, as well as making thorough reflective notes as soon as the interview was completed. It is a testament to her skills as an interviewer that Currer has managed to provide such a detailed and thoughtful account.

A vital skill for qualitative interviewers is the ability to reflect upon themselves as part of the research process. The researchers must be able to articulate the assumptions that might be influencing the design of the interview guide. They should also critically reflect while listening to the tape recordings of their interviews and reading the transcripts, not only to explore the informant's meanings but also to explore their own performance as a qualitative interviewer. The researchers should ask themselves questions such as:

- Was silence allowed?
- Were cues picked up?
- Were probes used?
- Were the participants given time and opportunity to develop ideas and take the interview into their own directions?
- How directive was I?

Guidance to the participant can be useful, but researchers must be aware of how directive their interview style might be. Whyte (1982) has devised a scale to help researchers identify directiveness in their interview style. The scale is from least (1) to most (6) directive:

- Making encouraging noises (1).
- Reflecting on remarks made by the participant (2).
- Probing on the last remark of the participant (3).
- Probing an idea preceding the last remark by the participant (4).
- Probing an idea expressed earlier in the interview (5).
- Introducing a new topic (6).

By keeping a reflexive research journal, the researchers can be systematic in their examination of the experience of being a qualitative interviewer, which should facilitate the emergence of new insights and deeper understanding of both the research topic and the research process. These insights might include reflections about how reactions to particular participants might have influenced the interview process. It is rare that the researcher will feel positively about all of the participants. Lincoln and Guba (1985) comment that writing about the frustrations and other emotional responses to the interview process can be a positively cathartic experience. The process of reflection can also help to identify ways of improving the interview guide. By recording any changes to the research process the researcher is keeping a useful record for subsequent audit trails to ensure the trustworthiness of the research process. The reflexive journal also provides the researcher with the opportunity to explore emergent themes from the data and to compare these themes with previous assumptions; it is intended to ensure that the final analysis is a reflection of the participants' meanings and beliefs about the phenomenon and not just an exercise in forcing the data into pre-existing categories. The process of reflexivity is complex and time-consuming and requires researchers to be honest and open to their own thoughts and feelings. Many health-care professionals should have relatively few problems with the process of being a reflexive researcher as so much emphasis is placed on the use of reflection within current health-care continuing professional development.

The qualitative interview experience

The aim of the qualitative interview is to explore the participant's own perceptions and meanings, and the researchers must attempt to avoid imposing their own structures and assumptions onto the participant's account. This requires the interviewer to be open and flexible, to allow ideas to emerge and not to allow pre-existing assumptions and ideas to dictate the nature of the interview. The researcher must be prepared to probe beneath the superficial, to be able to explore the phenomenon in depth and to be prepared to be surprised by the directions that the interview might take. He or she must clarify meanings and interpretations and feed these to the participants to make sure that it is their voice and not the researcher's assumptions and interpretations that are recorded. Interpretation can come late once the data has been analyzed and themes emerge. Clarification is important when the researcher and the individuals who are interviewed might use language differently. When a clinician is interviewing a patient, for instance, the clinician might use technical clinical language that the patient does not understand. Clarification is even more important when the interviewer and interviewee share a common language and terminology, such as a practitioner–researcher interviewing similar practitioners. Here there is an assumption of shared interpretations, but it is vital that the researcher clarifies the informants' meanings and assumptions, to ensure that words and ideas are not over-interpreting things that might not actually have been stated.

Patton (2002) suggests that good qualitative interview questions should be open-ended, neutral, sensitive and clear. He proposes six types of question and suggests that if the researcher is clear about the nature and purpose of each question, then the participant will be able to respond appropriately. Patton's (2002: 352) six question types are:

- Behavioural/experience.
- Opinions/values.
- Feelings/emotions.
- Knowledge.
- Sensory.
- Background.

It is often better to begin the interview with background information questions, which the participant should find easy to answer and then to progress to the more complex or sensitive questions as the interview relationship develops.

Within qualitative interviews it is rare for the researcher to have a rigid interview script. Rather a series of themes and prompts will form an interview schedule. These themes and prompts are used to initiate conversation around the phenomenon and can act as an *aide-mémoire* (Burgess 1982) for the researcher to check that key topics have been covered within the interview. Because of the conversational and lightly structured nature of the process it is possible to fall into a number of traps, the full reality of which only emerge when the researcher is transcribing the interview and playing back the recording of the conversation. These common traps and pitfalls include:

- Double-barrelled, or multiple questions, where the interviewer asks a number of questions, all related to the topic but all requiring thoughtful responses.
- Asking leading questions.
- Having a rigid interview script, this is often the trap for the novice researcher, who feels the need to have a detailed and structured guide to maintain some sense of control over a seemingly uncontrollable event.

- Using the guide as a script, which might lead to missing interesting, and useful, diversions if comments from the participants are not followed through. As McCracken (1988: 37) says, the interview guide provides a

  > rough travel itinerary with which to negotiate the interview. It does not specify precisely what will happen at every stage of the journey, how long each lay-over will last or where the investigator will be at any given moment, but it does establish a clear sense of the direction of the journey and the ground it will eventually cover.

- Not modifying the interview guide in the light of experiences in preceding interviews.
- Not asking probe questions that might give the respondent the opportunity to explore the topic further. Patton (2002) identifies four types of probe:
  - detail-orientated probes, the *who, where, what* and *how* questions;
  - elaboration probes, which are often the non-verbal cues used to encourage the respondent to keep talking;
  - clarification probes, involving restatement of an answer and reflecting back to the respondent what has been said;
  - contrast probes, which give the respondent 'something to push off against' (Patton 2002: 374).

Most qualitative interviews will take place in a face-to-face setting. However, it must not be forgotten that qualitative interviews can also take place over the telephone and via the medium of the Internet. Both of these settings have the disadvantage of not being able to access the non-verbal communication of the respondent, and may lead to confusion about the nature of pauses within the interview process. The advantages of these two settings are that it is possible to access people who are otherwise inaccessible due to distance [via the telephone] or due to hearing impairment, who might be able to converse fluently [via the medium of the Internet].

Interviews for different qualitative methodological approaches

While other chapters have explored a variety of qualitative methodological approaches in some detail, the task of this chapter is to explore interviewing as a data collection tool within some of those methodological approaches. It also aims to illustrate this exploration with examples from the research literature and to highlight key lessons that can be learnt about interviewing in general from the different methodological approaches. Not all researchers who use qualitative interviews as their data collection tool clearly identify which methodological approach they are using. This can lead to method/methodology slurring (May 1991). It is vital for the qualitative researcher to clearly locate her/his research within a philosophical and methodological position, so that the research can be seen as rigorous.

Ethnographic interviews (See chapter 10)

For ethnographers, interviews are only one data collection method in their data collection toolkit. For the ethnographer, observation, and particularly participant observation (Toren 1996), will be the primary data collection technique, while interviews will be used to explore and develop a deeper understanding of particular aspects of the culture being researched. These interviews may take the form of informal conversations with particular informants, where the researcher seeks opportunities to explore the nature of cultural understanding by asking, often naïve, questions about things that have been observed. The researcher may also make opportunities to interview participants more formally, although still within the semi-structured format of a qualitative interview, to ask them to explain observed behaviours or interactions. Often, where there are particular issues with language, the researcher may rely on one particular informant or 'guide', who might be interviewed on a regular basis in order to gain a deeper understanding of the observed culture. Whatever form the interviews take, the researcher must always be aware of the potential hazards and pitfalls of cross-cultural interviews:

> You don't have to be a woman to interview women, or a sumo wrestler to interview sumo wrestlers. But if you are going to cross social gaps and go where you are ignorant, you have to recognize and deal with cultural barriers to communication. And you have to accept that how you are seen by the person being interviewed will affect what is said (Rubin and Rubin 1995: 39).

The complexities of cross-cultural interviewing have already been touched on above, in the discussion of Currer's (1986) work. The issue of the researcher's credibility because of shared meanings (e.g. being a woman or a sumo wrestler) will be explored further in the discussion of feminist research approaches and researching people with learning disabilities.

Interviews in phenomenological research (See chapters 7 and 8)

For the researcher who decides to adopt a phenomenological approach, interviews will be the primary data collection tool. The goal of phenomenological research is to understand the lived experience from the perspective of the respondent. Therefore, interviews, which capture, in the respondent's own words, their experiences, must be the method of choice.

The phenomenological interview is often described as in-depth in structure, and will be the nearest to an unstructured interview. The researcher usually has one very open opening question, such as 'tell me about your experience of x'. This very open, unstructured style allows the respondent to present their experience not only in their own words but also in their own style. The researcher will probe and reflect back, allowing for both a description of the phenomenon and an exploration of its meaning to emerge. The researcher is non-directive, as the researcher does not want to contaminate (Jasper 1994) the data with her or his own assumptions. The technique, adopted by many phenomenologists, is that of bracketing their preconceptions and assumptions, although it is not within the scope of this chapter to engage in a discussion of this contentious topic. The skills of the phenomenological interview will include 'the use of refection, clarification, requests for examples and description and the conveyance of interest through listening techniques (Jasper 1994: 311), skills that all qualitative interviews might need.

Grounded theory interviewing (See chapter 9)

As with ethnography, for the researcher using a grounded theory methodological approach qualitative interviewing will be just one tool in her or his data collection toolkit. Indeed, Glaser and Strauss (1967) themselves encourage the use of a variety of data types and data collection methods.

Because the goal of any grounded theory study is to develop a theory, the first interviews in the study will be in-depth and loosely structured, to allow the breadth and variety of the social process under investigation to emerge. As the study progresses and theories begin to emerge, so the structure of the interviews will change to become more focused and semi-structured, so that specific aspects of the theory can be explored in more depth or validated. Knox's study of the meaningful social relationships of a group of people with learning disabilities (Knox *et al.* 2000), discussed below, shows how a series of interviews can be used. Each interview in the series was developed to explore relevant aspects for each participant and to discuss and expand the emergent theories.

One aspect of the research process, which differs, depending on the chosen research approach, is the timing of data analysis. Within phenomenological studies, although the recordings of each interview are transcribed immediately after the interview has taken place, data analysis is usually only begun once all of the data have been collected. Within grounded theory studies the process of analysis is ongoing, beginning as soon as the first data have been collected and repeated as any new data are gathered.

Feminist perspectives on interviews

Many of the strategies proposed and developed by feminist researchers in order to give women a relevant and appropriate voice can be adopted by any qualitative interviewer, particularly qualitative researchers interested in developing collaborative and participatory approaches to their research. The goal of feminist researchers has been to build a tradition of research *for* women, thus moving away from the oppressive and paternalistic traditions of researching *on* women. This approach has been highly influential in areas such as disability research, which is now attempting to redress the balance in favour of research *for* and *with* disabled people, as discussed below.

Oakley (1981) argued very strongly that the traditional view of interviewing, even qualitative interviewing, saw the interview as a one-way process, where the interviewer elicits information from the respondent but does not give any information in return. While the social nature of interviews as conversations is acknowledged, the personal meaning of the social interaction of interviewing and being interviewed is often ignored. These traditional methods create more problems for the researcher than they should, by dehumanizing and often alienating the people they interview. Thus creating the researcher's view of the phenomenon under investigating, rather than creating a shared meaning of the experience.

Oakley (1981) proposed a new model of interviewing that was based on feminist notions of collaboration, where the researcher and the researched worked together. Feminist interviewers aim for research relationships that are non-hierarchical and non-exploitative, where there is give and take between the participants and where the conversational process may develop into a lasting friendship. Arksey and Knight (1999) suggest that interviewers attempting to work within a feminist or collaborative perspective should utilize the following strategies:

- High levels of trust.
- Continual attention to ethical issues.
- Reciprocity.
- Equity of control of the interview process.
- Self-disclosure and personal involvement.
- Encouraging an active role for the interviewee.
- Requesting feedback on interview transcripts and data analysis.

Many feminist researchers and those influenced by this collaborative approach, such as disability and gay theorists and researchers, suggest that for an interview to be successful and to get a 'true' picture of the experience, there should be a shared culture between researcher and researched. They would contest Rubin and Rubin's (1995) notion that one didn't have to be a woman or a sumo wrestler to interview women or sumo wrestlers. By drawing on commonalities of language and experience the researcher is more likely to hear, and respond, to what is said, and what is not said. Without shared norms and values the collaborative approach might suffer and the researcher will not access the full richness of the lived experience. Researchers from other traditions, for example ethnographers, might argue that it is the very lack of shared norms and values that allows the researcher to ask naïve questions and to explore the taken-for-granted notions that might otherwise be ignored. However, as Knox et al. (2000) demonstrate (see below) the perceived credibility of a particular researcher, based on shared experiences, allows her to access the life-worlds of those participating in her research.

Interviews in different health-care contexts

Interviews are conversations, which require both the researcher and the participant to be able to communicate and interact at a level sufficient to provide meaningful data. This is based on the assumption that the phenomenon under investigation is capable of being articulated and made explicit (Patton 2002). It is also based on the assumption that the participants are capable of verbalizing and articulating in a meaningful way, their experiences, thoughts and feelings. Within some health-care contexts this may be challenging for the researcher. Respondents who have impairments of memory, concentration or attention span will require particular strategies if their voices are to be heard within qualitative research. Potential barriers to qualitative interviewing might include hearing impairments or language and communication impairments. However, as will be discussed, by creative use of interviewing strategies, it is possible to give a voice to the experiences of previously voiceless groups, such as people with learning disabilities.

People with learning (or intellectual) disabilities have been described as the poor relations of the research family (Ward and Flynn 1994). They have been researched *on* in order to test hypotheses or develop theoretical perspectives, all for the benefit of the researcher. However, qualitative research offers a different perspective, it provides opportunities to research *with* people with learning disabilities, by using a collaborative, participatory and emancipatory approach (Zarb 1992; Knox *et al.* 2000). This approach, however, requires a particularly sensitive and creative approach on the part of the researcher, as this exploration of the use of qualitative interviews with people with learning disabilities will demonstrate.

Knox *et al.* (2000) discuss the use of a grounded theory approach, with a series of in-depth interviews, to develop a theory of meaningful social relationships with a small group of people with learning disabilities. The study illustrates a number of issues pertinent to the discussion of the use of qualitative interviews in general as well as the particular case of interviewing people with learning disabilities. Knox *et al.* adopted aspects of a participatory approach to their research. The approach was not fully participatory, as the research participants were not involved in the original design of the study. However, the process used for the series of interviews did allow each respondent to influence their own research process. The use of a series of interviews is consistent with a grounded theory approach and allowed for both respondent validation of emergent themes and testing of the emergent theory. Each interview, which was termed 'the business' by the participants consistent of five distinct phases:

1. Checking back.
2. Agreeing content.
3. The interview.
4. Putting items onto the agenda for the next interview.
5. Transcription.

The process of agreeing the content of the interview allowed both the participant and the researcher to influence the nature of the interview, allowing individual interview guides to emerge for each of the six people involved. The researchers argue that this level of individuality was both participatory, because joint decisions were made, and allowed each participant's individual expertise and experience to be explored. By this process of ongoing negotiation of the content of the interviews, participants were also engaging in an ongoing process of informed consent, highlighting the issue that consent, within qualitative interviewing, is rarely a static and one-off event, but something that must be renegotiated throughout the research process. The use of a participatory approach, within this context, allowed the researchers to gain access to lived experience of this previously voiceless group; however, the participants were all living relatively independently in the community and were working, albeit in sheltered settings, and they were able to articulate their ideas.

Not all participants with learning disabilities are so articulate, as Booth and Booth (1996) point out. They argue that many people with learning disabilities might be seen as poor informants because of four particular problems:

1. Inarticulateness
2. Unresponsiveness
3. A concrete frame of reference
4. Problems with the concept of time

Inarticulateness is due to restricted language skills, which will be exacerbated by low self-esteem, learned helplessness and social isolation, all of which are common for people with learning disabilities. Unresponsiveness is not the inability to respond but the inability to respond to open questions, which is also linked to a concrete frame of reference, which will make abstract thought and reflection difficult. Any of these problems might imply that people with learning disabilities would make poor participants in qualitative interviewing.

Booth and Booth (1996) argue that it is possible to use qualitative interviews with apparently inarticulate individuals. They illustrate this with the story of 'Danny'. Despite the fact that during two-and-a-half hours' worth of interviews with Danny, over three separate interviews, he uttered only ten complete sentences and the longest sentence was five words long, they were able to create a picture of Danny's world. The interviews had an emerging structure. Different approaches were used to encourage responses. The most successful strategies were to use direct questions, which required single word responses and to use silences creatively. Silence within an interview can be interpreted in a number of ways: that the respondent has not understood the question, that the respondent is embarrassed by the question or that the respondent is unwilling to answer the question. By attempting to interpret Danny's silences the researcher was able to progress the interview and to piece together Danny's story. The use of a creative, if time-consuming, approach to qualitative interviewing allowed a voice to be given to previously ignored and voice-less people.

The nature of the researcher–researched relationship was also highlighted. The researcher was seen as a 'learner', while the person with a learning disability was seen as the 'expert', which was a novel experience for all the participants in the study by Knox and colleagues. The relationship was also allowed to develop over the series of interviews, so that the participant felt comfortable and able to allow the researcher into his world. Knox *et al.* argue that it was not the researcher's ability to ask probing questions that facilitated this access but her credibility as a parent of someone with a learning disability, as someone who had experienced marriage and divorce and as someone who was known to be an advocate for people with learning disabilities. This issue of credibility, trustworthiness and integrity based on perceptions of shared credentials highlights the complexity of the researcher–informant relationship within any qualitative interview setting, and reinforced the need for the researcher to be constantly reflexive about the research process.

Rigorous and trustworthy interviews

The issue of methodological rigour within qualitative research is one of the most frequently discussed and contested within the qualitative research community (see for example: Morse 1999; Sparkes 2001). However, there appear to be a number of strategies that qualitative interviewers might find useful as ways of ensuring and demonstrating the methodological rigour and trustworthiness of their interview processes, thus attempting to ensure that the voices of their participants are clearly heard and that the interview process is clearly articulated within the context of both the methodological and researcher's perspectives and assumptions.

(Some of the complexities of rigour and trustworthiness are discussed in Chapter 15.)

Advantages and weaknesses

Interviewing, as a qualitative data collection tool, has many strengths, including:

- The participants' own words can be captured.
- The interview can focus on issues salient to the participants, rather than being driven by the researcher's agenda.
- Clarification can be sought.
- They allow opportunities to probe and explore in depth.
- Non-verbal behaviours can be noted and recorded.
- The format of the interview is flexible.
- It requires little specialist equipment, only a tape-recorder.
- The process draws on existing skills of conversation and communication.

They also have limitations. The limitations of qualitative interviews include:

- They are time-consuming, especially in terms of transcription and analysis.
- The interview format will vary between participants.
- Reflexive and open interviewing is a complex skill, requiring practice.
- Interviews can only capture reconstructions of events rather than how people might actually behave.

- The interviewers must be able to reflect on the impact their class, gender and position might have on the interview process.

Problems of the 'interview society'

Interviews are often seen as the easy option for the novice qualitative researcher, who often does not fully appreciate the complexity of using interviews in qualitative research. Indeed, several writers see interviews as problematic. Kvale (1996: 292) maintains that interview research might neglect social interaction and action which needs observation studies. Interviews are staged; they do not take place in the real world and, unless they are informal, they are not 'naturally occurring' data sources. Interviews by themselves can also be a-theoretical and trivial. Atkinson and Silverman (1997: 309) are very critical of 'the interview society' in which interviews are used too often. Particularly critical of 'illness narratives', they question the romantic assumption that the interview 'offers the opportunity for an authentic gaze into the soul of another' (p. 305) and claim that it is no more authentic than any other type of social representation.

Silverman (2000) suggests that the open-ended interview might be seen as the gold standard of qualitative research methods, much as RCTs are the gold standard for quantitative methodology. However, he also cautions

> To what extent do our preferred research methods reflect careful weighing of the alternatives or simple responses to time and resource constraints or even an unthinking adoption of current fashions?
>
> (Silverman 2000: 290)

Conclusion

Interviews give a window on what participants think and how they report their feelings and actions. However, they do not capture actual behaviours and actions. They investigate perceptions of a phenomenon but might not explore the reality of the phenomenon itself.

Qualitative interviews are a valuable research tool; however, the qualitative interviewer must ensure that interviews are the *best* method for answering the particular question, and not just the most convenient or fashionable. The researcher must also ensure that the open-ended interview, as a data collection strategy, fits with the assumptions and perceptions of the chosen research methodological approach.

References

Arksey, H. and Knight, P. (1999) *Interviewing for Social Scientists*. London: Sage.

Atkinson, P. and Silverman, D. (1997) Kundera's immortality: The interview society and the invention of the self, *Qualitative Inquiry*, 3 (3): 304–325.

Booth, T. and Booth, W. (1996) Sounds of silence: narrative research with inarticulate subjects, *Disability & Society*, 11 (1): 55–69.

Britten, N. (1995) Qualitative interviews in medical research, *British Medical Journal*, 311: 251–253.

Burgess, R.G. (1982) *Field Research: A Sourcebook & Field Manual*. London: Allen & Unwin.

Burgess, R.G. (1984) *In the Field*. London: Allen & Unwin.

Currer, C. (1986) Concepts of mental well and ill being: the case of Pathan mothers in Britain. In Currer, C. and Stacey, M. (eds) *Concepts of Health, Illness and Disease: a Comparative Perspective*. Leamington Spa: Berg, 183–198.

Evans, A., Harraf, F., Donaldson, N. and Kalra, L. (2002) Randomized controlled study of stroke unit care versus stroke team care in different stroke subtypes, *Stroke*, 33 (2): 449–455.

Fleming, M.H. (1991a) Clinical reasoning in medicine compared with clinical reasoning in occupational therapy, *American Journal of Occupational Therapy*, 45 (11): 988–996.

Fleming, M.H. (1991b) The therapist with the three-track mind, *American Journal of Occupational Therapy*, 45 (11): 1007–1014.

Glaser, B.G. and Strauss, A.L. (1967) *The Discovery of Grounded Theory: Strategies for Qualitative Research*. Chicago: Aldine.

Jasper, M.A. (1994) Issues in phenomenology for researchers of nursing, *Journal of Advanced Nursing*, 21: 827–836.

Jones, S. (1985) Depth interviewing. In Walker, R. (ed.) *Applied Qualitative Research*. London: Gower, 45–55.

Knox, M., Mok, M. and Parmenter, T.R. (2000) Working with the experts: collaborative research with people with an intellectual disability, *Disability & Society*, 15 (1): 49–61.

Kvale, S. (1996) *InterViews: An Introduction to Qualitative Research Interviewing*. London: Sage.

Laliberte-Rudman, D. and Moll, S. (2001) In-depth interviewing. In Cook, J.V. (ed.) *Qualitative Research in Occupational Therapy: Strategies & Experiences*. Albany: Delmar, 24–75.

Leicester, M. and Lovell, T. (1997) Disability voice: educational experience and disability, *Disability & Society*, 12 (1): 111–118.

Lincoln, Y.S. and Guba, E.G. (1985) *Naturalistic Inquiry*. Newbury Park: Sage.

Maclean, N., Pound, P., Wolfe, C. and Rudd, A. (2000) Qualitative analysis of stroke patients' motivation for rehabilitation, *British Medical Journal*, 321 (7268): 1051–1054.

Maclean, N., Pound, P., Wolfe, C. and Rudd, A. (2002) The concept of patient motivation: a qualitative analysis of stroke professionals' attitudes, *Stroke*, 33 (2): 444–448.

Marshall, C. and Rossman, G.R. (1989) *Designing Qualitative Research*. Thousand Oaks: Sage.

Mason, J. (2002) *Qualitative Researching*, 2nd edn. London: Sage.

Mattingly, C. and Fleming, M.H. (1994) *Clinical Reasoning: Forms of Inquiry in a Therapeutic Practice*. Philadelphia: F.A. Davis.

May, K.A. (1991) Interview techniques in qualitative research: concerns and challenges. In Morse, J.M. (ed.) *Qualitative Nursing Research: a Contemporary Dialogue*. Newbury Park: Sage, 188–201.

McCracken, G. (1988) *The Long Interview*. Newbury Park: Sage.

Moll, S. and Cook, J.V. (1997) 'Doing' in mental health practice: therapists' beliefs about why it works, *American Journal of Occupational Therapy*, 51 (8): 662–670.

Morse, J. (1999) Myth #93: reliability and validity are not relevant to qualitative inquiry, *Qualitative Health Research*, 9 (6): 717–718.

Oakley, A. (1981) Interviewing women: a contradiction in terms. In Roberts, H. (ed.) *Doing Feminist Research*. London: Routledge, 30–61.

Patton, M.Q. (2002) *Qualitative Research & Evaluation Methods*, 3rd edn. Thousand Oaks: Sage.

Richards, H. and Emslie, C. (2000) The 'doctor' or the 'girl from the University'? Considering the influence of professional roles on qualitative interviewing, *Family Practice*, 17 (1): 71–75.

Robson, C. (2002) *Real World Research*, 2nd edn. Oxford: Blackwell.

Rubin, H.J. and Rubin, I.S. (1995) *Qualitative Interviewing: The Art of Hearing Data*. Thousand Oaks: Sage.

Silverman, D. (2000) *Doing Qualitative Research*. London: Sage.

Sparkes, A.C. (2001) Myth #94: qualitative health researchers will agree about validity, *Qualitative Health Research*, 11 (4): 538–552.

Stroke Unit Trialists' Collaboration (2004) Organised inpatient (stroke unit) care for stroke (Cochrane Review). In *The Cochrane Library*, Issue 1, Chichester, UK: John Wiley & Sons.

Taylor, M.C. (1990) *Concepts of Health among Occupational Therapy Students and Occupational Therapists*. University of Warwick: Unpublished Masters dissertation.

Taylor, M.C. (1999) *Occupational Therapists: Empowerors or Oppressors? A study of student occupational therapists' attitudes towards disabled people*. University of Warwick: Unpublished PhD thesis.

Taylor, M.C. (2001) Independence and empowerment: evidence from the student perspective, *British Journal of Occupational Therapy*, 64 (5): 245–252.

Taylor, S.J. and Bogdan, R. (1984) *Introduction to Qualitative Research Methods: The Search for Meanings*, 2nd edn. New York: John Wiley.

Toren, C. (1996) Ethnography: theoretical background. In Richardson, J.T.E. (ed.) *Handbook of Qualitative Research Methods for Psychology and the Social Sciences*. Leicester: BPS Books, 102–112.

Ward, L. and Flynn, M. (1994) What matters most: disability, research and empowerment. In Rioux, M. and Bach, M. (eds) *Disability is Not Measles: New Research Paradigms in Disability*. Ontario: Roeher Institute, 29–48.

Whyte, W.F. (1982) Interviewing in field research. In Burgess, R. (ed.) *Field Research: a Sourcebook & Field Manual*. London: Allen & Unwin, 111–122.

Zarb, G. (1992) On the road to Damascus: first steps towards changing the relations of disability research production, *Disability & Society*, 7 (2): 125–138.

4

JENNY KITZINGER

Focus group research[1]: using group dynamics to explore perceptions, experiences and understandings

Introduction

Focus group research is a very popular method across many academic disciplines and for professional practitioners, particularly within health research. Focus groups offer a very valuable alternative, or supplement, to other data collection techniques such as individual interviews, or participant observation. But what exactly is a focus group? Under what circumstances are they appropriate? What practical issues should be considered when running group discussions? How should they be analyzed? This chapter offers a basic introduction to some core issues in focus group research and highlights the rich potential of this data collection technique.

The principles of focus group research

What are focus groups?

Focus groups are group discussions organized to explore a particular set of issues. The group is focused in the sense that it involves some kind of collective activity – such as debating a particular set of questions, reflecting on common experiences or examining a single health education campaign. There is a strong tradition of various forms of 'group work' within health services research. The term 'focus group' is often used (and sometimes misused) for a wide variety of such work, and other terms are sometimes employed interchangeably. This can lead to extensive confusion. Before talking in depth about the type of work that can be defined as focus group research, it is therefore important to mention the other terms the reader may have encountered. Some researchers talk of '*nominal groups*' – groups specially convened by the researcher often for the purpose of ranking exercises with respect to (most frequently consumer/patient) concerns or priorities. Others use '*consensus groups*' – often set up by professional bodies in order to carry out specific tasks – or '*expert panels*', which bring together acknowledged experts or sometimes 'opinion leaders', who can be relied upon to bring to the discussion an in-depth knowledge of practice development, policy considerations or the research literature. '*Delphi groups*' build on this idea of harnessing existing expertise, but seek to combine 'expert panel' discussions with other research methods – most commonly involving experts in responding to the results of a survey or postal questionnaire.

In fact, any of these groups could be, but are not necessarily, examples of 'focus group research'. 'Focus group research' is a generic term for any research which studies how groups of people talk about an issue. Indeed, a defining feature of focus group research is using the interaction between research participants to generate data and giving attention to that interaction as part of the analysis. A focus group is 'a research encounter which aims to generate discussion on a particular topic or range of topics, with the emphasis being on interaction between participants' (Kitzinger 1994a: 103).

Using this definition it is clear, for example, that a nominal group could be treated as a focus group, but not if the researcher simply comes away with the final outcome of the ranking exercise as the 'findings'. She or he would also have to consider how the group members debated the ranking exercise and came to their 'consensus' (a process which is often far more revealing than the final outcome). Similarly any of the other sessions, such as the 'expert panel' might also be treated as a 'focus group', again as long as the researcher was not only interested in the final assertion of 'advice', but in the *processes* through which the participants debated the issues. The key issue in focus group research is to treat the interaction in the group (the exchange of ideas and experiences, use of rhetoric or anecdotes, shifts in agreement and disagreement) as an integral part of the data.

Apart from this there are no other golden rules which define focus groups. Focus groups can involve different group compositions (including strangers or friends, 'lay people' or professionals) and diverse group tasks (including brain-storming, ranking exercises or attempting to reach a consensus). Indeed, the creative use of focus groups could include developing – where appropriate – hybrids of the various group types on offer and using focus groups in multi-method studies as well as refining standalone group methods to address a wider range of issues.

When is it appropriate to use focus groups?

Focus groups are ideal for exploring people's talk, experiences, opinions, beliefs, wishes and concerns. The method is particularly useful for allowing participants to generate their own questions, frames and concepts and to pursue their own priorities on their own terms, in their own vocabulary. Group work also helps researchers tap into the many different forms of communication that people use in day-to-day interaction – including jokes, anecdotes, teasing, and arguing. Gaining access to such variety of communication is useful because people's knowledge and attitudes are not entirely encapsulated in reasoned responses to direct questions. Everyday forms of communication may tell us *as much*, if not *more*, about what people know or experience. In this sense focus groups reach the parts that other methods cannot reach: revealing dimensions of understanding that often remain untapped by more conventional data collection techniques. Focus groups also enable researchers to examine people's different perspectives as they operate within a social network. Crucially, group work explores how accounts are articulated, censured, opposed, and changed through social interaction and how this relates to peer communication and group norms. Indeed, depending on the researcher's theoretical approach, focus group data can go further and challenge the notion that opinions are attributes of participants at all rather than utterances produced in specific situations (see Myers and Macnaghten 1999).

Focus groups are often used to explore in depth the form of people's talk, or thoughts, or experiences, about an issue from a variety of practical or theoretical perspectives.

Focus groups can be used, for example, for:

- The development or evaluation of a health education campaign.
- The improvement of health services provision or outreach.
- In-depth exploration of the experience of a diagnosis, diseases or treatment.
- Examination of professional identities and role or responses to institutional changes (e.g. Barbour 1999).
- Analysis of the role of the mass media or broader cultural representations in shaping understandings of a disease (or profession, or stigmatized group) (e.g. Miller *et al.* 1998).
- Gaining insights into broad public understandings of and responses to, issues such as biomedical ethics, new biotechnologies, health services, health policies or health inequalities.

Some people worry that group work may be inappropriate for very sensitive topics such as sexually transmitted diseases or bereavement, but this is not necessarily true. Sometimes people may be more willing to talk openly about issues when in a group of people with similar experiences than they would be in a one-to-one interview (Farquhar and Das 1999; Kitzinger and Farquhar 1999). In fact, I have yet to see a research question where focus groups in some form would not be relevant, even if other data collection techniques are also used. However, when considering whether or not to use focus groups, it is worth thinking through what they offer *compared* to other data collection techniques, and what they might offer in *combination* with other data collection techniques.

Comparing focus groups to other qualitative data collection techniques

Focus group research is different from individual *interviews* because research participants talk to the researcher as a group, and most importantly, discuss the issues with one another. Focus groups differ from observation or ethnographic work; instead of observing spontaneous action and interaction in a natural setting the focus group is usually convened by the researcher (albeit often involving naturally occurring groups on their home territory), and the researcher prompts and focuses the discussion around a particular issue. Interviews may be more effective for tapping into individual biographies. Observation may be more appropriate for documenting social roles and formal organizations. Focus groups, however, are invaluable for examining how knowledge, ideas, story telling, self-presentation and linguistic exchanges operate within a given cultural context around specific topics – and this can include the narratives people tell about their own lives, and their experiences of social roles and formal organizations.

Comparing focus groups to quantitative data collection techniques

Focus groups are also very different from quantitative methods such as survey questionnaires because it is a qualitative technique – with all that implies about the quality of the data. Whereas large-scale surveys aim for representativeness, qualitative work may try to reflect the range of experience or opinion, and whereas surveys aim for breadth, qualitative work aims for depth. In general, large-scale questionnaires are more appropriate for obtaining quantitative information and explaining how many people 'hold' a certain (pre-defined) 'opinion'. However, focus groups are better for exploring how points of view are constructed and expressed. Thus, for example, while surveys repeatedly identify gaps between health knowledge and health behaviour, only qualitative methods, such as focus groups, can actually fill these gaps and explain why these occur.

Even these generalizations, however, should not be treated as if they were cast in stone, and combining different data collection techniques into a single project can be highly productive. No one data collection technique is inherently 'better' than another. It depends on the aims of the research question and on how each technique is employed in practice. Often it may also be useful to combine methods.

Combining focus groups with other research methods

Focus groups can be combined with in-depth ethnographic work or with interviews. Researchers have found, for example, that ethnographic work may help them develop more sensitive focus groups (Baker and Hinton 1999) or that interviews combined with focus groups gain access to different aspects of people's experience (Michell 1999). One cannot assume that people are more 'honest' in interviews or in groups, but they may talk in different ways or reveal different aspects of their experience (Baker and Hinton 1999; Michell 1999).

Focus groups can also be combined with questionnaires. This may be simply that focus group participants complete questionnaires before and/or after the session. This can help provide basic background information, and may offer participants opportunities to say things they would rather not reveal in the group, or to reflect on the experience of participating in the group afterwards. The questionnaire need not strictly be a 'quantitative' method if it includes open-ended questions and the analysis of responses is qualitative.

Focus groups can also be used in combination with more traditional large-scale surveys. Focus groups are often used to help design or interpret a major survey project. At the outset of such research, group work can be employed to help construct questionnaires: developing an understanding of key issues and refining the phrasing of specific questions (O'Brien 1993; Kitzinger 1994a). Focus groups can also provide fertile ground for eliciting anecdotal material and are therefore ideal 'seed beds' for 'germinating' vignettes for use in questionnaires. Focus groups are often useful in the latter stage of predominantly quantitative projects. They can help to tease out the reasons for surprising or anomalous findings and to explain the occurrence of 'outliers' identified – but not explained – by quantitative approaches, such as scattergrams or 'box and whisker plots'. Sometimes group work can not only complement data collected via other methods, but may actually challenge how such data are interpreted. My own study of public understandings of AIDS, for example, demonstrates how focus groups can suggest different ways of interpreting survey findings through revealing the 'readings', 'facts' and value systems that inform respondents' answers to survey questions (see Kitzinger 1994b).

What theoretical or political research perspectives are implied by the choice of focus groups as a data collection technique?

Focus groups can be used from a wide variety of theoretical perspectives with very different analytical tools. They are a data collection technique not an epistemo-logical or ontological straitjacket. The group discussion may be analyzed from straightforward positivist approaches, or approaches using phenomenology (see Chapters 7 and 8 in this volume), narrative analysis (Chapter 12) discourse or conversation analysis. They can also be used in very different types of research, framed by contrasting political agenda. Focus groups are used in traditional top–down research (and, indeed, are very popular within commercial marketing). However, they have also proved very fruitful in 'client centred', action research or feminist research (Wilkinson 1999). Focus group methods are popular with those concerned to 'empower' research participants because the participants can become an active part of the analysis process. Indeed, if the research brings together people for the purposes of the research, group participants may actually develop parti-cular perspectives as a consequence of talking with other people who have similar experiences. For example, group dynamics can allow for a shift from personal self-blaming psychological explanations ('I'm stupid not to have understood what the doctor was telling me'; 'I should have been stronger – I should have asked the right questions') to the exploration of structural solutions ('If we've all felt confused about what we've been told maybe having a leaflet would help or what about being able to take away a tape-recording of the consultation?').

Some researchers have also noted that group discussions can generate more critical comments than interviews (Watts and Ebbutt 1987). For example, Geis and his colleagues, in their study of the lovers of people with AIDS, found that there were more angry comments about the medical community in the group discussions than in the individual interviews: '... perhaps the synergism of the group "kept the anger going" and allowed each participant to reinforce another's vented feelings of frustration and rage ...' (Geis et al. 1986). Using a method that facilitates the expression of criticism and the exploration of different types of solutions is invaluable if one is seeking to improve services. Such a method is especially appropriate when working with particular disempowered 'patient' populations who are often reluctant to give negative feedback or may feel that any problems result from their own inadequacies. After childbirth, for example, many women may be grateful to have a healthy baby, and be unwilling to make criticisms of how they were treated when interviewed one-to-one, but may be more able to make constructive suggestions for improvements when involved in a group discussion (DiMatteo et al. 1993).

There is, however, nothing inherent about focus group work that will automatically make it 'empowering' – researchers have to think through the entire context of the research design, implementation, analysis and presentation to achieve this (Baker and Hinton 1999)

Planning a focus group study

The size of the group

A group, for the purposes of focus group research, could be three people or fifteen people. The smaller number, however, offers minimal opportunities for lively group interaction, and the larger number can have the same effect and leave very little time for individuals to contribute. A group between the size of four and eight is usually ideal. Often, however, it is necessary to over-recruit, as not everyone may be able to turn up on the day.

Group composition

Most researchers recommend aiming for some homogeneity within each group in order to capitalize on people's shared experiences. However, it can also be advantageous to bring together a diverse group (e.g. from a range of professions) in order to maximize exploration of different perspectives within a group setting. However, it is important to be aware of how hierarchy within the group may affect the data, for example, a nursing auxiliary is likely to be inhibited by the presence of a consultant from the same hospital.

Related to the above issue is the question of whether or not to work with people who already know each other. Market research texts tend to insist on focus groups being held with strangers in order to avoid both the 'polluting' and 'inhibiting' effect of existing relations between group members. However, many social science researchers prefer to work with pre-existing groups: people who are already acquainted through living, working, or socializing together. These are, after all, the networks in which people might normally discuss (or evade) the sorts of issues likely to be raised in the research session and the 'naturally-occurring' group is one of the most important contexts in which ideas are formed and decisions made. By using pre-existing groups, one is able to observe *fragments* of interactions which approximate to naturally occurring data (such as might have been collected by participant observation). An additional advantage is that friends and colleagues can relate each other's comments to actual incidents in their shared daily lives. They may challenge each other on contradictions between what they *profess* to believe and how they actually behave (e.g. 'how about that time you didn't use a glove while taking blood from a patient?').

Pre-existing groups are not, however, a prerequisite for successful focus group research. Indeed, many projects bring together people who might not otherwise meet. Studies into the experience of living in a particular tower block, having a particular illness, or winning the lottery, might involve people who are virtual strangers. Even in a study where it has been possible to recruit pre-existing groups, the researcher might want to intervene to bring together other participants who do not know each other and whose voices and common experiences might otherwise be muted or entirely excluded from the research. In some cases, too, researchers deliberately opt to observe the talk generated by strangers or set up one-off groups to ensure that participants will talk without fear of making revelations to members of their own social circle.

If pre-existing groups are chosen, consideration should be given to the types of networks used. For example, an investigation into school sex education pro-grammes could access the same 16-year-old boy through a variety of networks. He could participate in a focus group with his parents and sister; with a selection of his school friends or he could become involved in the research via a support group for gay teenagers. Each type of group may give a different perspective on this same young man's views and experiences.

Whether or not 'naturally occurring' groups are used it would be naïve to assume that group data are by definition 'natural' in the sense that such interac-tions would have occurred without the group being convened for this purpose. Rather than assuming that sessions inevitably reflect everyday interactions (although sometimes they will), the group should be used to encourage people to engage with one another, formulate their ideas and draw out the cognitive struc-tures that previously have not been articulated.

It is important to consider the appropriateness of group work for different study populations and to think about how to overcome potential difficulties. Group work can facilitate collecting information from people who cannot read or write. The 'safety in numbers' factor may also encourage the participation of those who are wary of an interviewer or who are anxious about talking (Lederman 1983). However, group work can compound difficulties in communication if each person has a different disability. In the study assessing residential care for the elderly, I conducted a focus group which included one person who had impaired hearing, another with senile dementia and a third with partial paralysis affecting her speech. This severely restricted interaction between research participants and confirmed some of the staff's predictions about the limitations of group work with this population. However, such problems could be resolved by thinking more carefully about the composition of the group and sometimes group participants could help to translate for each other. It should also be noted that some of the old people who might have been unable to sustain a one-to-one interview were able to take part in the group, contributing intermittently. Even some residents whom staff had suggested should be excluded from the research because they were 'unre-sponsive' eventually responded to the lively conversations generated by their co-residents and were able to contribute their point of view. Considerations of communication difficulties should not rule out group work but must be considered as a factor.

The number and range of groups

The number of groups conducted can consist of anything between just a couple of groups to over fifty groups, depending on the aims of the project and the resources available. Most studies involve just a few groups (between six and fifteen). Although it may be possible to work with a representative sample of a small population, most focus group studies use a theoretical sampling model whereby participants are selected to reflect a range of the total study population or to test particular hypotheses. If researchers are examining people's views on AIDS they might wish to include people who have tested HIV positive and those who have tested HIV negative; if exploring experiences of breast cancer researchers might wish to talk with women at different stages of their treatment, and include a group of men with breast cancer. If working with nurses they might wish to run groups with nurses at different points in the hierarchy. It is also important to reflect demographic diversity.

Imaginative sampling is crucial. Most people now recognize age, class or ethnicity as important variables. However, it is also worth considering other variables. For example, when exploring women's experiences of maternity care or cervical smears it may be advisable explicitly to include groups of lesbians or women who were sexually abused as children (Kitzinger 1990a).

Location of the focus group session

It helps to hold focus group sessions in a place easily accessible to potential participants (and familiar to them). However, sometimes it is useful to run sessions outside people's institutional setting, away from their place of work or institution, so that they can talk more freely and be away from interruptions or observation. The room should be comfortable, quiet (for recording purposes) and facilitate a relaxed atmosphere.

It'll be all right on the night ... or will it?

There is often an element of unpredictability to focus group research. However carefully it is planned, researchers may confront problems such as that the room they were planning to use has been double-booked or a loud disco is being held next door; sickness, transport or child-care problems can mean some people do not turn up. One can try to mitigate against some of these factors by researching the venue and making contingency plans. It is wise, for example, to over-recruit for the session to allow for non-attendance. It helps if the researcher can organize transport or child care. Alternatively sometimes researchers may also find people are participating in the group who had not been invited (someone may bring along a partner, mother-in-law or child), or is included by mistake. I have had the experience of facing a group of young men (contacted for me by an agency) who believed they were there to discuss football hooliganism. In fact, I wanted them to discuss child sexual abuse! In this situation it was important that I did not simply proceed with my agenda, although in the event the participants decided they would be prepared to discuss my topic of concern – with very interesting results. On another occasion I mistakenly included a short-term resident of a hospital unit for the elderly in a group discussion with long-term residents. In fact this proved invaluable – the resident who was soon due to return home – prompted far more critical discussion in this group than in the groups composed entirely of longer-term residents who adopted a more resigned and institutionalized attitude.

Do not worry if the focus group composition is not quite what you expect. Go ahead anyway (as long as there are no ethical problems) and reflect on this in your analysis and writing up.

Preparing material for the session

Documentation that the researcher will need to prepare in advance of running a focus group includes:

(a) the letter of invitation to participants, including a (very brief) outline of the research and what they can expect from the session, and
(b) guidelines for the researcher (or the session facilitator) outlining some questions that might be addressed by the group. In addition some researchers like to take along some group materials, prompts, games or exercises.

This can be as simple as a flip chart and pens, some newspaper headlines, a taking along an object. For example, Lai-fong Chiu and Deborah Knight took a speculum along to their focus group discussions about cervical smears and encouraged women to pass it around and comment on it. In another group, a woman spontaneously passed round her breast prosthesis, again generating fascinating data (see Wilkinson 1999). More structured exercises can include presenting the group with a series of statements on large cards. The group members are asked collectively to sort these cards into different piles depending on, for example, their degree of agreement or disagreement with that point of view or the importance they assign to that particular aspect of service. For example, I have used such cards to explore public understandings of HIV transmission (placing statements about 'types' of people into different risk categories), old people's experiences of residential care (assigning degrees of importance to different statements about the quality of their care) and midwives' views of their professional responsibilities (placing a series of statements about midwives' roles along an agree–disagree continuum). Such exercises encourage participants to concentrate on one another (rather than on the group facilitator) and force them to explain their different perspectives. The final layout of the cards is less important than the discussion that it generates. For further discussion of this technique see Kitzinger (1990b). Researchers may also use such exercises as a way of checking out their own assessment of what has emerged from the group. In this case it is best to take along a series of blank cards and only fill them out towards the end of the session, using statements generated during the course of the discussion.

Reflecting on some ethical issues

As with all research it is important to consider the ethics of what the researcher is doing. For example: have research participants given their informed consent and will the information they give be treated with respect and confidentiality? Group work poses more challenges than individual interviews because gatekeepers may have not passed on information and, unlike interviewees, focus group participants cannot be given an absolute guarantee that confidences shared in the group will be respected. Another issue is that group members may voice opinions that are upsetting to other participants (e.g. in one group I ran, the suggestion that incest survivors should be sterilized because they were deemed to be 'unfit parents'). A related problem is that participants may actually provide each other with misinformation during the course of the group, information that may be implicitly legitimized by the presence of the researcher. It is inappropriate simply to walk away from a group after having silently listened to people convincing each other that HIV can be transmitted by casual contact or that anal intercourse is safer than vaginal intercourse. In such cases the researcher has a responsibility to provide accurate information.

Such ethical issues can be addressed through attempting to set ground rules prior to the session, and through debriefing and supplying literature after the session. During the course of the session itself it may very occasionally be necessary to intervene. (For a more extensive discussion see Kitzinger and Farquhar (1999)).

Running the session

Sessions should be relaxed: refreshments and sitting round in a circle will help to establish the right atmosphere. Sessions may last around one or two hours (or extend into a whole afternoon or a *series* of meetings). The facilitator should explain that the aim of focus groups is to encourage people to talk to each other rather than to address themselves to the researcher. It helps to start by going round the table asking people to state their name (for the tape and for voice recognition). The facilitator may wish to start with group 'games' and may wish to take a back seat at first, allowing for a type of 'structured eavesdropping'. Later on in the session, however, the researcher can adopt a more interventionist style: urging debate to continue beyond the stage it might otherwise have ended and encouraging them to discuss the inconsistencies both between participants and within their own thinking. Disagreements within groups can be used to encourage participants to elucidate their point of view and to clarify why they think as they do. Differences between individual one-off interviews have to be analyzed by the researchers through armchair theorizing; differences between members of focus groups should be explored *in situ* with the help of the research participants.

Recording the discussion

Ideally the group's discussions should be tape-recorded, and some researchers even like to videotape sessions. How the session is recorded will have a major impact on how and what can be analyzed. At the very least it is vital to take careful notes and researchers may find it useful to involve the group in noting key issues on a flip chart. Some researchers would find this record of a session totally inadequate for their purposes and, indeed, insist on a full transcript, even, if a formal conversation analysis is planned, recording every pause and hesitation.

Analysis and writing up

Analyzing focus groups is basically the same as analyzing any other qualitative self-report data (see Britten 1996; Mays and Pope 1996). At the very least, the researcher draws together and compares discussions of similar themes and examines how these relate to the variables within the sample population. In general, it is not appropriate to give percentages in reports of focus group data, and it is important to try to distinguish between individual opinions expressed in spite of the group, and the actual group consensus. As in all qualitative analysis, deviant case analysis is important: attention must be given to minority opinions and examples which do not fit with the researcher's overall theory and attention given to silenced voices.

The only distinct feature of working with focus group data is the need to indicate the impact of the group dynamic and analyze the sessions in ways that take full advantage of the interaction between research participants. When coding the script of a group discussion it is worth employing special categories for certain types of narrative such as jokes and anecdotes, and types of interaction, such as 'questions', 'deferring to the opinion of others', 'censorship' or 'changes of mind'.

A focus group research report that is true to its data should also usually include at least some illustrations of the talk *between* participants, rather than simply presenting isolated quotations taken out of context. They may also want to track how individual voices weave through the broader group discussion. Figures 4.1 and 4.2 present extracts from different focus group sessions from two different studies. Obviously, each one is only an extract from a much lengthier discussion and it is taken out of social context. However, what does the researcher think is going on here? What insights does this discussion provide?

Each of the extracts shown in Figures 4.1 and 4.2 could be approached in different ways. There is no definite rule beyond this about how to approach focus group data. The method of analysis will depend on the theoretical perspective. A conversation analyst, who treats talk as action, will be interested in every intonation and will analyze the (very detailed) transcript as no more, and no less, than talk. (The quality of the above transcription would be inadequate for this sort of analysis.) Discourse analysts will be interested in the discourses employed; researchers coming from other approaches will see the talk as accessing something else (feelings, experiences, attitudes, group norms).

Figure 4.1 Extract from a focus group discussion with elderly people in hospital residential care evaluating the service and seeking suggestions for improvements. For ease of reading one participant's comments, Bessy's, have been highlighted in bold

---

Facilitator: If you have any problems or worries who do you talk to?

F3: We would talk to the sister I would think, but I've never really had any problems, have you?

Bessy: Well, just I wanted to go home.

F3: Well, we all do, don't we, but we are here [. . .]

Facilitator: What are the sort of things you miss? [. . .]

Bessy: I have lost all my friends. I've been shifted about so much [. . .]

f?: We are friendly, it is up to yourself . . .

Bessy: The neighbours [at the previous smaller unit] were really great . . . before we came here, well you can't make the same neighbourliness in a place like this.

f?: Well I think it is up to yourself how you mix with people.

Bessy: It is, there is nothing wrong with it really, it's just eh . . . it's hard to get used to [. . .]

Facilitator: I have a few words [on cards] here I would like you to comment on [. . .] Let me choose one that you brought up earlier, **Bessy** . . . 'Independence'.

Bessy: Yes.

Facilitator: That's important to you then?

Bessy: Oh yes . . . oh yes, _very_ much so.

Facilitator: And are there things that make you feel independent?

Bessy: [There's] an unwritten law that you stay here, that, em, your independence, well, I couldn't say anything more . . . I like to be independent . . . but em . . . yes. [. . .]

Facilitator: Are there things that make you feel that you are _not_ independent . . .?

Bessy: Get out of here . . . no, no . . . it's not a bad place to be in [. . .] I'm as happy as the rest. It's just . . . where dignity is concerned, I don't know.

F2: Well, you never use your dignity now, so much.

Conclusion

This chapter has presented the factors to consider when designing or evaluating a focus group study. In particular, it has drawn attention to the overt exploitation and exploration of interactions in focus group discussion. Interaction between participants can be used to achieve seven main aims:

1. To highlight the _participants'_ attitudes, priorities, language and framework of understanding.
2. To encourage research participants to generate and explore their own questions and develop their own analysis of common experiences.
3. To encourage a variety of communication from participants – tapping into a wide range and form of understanding.
4. To help to identify group norms/cultural values.
5. To provide insight into the operation of group social processes in the

Figure 4.2 This discussion took place in a community with very low rates of breastfeeding and involved a group of teenage mothers. All the young mothers in this group used formula milk and talked about breastfeeding as rather disgusting. Samantha (highlighted in bold) presented a rather different attitude (she was also the only member of the group who had not yet given birth)

F: There was a woman in the travel agent that was breastfeeding in front of a guy and all that.

Samantha: If a guy it going to get thingmy when he sees a women pull her breast out then he is not much a guy is he.

F: Listen to you, Samantha!

Samantha: But he is not, if he is going to get all flustered and that over a woman feeding a baby. [...] I think I am going to do it [breastfeed]. [...] It was my boyfriend that said about it because he was breastfed.

F3: Because he wants a better look at your breast more often! [...]

F4: What is the point in hurting yourself?

F1: You end up bottle-feeding anyway.

Samantha: I was told if I breastfeed my baby then my baby might not get asthma.

Facilitator: Right.

Samantha: Less chance than there would be if I bottle-fed.

F3: If it is going to get asthma it is going to get asthma.

F6: That's right.

Facilitator: Can I just ask you why you are maybe going to try breastfeeding?

F1: She just wants to be different.

Samantha: For a better bond. I don't know. I just read up on it and I was thinking about trying it out because it [breastfeeding] can improve its sight and improve its abilities and all that crap.

[Note: We kept in touch with Samantha, in the event she did not breastfeed her baby.] (See: Henderson *et al.* 2000.)

articulation of knowledge (e.g. through the examination of what information is censured or muted within the group).

6. To encourage open conversation without embarrassing participants and to permit the expression of criticism.

7. Generally to facilitate the expression of ideas and experiences that might be left underdeveloped in an interview and to illuminate the research participants' perspectives through the debate within the group.

This chapter is not arguing that group data are either more or less authentic than data collected by other methods; instead it is illustrating how focus group research may be the most appropriate method for researching particular types of question, and it is often a useful component of any project. Focus groups are not an easy option. The data they generate can be as cumbersome as they are rich and complex. Yet the method is basically straightforward and need not be intimidating for either the researcher or the researched. Perhaps the very best way of working out whether or not focus groups might be appropriate in any particular study is to try them out in practice.

References

Baker, R. and Hinton, R. (1999) Do focus groups facilitate meaningful participation in social research? In Barbour, R. and Kitzinger, J. (eds) (1999) *Developing Focus Group Research: Politics, Theory and Practice.* London: Sage, 79–98.

Barbour, R. (1999) Are focus groups an appropriate tool for studying organizational change? In Barbour, R. and Kitzinger, J. (eds) (1999) *Developing Focus Group Research: politics, theory and practice.* London: Sage, 113–126.

Barbour, R. and Kitzinger, J. (eds) (1999) *Developing Focus Group Research: politics, theory and practice.* London: Sage.

Britten, N. (1996) Qualitative interviews in medical research. In Mays, N. and Pope, C. (eds) *Qualitative Research in Health Care.* London: BMJ Publishing Group, 28–35.

DiMatteo, M., Kahn, K. and Berry, S. (1993) Narratives of birth and the postpartum: an analysis of the focus group responses of new mothers, *Birth,* 20 (4): 204.

Farquhar, C. and Das, R. (1999) Are focus group suitable for 'sensitive topics?' In Barbour, R. and Kitzinger, J., (eds) *Developing Focus Group Research: politics, theory and practice.* London: Sage, 47–63.

Geis, S., Fuller, R. and Rush, J. (1986) Lovers of AIDS victims; psychosocial stresses and counselling needs, *Death Studies,* 10: 43–53.

Henderson, L., Kitzinger, J. and Green, J. (2000) Representing infant feeding: content analysis of British media portrayals of bottle feeding and breast feeding, *British Medical Journal,* 321 (7270): 1196–1198.

Kitzinger, J. (1990a) Recalling the pain: incest survivors' experiences of obstetrics and gynaecology, *Nursing Times,* 86 (3): 38–40.

Kitzinger, J. (1990b) Audience understanding AIDS: a discussion of methods, *Sociology of Health and Illness,* 12 (3): 319–335.

Kitzinger, J. (1994a) The methodology of focus groups: the importance of interactions between research participants, *Sociology of Health and Illness,* 16 (1): 103–121.

Kitzinger, J. (1994b) Focus groups: method or madness? In Boulton, M. (ed.) *Challenge and Innovation: Methodological Advances in Social Research on HIV/AIDS.* London: Taylor & Francis, 159–175.

Kitzinger, J. and Farquhar, C. (1999) The analytical potential of 'sensitive moments' in focus group discussions. In Barbour, R. and Kitzinger, J., (eds) *Developing Focus Group Research: politics, theory and practice.* London: Sage, 156–172.

Lederman, L. (1983) High apprehensives talk about communication apprehension and its effects on their behaviour, *Communication Quarterly,* 31: 233–237.

Mays, N. and Pope, C. (1996) Rigour and qualitative research. In Mays, N. and Pope, C. (eds) *Qualitative Research in Health Care.* BMJ Publishing Group, 10–19.

Michell, L. (1999) Combining focus groups and interviews: telling how it is; telling how it feels. In Barbour, R. and Kitzinger, J., (eds) *Developing Focus Group Research: politics, theory and practice.* London: Sage, 36–46.

Miller, D., Kitzinger, J., Williams, K. and Beharrell, P. (1998) *The Circuit of Mass Communication: media strategies, representation and audience reception in the AIDS crisis.* London: Sage.

Myers, G. and Macnaghten, P. (1999) Can focus groups be analysed as talk? In Barbour, R. and Kitzinger, J., (eds) *Developing Focus Group Research: politics, theory and practice.* London: Sage, 173–185.

O'Brien, K. (1993) Improving survey questionnaires through focus groups. In Morgan, D. (ed.) *Successful Focus Groups: Advancing the State of the Art.* London: Sage, 105–118.

Watts, M. and Ebbutt, D. (1987) More than the sum of the parts: research methods in group interviewing, *British Educational Research Journal*, 13 (1): 25–34.

Wilkinson, S. (1999) How useful are focus groups in feminist research? In Barbour, R. and Kitzinger, J., (eds) *Developing Focus Group Research: politics, theory and practice*. London: Sage, 64–78.

Note

[1] Parts of this chapter first appeared in Barbour, R. and Kitzinger, J. (1999) *Developing Focus Group Research*, Sage; and in Kitzinger, J. (1995) Introducing focus groups: A guide for medical professionals, *British Medical Journal*, 29 July 1995, vol. 311, no. 7000, 299–302.

5

STEPHEN WALLACE

Observing method: recognizing the significance of belief, discipline, position and documentation in observational studies

Introduction: believing is seeing?

The current wave of 'reality television' shows us just how engaging and revealing the processes of observation may be. Every night viewers are provided with high-tech observations of a whole range of human actors in different contexts. In the case of television, these observations are provided as much for entertainment as for any other purpose. But what is clear is that such observational data greatly interest lay communities, if viewer rating-scales are to be believed.

It is just as revealing when we consider how much professional work is dependent upon the powers of observation. Nurses take frequent observations as part of their routine work on the ward. Mental health service users and their environs are closely observed by psychologists and social workers to determine diagnoses and therapies. Regular and intensive observations taken by midwives in the birthing suite (or the labour ward) form part of the routine work of birthing, and physicians in general practice initially collect both patient reports of illness (symptoms) and make their own observations of clinical 'signs'. So it should come as no surprise to learn that observational methods, which are 'a royal road' in the routine activities of these professionals, take such a prominent place in their research activities as well.

The phrase 'Too much information!' from a recent Tarantino film now has a cultural meaning which is replete with normative properties; however, it does suggest the very problem faced by the researcher who wants to investigate any ongoing life-world. Sanger (1996) re-describes the 'whirring, buzzing confusion' of an information-rich environment as the problem of social noise. It is in just such a chaotic informational field, that the observer is not just expected to perform competently as a member of the tribe but is also expected to extract some coherent meanings from this field, and 'bring them back' for later use. It is well to remember that the very act of observation both loses and adds dimensions which are often extremely difficult to identify, or even specify explicitly. The expert observer knows well of the tension between the stresses of maintaining the most natural and open categorical attitude in the midst of a sea of stimuli, and the relative comfort of sorting these chaotic observations into trusted and well-used categories. It seems that it's hard for the observer to maintain both a sense of relaxation and competence in the field, while at the same time being ever alert and open to the possibilities of novel observations and the subsequent demand for the generation of new categories.

While it may sound obvious to say that 'seeing is believing', it is the very problem of identifying and naming what one sees that is at the heart of observation. And it might be more accurate to suggest that skilled observers see what they believe, rather than believe what they see. It is hard to imagine the collection of data without a belief in what one observes; yet up until the time of Popper (1992), it was commonly believed, at least in scientific circles, that the acts of seeing or observation were uncontaminated by theoretical considerations. Popper argued that all observations were dependent upon some theory of just what it was one was observing, and described them as 'theory-laden' – a fact which makes the strategy of theoretical sampling quite problematic as well. He argued that even in the most rigorously controlled and designed scientific studies, we saw what we believed, rather than simply believed what we saw. Recently Collins suggested that observational 'beliefs' are very much premised now upon the methods or technologies used to collect data, which in turn rely primarily upon social conventions and practices (see Collins 1985). While others would argue that the problems of observation can be resolved by increasing dependence on technology, many micro-studies of such technological observations show how the problems of observation are simply shifted further up the belief chain, rather than resolved by this move (see also Latour 1986).

One particular pay-off that is accomplished through the foregrounding of belief as the foundation of observation is that one immediately has to recognize the contingent and social nature of observation. If all observations are premised upon socially-mediated value and belief systems, then there is no possibility of value-free or belief-free observations. And this is an important starting point for all those making and reading observational studies.

Sanger (1996) has written a field guide to observation in which he claims that observation arises from the concept of 'otherness'. Given the socially-saturated nature of observation, however, the prospect of unproblematic boundaries, even between the 'observed' and an 'observer', appears risky and raises all sorts of resonances about the nature and problems of objectivity. Suffice it to say here that various social worlds import particular and local commitments to their routine social–material practices (including observations) which need to be recognized both by members and their audiences. So it can never be assumed that the semiotic boundaries 'observed' by one social world are 'observed' by another, at least till some evidence of such observational solidarity is obtained. Jorgensen (1989) suggests that questions of 'otherness', which ask insiders to compare and contrast the experience of their own social world with other social worlds, can be quite a fertile approach in observational studies.

Regarding method

Observations are often supplemented and complemented by conversations with social actors that ask them to explain meanings, procedures, and experiences which have been observed and perhaps not fully understood. The form of these questions is important, as the traditional search for 'rational action' is unlikely to yield fruitful results. So the most open kinds of questions are preferred as they tend to generate both more fulsome responses and a cascade of other questions. Following Jorgensen, I would propose, especially in later stages of enquiry when some trust and rapport has been developed with the members of the social world, that questions which ask how things might have been otherwise, even within the same social world, with the same set of participants, are very fruitful (and, in fact, Sanger suggests that skilled researchers can observe 'absences' as well as instances). It is often very useful to collect or even examine documents and artefacts of significance to the social world. Clark and Fujimura (1992) warn us of the dangers of 'cleaning up' data, especially when our observations seem inconsistent (sometimes with other data). Again I find such paradoxes and inconsistencies sometimes the most fascinating aspects of such micro-studies of any social world.

While interviews have become commonly-used tools of qualitative research, observations have always played an important part in human inquiry, especially in ethnographic studies. One of the major problems of all observational research is the problem of reactance, the influence of the process of observation upon the observed. While the term 'non-reactive' has been commonly applied to measures (see Webb et al. (1996)) the term 'reactance' is used here in preference to 'reactivity' following Stangor's (2003) discussion. Reactance consists of one of the major threats to internal validity. Some of the first significant findings from ecological studies of actors performing their mundane work in their own milieu (Roethlisberger and Dickson 1939) showed very tellingly just how 'reactive' such naturalistic observation might become. The 'Hawthorne Effect', as it came to be known, attempted to describe the complex link between the actors' motives of self-presentation (see Goffman (1959)) and the valid observation of mundane performances.

The work of Foucault (1980) has recently revealed other dimensions involved in surveillance which might also be seen to threaten internal validity. Although there has been considerable discussion in the professional literature about the ethics of observation, Foucault's work has drawn our attention, not only to the proximal aspects attendant in all observation, but also to the more distal and political implications that arise when actors are observed in their social world. Not surprisingly, people these days are concerned about how such data might be used in future.

While this is not the place for a detailed discussion of the importance of validity and reliability in observational methods, suffice it to say that the usual canons of controlled observation are unlikely to be helpful in naturalistic studies of relatively inaccessible social worlds. So what I am suggesting in general terms is a somewhat backward view of reliability and validity, which starts with the objective of how best to observe the social world naturalistically, rather than in a controlled manner. In the kind of naturalistic participant observation I discuss here, the social worlds are observed in their natural settings and contexts, with as little intrusion (or control) as possible emanating from the observer. So the very notion of controlling one's observations is anathematic to participant observation, and the downstream notions of reliability and validity take on a different meaning. The term 'ecological validity' suggests that, rather than aiming for reliability or other surrogates of validity, one aims to conduct intensive, extensive and non-reactive observations in the social world of interest which generate understanding and meaning of the social world from the perspective of the insider, rather than some objective world view (see Wallace 1999).

The issue of sampling is always contentious in observational studies, especially of the qualitative kind. And the problem of how many informants and sites to observe, over what time period, always requires careful consideration. While the processes of observational data collection and analysis could continue (in principle at least) forever, the very artificiality of timelines and deadlines often creates its own necessary, even if entirely arbitrary, end-points (DeWalt and DeWalt 2002).

In observational studies, the problem of sampling could be seen, not just as a routine decision about the size of sample, but rather a matter of 'proper specification' of an adequate and appropriate group of informants who inhabit, are willing and able to inform researchers about particular social worlds (DeWalt and DeWalt 2002). Almost invariably, informants for observational studies are selected (and select themselves) through an inchoate process of 'opportunistic' or 'convenience' sampling, despite the best planning, intentions and rationalizations. This emergent character of 'non-probability' sampling can often appear offensive and ill-disciplined when compared to modern views of method, but it is precisely this methodological flexibility and contingency which gives many qualitative research approaches their unique strengths and capacities. One problematic aspect of such an approach is the issue of data sufficiency. How do we know when we have collected enough data, observed 'typical' examples of mundane performances in the life-world, explored enough domains of the social world of interest? While it may again not be an entirely satisfactory response, the best response that may be offered is the imperative of data 'saturation'; the researcher's judgement that a specified empirical 'understanding' is unlikely to be further elaborated or clarified by the gathering of more data.

Questions of sampling are also made more complex by the problem of the relative visibility and accessibility of various social worlds. People and communities involved in unusual, antisocial, or undesirable behaviour are often difficult for researchers to access and observe. When such behaviours are also criminal, or of themselves conducted in secret or private contexts, the difficulties of any 'ecological' kind of research become considerable. Drug users, who are one of the most 'invisible' groups, have become a favoured population for ethnographic researchers like Agar (1986). Such 'hidden' populations, have proved particularly difficult to research from a conventional viewpoint, and so have often shown the particular advantages of ethnographic methods (see Panagopoulos 2002). But even when the sampling issues have been resolved, such observational studies raise another raft of ethical issues.

Observational studies are well known to be replete with ethical content. Leaving aside the heavy burden of research governance which increasingly embraces wider dimensions of research activity, some particular ethical issues arise in observational studies. DeWalt and DeWalt (2002) discuss the problems that arise when researchers decide to intervene in the very social world they are studying. It is reasonably easy to see how methodological confounds might arise when a researcher makes such a decision. And the resulting tension may be seen as adjudicable on the basis of the balance between ethical and methodological demands.

Of more concern is the symmetric problem of *not intervening*, which creates the first of several unrecognized ethical/methodological dilemmas which may be seen to arise over the conduct of routine observational studies. Whereas the action of intervening in the social world clearly compromises both the methodological and political neutrality of the observer, the alternative ethical problem of non-intervention at least preserves the methodological integrity of the researcher's position, as well as the political ecology to a large degree. But it leaves entirely aside the responsibility – if there can be one – and ethical duty of the researcher to act to prevent unethical action, in this case, in the research field. While most ethical duties are seen to be codified in advance by the relevant professional bodies, the informed consent protocol and the research brief, some experiential reports of experienced researchers suggest that this dilemma occurs quite frequently and results in quite distressing outcomes for some researchers.

More benignly, the second dilemma, which I will call 'the dilemma of informed consent', proposes that the data gained from participant observation following the strictest regimes of research governance are probably most valid when participants are *least* aware that it is going on. It is further argued that the experienced researcher has a much better idea than any participant of how such revealing and irreflexive 'natural' behaviours generally emerge over the course of a participant observation, yet this is rarely explicitly discussed in most informed consent protocols.

The third dilemma (of 'anonymity') proposes again that the success of imperative for descriptive 'thickness' – a hallmark of methodological virtue in observational studies – has the undesirable effect of making the identification of informants, whose words and action have been carefully documented in observational studies, progressively more likely, especially to members of that social world. It should be obvious that the demand for anonymity may mean that the kind of detail, specificity and thickness so valued in observational studies, will in all likelihood need to be forsaken in the interests of the ethical mandate for anonymity.

Covert observations, which are much less frequent nowadays due to the difficulty of acquiring ethical clearance for such studies, also raise many methodological and ethical issues of concern to observational researchers. The failure to acquire relevant informed consent is as ethically problematic in these kinds of observational studies, as is the option of providing misleading, incomplete or deliberately deceptive information to potential participants or informants. And while many attempts have been made to overcome some of these problems (from the 'breaching' experiments of the ethnomethodologists, to the one-way mirrors of the psychologists), they remain major problems of observational studies.

Positioning the observer

It is important to note that the observations conducted in qualitative studies usually take place in the natural settings of the social world of interest, and are often conducted by non-members of that social world. So there is a special attempt in most qualitative studies to gather not only traditional 'etic' data from the context in which the social members perform, but also to gain some understanding and insight into the 'emic' perspectives of those members. One observational technique especially devised for qualitative methodology involves the observer progressively becoming a member of the tribe and collecting observations through a skilled performance of participation in the social world – this is called participant observation.

In the first place, Sanger (1996) advises that one's presence in the field situation needs to be fully explained to the research participants. Ideally those negotiations with the 'members' should have been successfully completed before one commences observations. On each occasion when the participants enter 'the field' it is important for the observer to enter in the same way as the participants, and at the same time. It is important to choose a position where it is possible to observe the greatest range of interactions, but a position which allows some interpretation or ambiguity about the role one is taking. Sanger advises limiting eye contact with participants, and suggests an observational style which distributes one's gaze across the participants. He advises observers to wear clothing appropriate to the context, and try to adopt a common body position whereby the observer appears to be undertaking a similar or coordinated activity to the participants being observed. The observer should show only a moderate degree of interest in the circumstances and proceedings being observed.

On entering the research field for the first time there are many things to observe. While human action may appear in principle to be the 'figure' in the research 'ground', there is much value in observing the material, geographic, temporal and spatial dimensions of the research field. For example, Jorgensen (1989) suggests that quantitative data about the numbers of human actors, and their ages, and the gender and ethnic ratios may well yield useful introductory data. I would also countenance the development of the general curiosity and eclecticism about the kind of data gathered as 'significance', is a problematic concept in observation. Roland Barthes' (1982) studies of photography reveal that either 'figure' or 'ground' may be examined closely to produce interesting and useful knowledge.

It is well to remember that all human action occurs in the social field, and the research act is no different. So participant observers should not be surprised when the actors in the social field appear to be exercising both a welcome and unwelcome influence upon them. Again, the methodological position of this research tradition recognizes explicitly the reflexivity of the research act. And rather than this being a methodological problem which must be resolved, the documented

LIBRARY
EDUCATION CENTRE
PRINCESS ROYAL HOSPITAL

observations of the researcher's experience of reflexivity becomes data for the study, rather than extraneous research 'noise' which must be explained away (see Woolgar 1988).

As Spradley's (1970) work showed, the social world of the 'urban nomads' is often described differently by different participants (who themselves constitute disparate social worlds) outside the social world of interest. Various professional groups will adopt particular analytic terms which say as much about the 'labellers' as those labelled. 'Insiders' tend to make finer internal distinctions between the constituent social worlds that comprise the larger social world, to distinguish each from the other. Spradley suggests that a participant observer needs at least to recognize these distinctive sub-labels, as use of this terminology signifies 'insider' status.

Jorgensen (1989) insists that the development of rapport is necessary to perform competently as a participant observer. Such competent performance may be signalled to members through the use of insider language, although the mere use of their terminology would not be sufficient to indicate the level of 'verstehen' required for such rapport to develop. While the use of appropriate self-disclosure is also a reliable method for generating rapport, such disclosures need to be tempered by the demands for ecological validity (see Banister et al. 1994), which means that disclosures need to be framed so as to minimally shape and intrude upon the research setting. It should be obvious then that participant observation might not be a method of choice when the researcher holds negative views about the social world of interest and its members. On the other hand it would be also disabling, from the research perspective, if participant observers imported strong emotional attachments and investments in the social world they were researching.

Being there – the participant observer

Anselm Strauss has been a very influential figure in much social science research. Aside from coining the very useful term 'social world' and developing a major theory around this term, he is also credited, with Barney Glaser, of developing the 'grounded theory' approach which emerged from, and ultimately depends upon, participant observation (see Glaser and Strauss 1967).

One aspect which characterizes participant observation from other research approaches is its emphasis on observing the routine and mundane performances of a particular social world in its natural setting, and its insistence on understanding such performances from an insider (or emic) perspective. Depending upon the circumstances, participant observation may make some or all of the following demands upon researchers. The participant observer may be expected to live in the context for an extended period of time and to learn and use the local language and dialect. They might be expected to participate actively in a wide range of the daily routine (and even extraordinary activities) with their participants. Participant observers are expected to use everyday conversation as an interview technique, and often spend long periods 'hanging out' in the social world, especially during recreation or leisure activities. While this may sound rather an attractive way to spend one's time, the demands of participant research can test even the most diligent investigator.

DeWalt and DeWalt (2002) suggest that one of the particular advantages of participant observation is that it allows the tacit aspects of culture, which largely remain outside our awareness, to be noticed, noted, and analyzed in some depth. While it is generally considered that Bronislaw Malinowski first described in the 1920s the research approach we now know as participant observation, it has since become almost the method of choice in anthropology and ethnographic fieldwork. Margaret Mead is perhaps one of the best known, if controversial figures, to use participant observation methods in field studies. She described her method as 'speech in action', which was notable at the time, not only because she chose to study a living culture through direct participation, but because she chose a very narrow and particular focus for her studies, which was unusual for anthropology at that time (see Mead 1928). Mead's work has been criticized recently by other sociologists such as Derek Freeman, and it is worth noting that the evidence he adduces to contest her claims and substantiate his claim that her work should be disregarded relies upon exactly the same kind of 'speech in action'. Although Freeman could hardly describe his participation in Samoan culture as at the same level of immersion and duration as Mead (see DeWalt and DeWalt 2002), he insists on methodological privilege for his data, despite his work being methodologically challenged (see Wallace 1999).

While it may sound simple to suggest that participant observers merely select and gain entry to particular settings which they then observe routinely, it is both methodologically and practically significant how such a setting is accessed by observers. Rather than considering particular observational arrangements as examples of sample bias (which need to be remedied by representative sampling or randomization), the participant observer recognizes that at particular times some observational settings present themselves conveniently, and others become more difficult to access. This kind of convenience sampling is sometimes called 'judgemental' sampling, as it makes no pretensions of representativeness or probability sampling. And over the course of observation, the arrangements for access often change quite unpredictably. This requires that participant observers need to be flexible about the entry point into the research field, and the role they may play within it. Such flexibility will enable the observer to scope a wide range of phenomena, and be sensitive to new research opportunities.

Before starting out on a participant observation study it is important to be able to demonstrate that one is familiar with existing literature on the topic and the social world in question. One should ascertain that the research site is appropriate to inform or interrogate the existing literature and that the chosen theoretical approach is appropriate. The methods chosen should be conducive to the theoretical approach, the research setting and informants. Lastly, but just as importantly, it is crucial that the investigator is competent to fulfil all the above requirements.

It is obvious that there is no complete and consistent set of rules to follow in the observational field, and this is especially true when one undertakes participant observation. Jorgensen (1989) has written a dedicated book on just such a topic, and he is at great pains to show how participant observation requires more than the craft of skilled observation. Like many other methods in the qualitative tradition, both the aims and particular strategies of participant observation emerge over the course of their study, rather than are predetermined at the outset. Jorgensen sees participant observation as a distinctly useful method to understand the lived world of particular social actors. While Howard Becker was one of the early researchers to engage in participant observation over forty years ago, this method of social inquiry has become especially popular, even if it is now unlikely to be welcomed by the current imperatives of research governance.

Jorgensen (1989) describes different degrees of participation for the observer and suggests that the level of 'immersion' should be determined by the demands of the research situation, and the resources of the observer, and may indeed shift over the course of the observational period. It is quite clear that the more 'outside' the participant observer is seen by members of the social world, the more it is likely that 'insiders' will respond to demand characteristics like social desirability. One of the dangers of adopting a very 'inside' participant position, is the risk of 'capture', such as happened in the classic study of religious prophecy by Festinger *et al.* (1956). In this graduate students ended up as members of a religious cult they were studying, rather than writing up their observational data. This phenomenon is sometimes described as 'going native'. In the alcoholism field, this problem is sometimes resolved through the use of recovering alcoholics as participant observers (DeWalt and DeWalt call them 'native' ethnographers); as such researchers are often accorded the dual status of 'insider' (having once been 'active' alcoholics) and 'outsider' who is now performing a non-alcoholic, research role. DeWalt and DeWalt (2002) call participant observers 'native ethnographers'. While the task of establishing and maintaining an appropriate balance between participant and observer sounds very difficult, it is worth remembering that in our mundane life-worlds we routinely adopt multiple roles and perform quite competently and smoothly as 'inside' members and 'outside' observers across an enormous number and range of social worlds. One's supervisor can be especially helpful when the task of participant observation creates any such role confusion and performance anxiety.

As Jorgensen (1989) has argued, participant observation is especially useful when it is believed that there are differences between the views of insiders and outsiders, as often happens when the social practice of various social groups, or the very appearance of such a group itself, is barely visible to outsiders. This might suggest that the data derived from participant observation are rarely likely to yield the kind of nomothetic, mainstream data characteristically produced by more positivistic methods which are routinely employed within the social sciences, such as questionnaires, interviews, and other archival documents.

Participant observation is also more likely to yield the thick and rich data to provide the *verstehen*, or understanding of a social world from the perspective of the members inside that social world. As Jorgensen (1989: 15) says 'the methodology of participant observation seeks to uncover, make accessible, and reveal the meanings (realities) people use to make sense out of their daily lives.' While most studies using participant observation have 'studied down' (as Mary

Douglas has said) some of the most fascinating of these studies have been conducted by social scientists observing the mundane social world of other scientists. Perhaps one of the most revealing of these participant observation studies is one conducted by Latour and Woolgar (1979) at the Salk Research Institute.

One advantage of such an approach is that, over time, it renders the appearance of the observer as much less 'reactive' (or obtrusive) in the observational field and thereby increases the probability of internally valid observations. It is argued that participant observation studies are especially valuable on account of their preservation of ecological validity, precisely because the inquiries can be said to be conducted by 'members' with other members in the lived social world of interest. It might also be said that the peculiar position of the participant/observer is a delicate balance between behaving as a culturally competent member of the tribe, and maintaining sufficient 'strangeness' to recognize and construct analytic utility.

This task is made considerably easier through the compilation of an index of key linguistic and discursive resources deployed in this social world. Such resources will give a very clear insight into some of the key actors and social worlds of interest to these actors, as well as some indication of the power relations which obtain between them. For example, white, western, participant observers conducting studies in New Zealand soon learn that they are described by the indigenous Maori people as *pakeha*.

It is not always immediately obvious what benefits might be obtained by members of the social world which is being observed. And this can prove a problematic issue in terms of ethical governance of research. It is well to remember that all social situations involve elements of exchange, and in the absence of explicit arrangements, the researcher should pay close attention to the benefits acquired or expected from their research participants.

DeWalt and DeWalt (2002) warn about the role of cultural gatekeepers and their role in shaping the research activity by directing the researcher towards certain informants and contexts, and away from others. They claim that it is usually undesirable in a participant observation study to rely upon these 'field sponsors', who, although they are able to join diverse social worlds together in a seemingly helpful way, may be deviants who may also limit access to particular aspects of the social world due to their status.

Of course, major problems can arise when conducting participatory inquiry into social worlds where many of the practices are illegal, and many of the actors behave in socially undesirable ways (see Rosenhahn 1996). Leaving aside the ethical difficulties of conducting such research, the personal safety of such participant observers is always of concern. The 'embeddedness' of participation may vary across observers and social worlds, and the level of explicit knowledge about the role of the observer is also likely to vary across members of each social world.

Participant observation makes huge demands upon the researcher, especially its demand for the researcher to learn how to 'walk the walk' and 'talk the talk'. It is inescapable that there will be a gradient of comfort from the early days to the last days of a participant observation study and this is partly due to the dynamic tension and strain between participation (which implies emotional involvement) and observation (which requires some detachment).

Recording, analyzing and documenting

These days there are a number of technological devices which may assist observers in their task. Whereas tape or video recording may present various degrees of 'faithful' representation of the research field, they also import their own reactance into the field, and require appropriate levels of consent. What needs to be considered is that such technological devices are only and always aids, and can never be considered as substitutes for the human observer. It is indeed ironic that the fastest growing domain for computer-based data analysis is just in the research area where human inquiry finds its most sensitive expression. One of the factors that such technologies preserve is the 'observational ecology', in that they construct a certain symmetry between the observed and the observer, in that the 'observer' like the 'observed', is not (at least at the time of data collection) quarantined and immune from the observational 'gaze'. But what it does introduce into the observational field is a 'third' (non-human) actor; the technological observer. So while some aspects of the ecology remain undisturbed by the use of such technological devices, other aspects are clearly reconfigured by the use of such devices. Given all these factors, it is suggested that the mini-disc recorder, with its capacity for rapid download onto a computer for later analysis, its smaller size (and hence its relatively unobtrusive nature), and its capacity for later 'marking' for particular analysis, would be the recording instrument of choice in most observational studies these days.

Many researchers agonize over the documentation of their work, especially with regard to the question of when the writing-up and documentation process should begin. According to Wolcott (1999), the answer is simple; it is exactly the right time to start writing 'if you have not begun to write'. The iterative and recursive nature of data analysis seems to suggest that one should neither be too cautious about recording the early observations, not too reliant upon their significance at a later point of the study. After all, it might be expected that first observations both inform and interrogate later observations and vice versa. Ideally this process could go on forever, but due to the limited temporal window of opportunity for participant observation, the data at least are contained in some way.

It should be obvious that the detail, extensiveness and richness of one's fieldnotes are crucial aspects of observational studies. 'Thick descriptions' usually begin with thick fieldnotes. Malinowski, who was a pioneer of participant observation, was also one of the first to insist upon thorough, detailed, and highly organized field maps (Malinowski 1961). This view is still held by more recent writers (Sanger 1996; DeWalt and DeWalt 2002) who still urge the use of a wide range of graphic material in the fieldnotes such as diagrams and other graphic media. Such notes provide not only a crucial record of the social life that one observed at a particular point, but an invaluable series of reference points to guide and inform the data analysis. It is always better to write more than less in one's fieldnotes. DeWalt and DeWalt (2002) argue that time required to write sufficient and adequate fieldnotes is usually much greater than time to make the observations on which they are based. As a rough guide, it is probably useful to spend as much time writing the notes as making the observations. It is always better to try to complete each fieldnote writing session as soon as possible after the observations (DeWalt and DeWalt 2002), and certainly no more than three days after. If it is possible, it is useful to have an unobtrusive method of recording shorter notes *in situ*. Such jottings can either be transcribed directly or pasted in one's field journal.

So it is hard to exaggerate the importance of fieldnotes. Every responsible researcher is expected to record their observations in fieldnotes which should be organized chronologically. One of the best ways to do this is through the use of a bound 'journal' (of blank lined pages) which hold all the notes securely together in a sequential way. This journal should be supplemented with the diary, which simply signposts events and contacts and places, and agendas to be completed. DeWalt and DeWalt (2002) suggest a number of supplementary devices like 'jot notes' which again are best kept in a little pocket notebook, and which contain the briefest form of fieldnotes especially those which need to be taken down immediately in the field. DeWalt and DeWalt also mention 'head notes', which are undocumented memories, intuitions, and attempts to make the tacit explicit.

DeWalt and DeWalt (2002) have reported a tendency for the quality and quantity of fieldnotes to decrease as the researcher gains increasing familiarity with the research contexts. This is particularly unfortunate, as the number of 'breakdowns' (incomplete information recorded in fieldnotes) which tend to increase over the course of the study, can be indicative of confusions, paradoxes and partial observations, all of which beg further analysis.

It is important to remember that fieldnotes are always both data and analysis; they are never 'pure inscriptions'. Throughout the entire course of the study, observers should report regularities as well as conventions, and exceptions, as much as variations. While most fieldnotes, especially in the early stages, consist of *a priori*, etic categories and operational definitions, it is important that fieldnotes begin the process of (or at least suggest) some kind of meta-analytic categorization and discussion, which will become one's formal data analysis.

In terms of analyzing observational data, many researchers like Sanger suggest that the generation of analytic categories should proceed in a funnel-like way from the very broad to the quite narrow. Sanger calls this 'progressive focussing'. In my own work I found it useful to proceed in this way while attempting to keep an eye out for outlier categories and discrepant cases. While this peripheral sensitivity may be useful, I have found that another technique is even more useful. After some intensive work on developing what I see as the sensitizing concepts, I find it useful to leave my analysis behind for some time, and when I return, re-read the basic observational data, to see what emerges on a fresh reading. This can often generate surprising and new sensitizing concepts, which enrich my initial analysis, even if they make it somewhat more complex, and require me to do some rewriting.

The notion of sensitizing concepts, which was developed by Herbert Blumer in the 1950s, is especially helpful in analyzing observational data (see Blumer 1969). While there are some advantages in using operational definitions in some observational studies, especially when the observation phenomenon of interest is easily bounded and defined (such as an episode of hand-washing at a basin, using specified products) and one clearly wants to focus on episodes of such a micro-behaviour for specific reasons, such operational definitions are either useless or unhelpful in attempting to grasp the fullness of the life-world, especially in exploratory studies. So sensitizing concepts 'serve to alert the user to the general character of the empirical world, by providing the hints and suggestions illustrated by actual empirical cases' (Jorgensen 1989: 112). Theory then 'serves as a useful and practical guide to research'. The advantage of sensitizing concepts is that they provide an initial theoretical starting point for the researcher, which guides the initial set of observations, and assists the researcher to initiate a theoretically driven inquiry, while at the same time setting off an inquiry into that theorization, on the basis of empirical observations. Sensitizing concepts are very useful devices in observational studies (and in other data collection procedures), as they embody sufficient structure to assist the work to proceed, as well as sufficient flexibility and malleability to be transformed over the course of inquiry; they work in similar ways to the method of constant comparison as outlined by Glaser and Strauss (1967). They can be used, for example, to describe unique cases relevant to each social world, as well as generally acceptable concepts across a social world, and to describe the connectedness of phenomena within a social world. They can be subjected to testing improvement, revision and refinement, if not outright rejection. Their validity is usually verified through careful studies of empirical cases. Skilled users of sensitizing concepts would expect and welcome a growing sensitivity over time to the phenomena that they were observing, through the very use of these concepts.

Data analysis is a process that always involves a complex and interweaving set of analyses and syntheses. That is to say, one always tries to break down a complex and detailed flow of social life into much narrower, static, descriptive categories. On the other hand, one also tries to link a number of these micro-dimensions together to make larger, more thematic units. While the downside is there are very few rules or guidelines to help with this process, the advantage is that this creative process can be very rewarding, and usually quite illuminating. This process is facilitated enormously by having a prior and close familiarity with the theoretical and empirical literature on the subject of inquiry, and the social worlds of interest. Obviously, a close familiarity with observational data is also essential to assist this analytic and synthetic process. While it is useful sometimes to apply some of the labels (sensitizing concepts) that your participants use in their social world, it is always worth remembering that the researcher's ('stranger') understanding of these concepts is unlikely to correspond entirely with their ('member') understanding of these concepts. Equally, it is perfectly acceptable for the researcher to adopt labels and concepts from other social worlds, and use them in a way which is functional for his or her (and the audience's) purposes, so long as it is an attempt to make clear just how these concepts are used.

Becker (1986) who has been a pioneer in many domains of social science research, especially participant observation, has offered some general advice to the researcher struggling with the writing-up phase of their participant observations. He advises the use of active rather than passive verbs and the economical use of words, while avoiding repetition. He favours concrete and specific descriptions rather than abstract and general ones, and suggests examples and illustrations are always helpful in this regard. While he doesn't speak against the use of metaphors, he does caution careful and serious use of metaphors. It is worth adding that metaphors should always clarify and strengthen other (metaphorical on non-metaphorical) text. So the use of mixed metaphors, on metaphors which compete with more literal or prosaic descriptions, should be avoided.

Conclusion

The whole process of observation relies so heavily upon a set of, often un-acknowledged, philosophical assumptions. It seems that we see what we believe rather than believe what we see. As there appears to be no methodological way out of this dilemma, the best we might hope for are clear expressions of our underlying philosophy and adequately specified and expressed observation statements.

Observation can be seen not only as a useful method in its own right but as a valuable complement to other data-gathering procedures. This is not to say that observation could or should provide the final word or 'gold standard' method, but rather that it has the capacity to provide data which may test, inform or interrogate data generated by other means. Observation is especially useful in ethnographic studies, and many such studies use the method of participant observation. But observational data need to be considered as problematic as any data generated by any methodology, as particular issues of sampling, reactance and ethics are rarely resolved easily. There is much to be considered by the researcher planning to conduct observational studies, especially in the field, and the skills required to successfully conduct observational studies is considerable, and is usually acquired after extensive experience and reflection.

Observational methods have the potential to generate huge amounts of data which must be adequately stored initially and analyzed later, to justify the considerable costs of doing observational research. While there are many ways of recording observational data, the interplay between data-gathering and analysis is always somewhat problematic in observational studies. Although challenging in many ways, the process of collecting and analyzing observational data is both rewarding and revealing for the social and human sciences.

References

Agar, M. (1986) Speaking of Ethnography. Sage University Paper series on Qualitative Research Methods, Vol. 2. Beverly Hills, CA: Sage.

Banister, P., Burman, E., Parker, I., Taylor, M. and Tindall, C. (1994) Qualitative Methods in Psychology: A Research Guide. Buckingham: Open University Press.

Bathes, R. (1982) Camera Lucida. London: Jonathan Cape.

Becker, H.S. (1986) Writing for Social Scientists. Chicago: University of Chicago Press.

Blumer, H. (1969) Symbolic Interactionism. Englewood Cliffs, NJ: Prentice Hall.

Clarke, A.E. and Fujimura, J.H. (1992) Co Constructing Tools, Jobs, and Rightness. In Clarke, A.E. and Fujimura, J.H. (eds) The Right Tools for the Job: At Work in Twentieth Century Life Sciences. New Jersey: Princeton University Press.

Collins, H.M. (1985) Changing Order: Replication and Induction in Scientific Practice. London: Sage.

DeWalt, K.M. and DeWalt, B.R. (2002) *Participant Observation: A Guide for Fieldworkers.* Walnut Creek, CA: Altamira Press.

Festinger, L., Riecken, H.W. and Schachter, S. (1956) *When Prophecy Fails.* Minneapolis: University of Minnesota Press.

Foucault, M. (1980) *Power and Knowledge: Selected Interviews and Other Writings 1972–77.* New York: Pantheon.

Glaser, B.G. and Strauss, A. (1967) *The Discovery of Grounded Theory: Strategies for Qualitative Research.* Chicago: Aldine.

Goffman, E. (1959) *The Presentation of Self in Everyday Life.* Garden City, NY: Doubleday.

Jorgensen, D.L. (1989) *Participant Observation: A Methodology for Human Studies.* London: Sage.

Latour, B. (1986) Visualisation and Cognition in Knowledge and Society: Studies in the Sociology of Culture Past and Present, Vol. 6. In Kuclick, H. (ed.), *Knowledge and Society: Studies in the Sociology of Science, Past and Present.* Vol. 6. Greenwich: JAI Press, 1–40.

Latour, B. and Woolgar, S. (1979) *Laboratory Life.* Beverly Hills, CA: Sage.

Malinowski, B. (1961) *Argonauts of the Western Pacific.* New York: Dutton.

Mead, M. (1928) *Coming of Age in Samoa.* New York: William Morrow.

Panagopoulos, I. (2002) *Risk and Harm Reduction Among Recreational Ecstasy Users.* Unpublished PhD thesis, Deakin University Melbourne, Australia.

Popper, K.R. (1992) *Conjectures and Refutations.* London: Routledge.

Roethlisberger, F.J. and Dickson, W.J. (1939) *Management and the Worker.* Cambridge, MA: Harvard University Press.

Rosenhahn, D. (1996) Being Sane in Insane Places. In Rubington, E. and Weinberg, M. (eds) *Deviance: The Interactionist Perspective,* 6th edn. Boston: Allyn and Bacon.

Sanger, J. (1996) *The Compleat Observer? A Field Research Guide to Observation.* London: The Falmer Press.

Spradley, J.P. (1970) *You Owe Yourself a Drunk: An Ethnography of Urban Nomads.* Boston: Brown.

Stangor, C. (2003) *Social Groups in Action and Interaction.* New York: Psychology Press.

Strauss, A.L. (1987) *Qualitative Analysis for Social Scientists.* New York: Cambridge University Press.

Wallace, S. (1999) *Controlling Alcoholism: Technologies of Trust in a Struggle for Scientific Authority.* Unpublished PhD thesis, University of Melbourne, Melbourne.

Webb, E.J., Campbell, D.T., Schwartz, R.D. and Sechrest, L. (1996) *Unobtrusive Measures: Nonreactive Research in the Social Sciences.* Chicago: Rand-McNally.

Wolcott, H. (1999) *Ethnography: A Way of Seeing.* Walnut Creek, CA: AltaMira Press.

Woolgar, S. (1988) *Knowledge and Reflexivity: New Frontiers in the Sociology of Knowledge.* Newbury Park: Sage.

PART 3

Choosing an approach

Which kind of approach to choose

There is no one right way to investigate the social world. The uncovering of meanings, experiences, emotions and thoughts usually demand a qualitative approach. The choice of approach depends mainly on the research question that the researcher wishes to explore and the aims that are being pursued, but the epistemological stance, skill and even the personality of the researcher also affect it. Many qualitative approaches share common elements and are based on a similar stance to research. They all focus on human beings, their experience and their social and personal worlds.

Chapters 7 to 14 include some guidelines to data collection and analysis in each approach under discussion, but this is not the main concern of the contributors. Writers give major examples of these qualitative approaches.

Chapter 6 by **Immy Holloway** and **Les Todres** centres on the *status of method* and the three main approaches in qualitative inquiry. They argue that an essential tension exists between flexibility of method and its consistency and coherence. The differences between approaches are investigated. Holloway and Todres suggest that researchers be context-sensitive and thoughtful when choosing an approach as well as being mindful of its distinctive features.

In Chapter 7 **Les Todres** describes *descriptive phenomenology* in its philosophical context, tracing its origins to the ideas of Husserl. Todres explains the meaning of the key ideas and their modification or development by Husserl's followers. He then discusses how descriptive phenomenology has become a research approach, and in particular how Giorgi has developed this 'scientific practice' of descriptive phenomenology. It is stated that descriptive phenomenology can humanize health and social care.

Interpretive or *hermeneutic phenomenology* is the 'science of interpretation of texts'. In Chapter 8 **Frances Rapport** traces its origin not only to the interpretation of religious texts but also to the thoughts and writings of the philosophers Brentano, Husserl and Heidegger, developed later by Gadamer with his emphasis on language and historicity. Rapport lists and analyzes the main features of hermeneutic phenomenology and tells the researcher how it can be distinguished from descriptive phenomenology and other qualitative approaches.

One of the most systematic ways of qualitative research is adopting the approach of *grounded theory*. **Rosalind Bluff** (Chapter 9) considers its nature and basis in symbolic interactionism, and how the method is applied to health-care settings and professional education. She marks certain distinctions between Straussian and Glaserian perspectives on grounded theory. Practical guidelines are discussed in some detail. Finally, Bluff describes how to evaluate a grounded theory study and demonstrates its implications for practice.

As health professionals, anthropologists and academics, **Siobhan Sharkey** and **John Larsen** have a special interest in *ethnography*. In Chapter 10 they describe how this method, in particular, centres on culture and subcultures which, of course, includes values norms and rules as well as conflicting perspectives in the field of health care. In the course of Chapter 10 they guide researchers through the process of developing an ethnography – a piece of ethnographic writing. They also demonstrate the significance of ethnography for practice.

Andrew C. Sparkes (Chapter 11) shows how *narrative research* has been developed throughout the last fifteen years. He stresses the value and contribution of this research to clinical practice, especially when describing the reality of the storytellers and how they perceive their illness or problem, how it becomes part of their identity, and how others react to them. He also discusses the structure and form of narratives. Health professionals embrace this approach because of its immediacy and vivacity.

Action research (AR) is one of the most practical and useful methods in qualitative health research. It is a tool to bring about change and generate knowledge. In Chapter 12 **Dawn Freshwater** explains Lewin's action research cycle of planning, taking action, observing and reflecting. She also seeks the origin of AR and describes its processes. In critical reflection on the method, she demonstrates that through application of 'pragmatic epistemology', AR bridges the theory–practice gap and assists professionals in researching their own practice.

Much qualitative research in the health-care arena is concerned with evaluating programmes and processes. *Evaluation research* has only recently gained a distinctive place in the field of qualitative inquiry, rather than being treated as a collection of information. In Chapter 13 **Kate Galvin** describes qualitative evaluation frameworks and explores evidence in the context of developing policy and practice. She lists and explains the key features of evaluation research and its different branches. Galvin also discusses its utility in policy and practice although she also uncovers the difficulties inherent in it, as it is a 'deeply political' process.

Debbie Kralik takes a *feminist stance to research* in Chapter 14. Within the health-care field, this way of looking at inquiry exemplifies one of the main characteristics of much qualitative research, namely the equality of the researcher and the other participants in the process. She also stresses the 'affirmation' of women's experiences and thoughts, in order that women acquire more power than they have hitherto had. There is an explication of the common principles that guide the feminist stance, and how this is grounded in feminist theory.

Immy Holloway closes this section in Chapter 15 by an attempt to explain the distinctive character of *writing qualitatively*. Instead of presenting a dry 'report', qualitative researchers give an account in story form (or sometimes in poetic or other form of presentation) to bring to the reader a portrayal of the world of the participants and a description of the phenomena within it. This account includes the perspectives of the participants as well as those of the researcher. Participants, researcher and reader of the research together transform the account into more than the sum of its parts.

All the writers are passionate about qualitative research; they see it as a way to explore important phenomena and make people's experiences explicit and central to the health-care and educational process. Each approach has its own way of addressing and answering questions and of proceeding through data collection and analysis and exploring meaning; nevertheless, they are focused not only on the shared social reality but also on the uniqueness of human beings.

6

IMMY HOLLOWAY AND LES TODRES
The status of method: flexibility, consistency and coherence[1]

Introduction

There is considerable overlap in terms of procedures and techniques in different approaches to qualitative research. These approaches often share a broad philosophy such as person-centredness and a certain open-ended starting point. Researchers using these approaches, generally adopt a critical stance towards positivist perspectives and search for meaning in the accounts and/or actions of participants. This is due to 'disenchantment' with earlier, more traditional approaches and their failure to capture the experiences and perspectives of the people whose lives, thoughts and feelings are being explored. There is also a shared concern for attention to the various kinds of context within which the research takes place, for example, a sensitivity towards the social and political as well as a heightened awareness of ethical issues involved in such study.

Such overlap of epistemological, aesthetic, ethical and procedural concerns can encourage a fairly generic view of qualitative research – a 'family' approach in which the similarities are considered more important than the differences, and where the notion of *flexibility* becomes an important value and quest. This is demonstrated both in older and in recent texts (see for instance Potter 1996; Crabtree and Miller 1999; Bryman 2001).

However, there is another point of view, concerned with how such flexibility can lead to inconsistency and a lack of coherence. In this view, such 'method slurring' (Baker *et al.* 1992) and interchangeability can dilute the value of consistently pursuing the integrity of a particular approach from beginning to end – from its philosophical underpinnings to the specificity of the subtle nuances that it may adopt in its methodological procedures.

The present chapter attempts to show that it is possible to transcend these tensions and include these concerns in a third position that can allow flexibility as well as consistency and coherence. This third position is a more differentiated one in which an understanding of purposes and relative appropriateness of procedures leads to greater specificity about what can be mixed and what cannot. We are arguing for *this* concept of *appropriateness* rather than *method for method's sake* on the one hand, or the *flight from method* on the other. The chapter thus aims to clarify the conceptual tools that qualitative researchers may need for informed choices. A diagrammatic table is provided (p. 94) which summarizes three types of qualitative research. This forms the basis for a consideration of how to regard both the common and distinctive characteristics of these different approaches as a basis for appropriate choice and application. The three approaches were chosen as illustrations to demonstrate the kinds of distinctions and dimensions that could be fruitfully considered in relation to other approaches as well. Further, the diagram is followed by a brief exposition of each of the three approaches in such a way as to shed some light on the following two questions:

1. What kind of consistency and coherence is important within each approach?
2. What kind of flexibility is possible within and between each approach?

It is thus hoped that the table and discussion will contribute to the debate about the growing need to think comparatively 'between' approaches when engaged in qualitative research design and practice. We are aware that the differences between approaches become exaggerated, but this might achieve greater clarity in the argument.

Exploration of the tension between flexibility and coherence

Researchers who focus on the generic approach raise the notion of 'flexibility' to prime consideration, and many suggest 'doing what works'. This approach does have some philosophical precedent in the old Greek idea that the 'object deter-mines the method by which it is approached' (Kisiel 1985: 6). Indeed, Gadamer (1975) in his book *Truth and Method* was a strong proponent of the view that no abstract method could predetermine an approach to study. Such philosophical consistency, however, has not historically informed the development of a generic approach to any remarkable degree. Rather the generic trend has arisen out of very pragmatic concerns. Much of this is due to the early history of qualitative research when specific approaches had not been established nor developed in any depth.

Qualitative methodology has been developed rather rapidly in the last two decades. While health researchers often chose to carry out qualitative research in the past without attaching a label, they now often adopt a specific approach, such as grounded theory, phenomenology, ethnography or other forms of qualitative inquiry. The term 'approach' is used here to differentiate it from the narrower term 'methods'. It indicates a coherent epistemological viewpoint about the nature of enquiry, the kind of knowledge that is discovered or produced and the kind of methodological strategies that are consistent with this (Giorgi 1970). Giorgi dis-cusses this in relation to phenomenology; Strauss (1987) and Brewer (2000) also claim that grounded theory and ethnography respectively are 'styles' of research rather than research methods; hence the term 'approach' used in this chapter seems more appropriate than 'methods'.

This chapter will contain a discussion of these issues in three commonly used approaches as illustrations: phenomenology, grounded theory and ethnography. We wish to acknowledge the need for flexibility in at least two ways:

1. To respect as much as possible the primacy of the topic or phenomenon to be studied and the range of possible research questions by finding a methodological approach and strategy that can serve such inquiry. This means not being too attached to method for method's sake – a kind of reductionism. Janesick (2000) calls it 'methodolatry', an obsession with method as opposed to contents and substance.

2. To acknowledge that a number of qualitative research strategies and skills are generic, such as interviewing, thematizing meanings, and the kind of writing that finds a balance between narrative and illustration.

However, although there is some overlap, there are distinctions and differences in the nature of qualitative approaches; in history, strategies, epistemology and ontology. Bailey (1997) gives an interesting analogy: although familiar drugs in a generic group are often interchangeable and used in the treatment of similar conditions (she mentions Aspirin, Bufferin and Tylenol as examples of analgesics), they have nevertheless unique chemical compositions and therapeutic indicators. They might be compared to various styles of qualitative inquiry. The analogy is not complete, however, and not wholly appropriate. Although there are generic elements between approaches, they are rooted in a number of distinct disciplines and world views, which can be illustrated in our examples.

Novice researchers will find difficulty not only in the meanings of the various terms and the specific language used but also in distinguishing between different approaches; for instance the concepts of *life-world* and *social reality*. On the other hand, similar terms can have somewhat different meanings; for instance the notion of *experience*. Although we do not wish to support 'methodolatry', we take the position that a distinctive approach does lead to greater clarity about the nature of the phenomenon to be explored, the questions posed and the ways researchers answer questions and communicate their findings. Data collection, analysis and report writing are distinct and depend on the choice of approach. Indeed the very aim of each approach is different, and trustworthiness is established in different ways. The style of each is also distinct; for instance, some approaches are more formal than others. Each form of inquiry even has its own vocabulary as Creswell (1998) demonstrates. A framework for the differences can be established.

Not only do all the above influence the specific research approach, but researchers as individuals also affect the choice of method, with their various personalities and background as well as their work environment, socialization and culture. For instance, regardless of topic area, a researcher with an in-depth interest in a particular phenomenon who is reflective and inner-directed would choose a distinctly different approach to one who is centred on social interaction and group behaviour. Knafl (1994: 210), in a dialogue on method, speaks of 'the fit between the method, the person and the style'. Most researchers modify or adapt the chosen approach to suit their own perception of the topic area and their preferences even when they claim to stay true to the method and the data. Personal style, although important, is only one consideration; more than this is, of course, involved. An inquiry that focuses on a culture or subculture with its beliefs, norms and routines differs from that which analyzes language as text. Alvesson and Sköldberg (2000: 11), while stressing the importance of epistemological and theoretical starting points, state: 'What constitutes an interesting and manageable research problem depends on the researcher's fundamental stance on methodological questions in the broad sense'; in other words, on his or her ideology. This, in turn, is determined, or at least influenced, by the researcher's professional education and earlier induction to the research process.

There have been a number of books and authors who present the issues of qualitative research as if they were presenting a generic approach to the subject. Books, such as the text by Kvale (1996) entitled *InterViews*, give the reader the impression that they will be reading a text that provides a generic approach to qualitative research, and that the various distinctive approaches will either be integrated or included. However, when one engages with the text, it is often discovered that a consistent approach is taken, such as phenomenology, and that this is equated with qualitative research in general. The problem with this unarticulated equation is that there is little acknowledgement that other approaches address different kinds and levels of questions and take a different stance on the kind of phenomena that it is focused upon. We thus take the view that a generic approach to qualitative research is, on the one hand, unsophisticated as qualitative inquiry has matured and become more specific; on the other, it is premature and more discussion and debate is needed before a more integrative and inclusive approach could be justified.

The need for consistency and coherence becomes clearer if one considers the danger of what has been called 'method-slurring' (Baker *et al.* 1992). This is the problem of blurring distinctions between qualitative approaches. Each approach has to demonstrate consistency with its foundations and will reflect them in the data collection, analysis and knowledge claim.

From the above analysis one can see that it may be important to acknowledge that specific approaches such as phenomenology or grounded theory have distinctive features on a number of levels such as the type of question they are suited to answer, the kinds of data collection that are consistent with this, and also the kinds of analysis and presentation of results that fit with this approach – such 'goodness of fit' or logical staged linking can be referred to as 'consistency'.

If such consistency occurs then the whole thing 'hangs together' as coherent; that is, the kind of knowledge generated in the results or presentation section does what it said it would do under the aims of the project. In order to consider these criteria of consistency and coherence in greater detail we will need to look at the distinctive differences between qualitative approaches. We have chosen three approaches as illustrations and Table 6.1 emphasizes their differences in terms of the following criteria: the aims of the research approach, its roots in different disciplines and ideologies, the knowledge claims linked to it and, to a lesser extent, the data collection and analysis specific to each approach.

Table 6.1 Dimensions to evaluate the status of method

Dimensions	Phenomenology	Grounded theory	Ethnography
Goal	Describe, interpret and understand the meanings of experiences at both a general and unique level.	Develop a theory of how individuals and groups make meaning together and interact with each other; of how particular concepts and activities fit together and can explain what happens.	Describe, interpret, and understand the characteristics of a particular social setting with all its cultural diversity and multiplicity of voices.
Research question	What is the structure of this particular experience? What is it like to be or experience a particular situation?	What theory can be formulated from real world events and experiences to explain this social phenomenon?	How are people positioned in a particular social context and how do they interact with each other, especially with significant others? What are the power relationships within the setting?
Data gathering	Focused on the depth of a particular experience; interviews, narratives – anything that is able to describe the qualities of experiences that were lived through.	Open-ended beyond a general direction – breadth and depth at different phases; a variety of methods in which the questions may change at different stages depending on the data that are emerging and clues from the literature. Progressive focusing.	Through intensive fieldwork – participant observation and interviews – of key informants who are experts on the social setting and have rich knowledge of it. Also through visual data.
Analysis	Thematic analysis which clarifies the meanings by moving back and forth between whole meanings and part meanings.	Use the analysis to inspire a creative and plausible theory; constant comparison and organizing the data into useful conceptual patterns by codes and categories. Construct and build credible models.	Coding and building patterns. Searching for the main building blocks of local culture and its themes.

Dimensions	Phenomenology	Grounded theory	Ethnography
Presentation of results	Different levels depending on audience and purpose: a description of the essence (structure) of the experience, its 'bare bones'; followed by how each theme occurs in different and unique ways; sometimes, a more poetic and narrative account which communicates what the experience is like (its textures). Combinations of these.	A descriptive outline of the elements of the model and how they interact and fit together to form an explanatory theory that accounts for the range of the data collected. Often a diagram that represents these elements and relationships; followed by an exploration of the themes and concepts in relationship to both specific data examples as well as relevant literature.	An ethnography – the story of people in their social and cultural context describing behaviour, activities, and social relations and the way they perceive their position in the setting under study and society.
Knowledge claim	Transferable general qualities (essences) of what makes the experience what it is; description of unique contexts. Empathic understanding.	A plausible theory that can be applied and tested in other contexts. An explanatory model.	Knowledge about people within a setting or situation and the way in which they relate to others and perceive themselves.
Historical background	Philosophy, psychology.	Sociology and social psychology.	Social and cultural anthropology

Distinctions between approaches

Here we give an overview of the main elements of three approaches.

Phenomenology

Phenomenology has as its focus the faithful description of how experiential phenomena such as 'becoming a patient', or 'learning how to use medical skills' happen. Through paying careful attention to how such phenomena occur in unique and concrete contexts, it hopes to reveal in linguistic terms the essential features of a phenomenon – what we can say that captures it in its most general sense, and also what we can say about how it may vary from situation to situation. These variations help us to formulate 'essences' that may be judged by communities of readers as giving relevant and transferable insights into what an experience may be like through clarification of its essential structures and textures. It thus fosters intersubjective understanding into the human condition. Following from this, the kind of coherence and consistency that is important within this approach can be expressed as follows:

- It formulates a research question that asks participants to narrate actual experiences that they have lived through. It is primarily from these concrete descriptions of 'lived experiences' rather than from the participants' views, beliefs or conclusions that the researcher draws on in order to pursue the analysis. The methods of 'data collection' thus need to be consistent with an intention to gather descriptions of participants' experiences that are internally meaningful without reference to external theories or preconceived directions beyond the request to describe the experience as fully as possible. If interviewing for this purpose, the researcher requires an interviewing style that is different from that of a semi-structured interview. Data collection thus focuses on the specific 'time when . . .' or 'the situation in which . . .' and the internal coherence of 'what appears' is honoured as closely as possible at this stage.

- The methods of data analysis need to be consistent with a phenomenological or hermeneutic understanding that 'part meanings' within a text or experiential narrative can only be understood in terms of the role they play within the 'whole' sense of the text. To be coherent within this approach, the analysis needs a strategy that is mindful of a 'back and forth' movement between particular meanings and the sense of the text or experience as a whole. A 'part meaning' is thus not given more value just because it occurs more times. This is why the term 'content analysis' is avoided and the term 'constituent' is often used in order to indicate a concern with how the 'part meanings' function together and interactively make up the whole. The danger of computer-aided analysis packages is that they can divert attention in a way that over-emphasizes a concern with the 'parts' and obscures the intuition of the 'whole'. The philosophical depth of this distinction lies in Husserl's notion that meanings need to be holistically intuited and cannot merely be put together in a kind of additive or quantifiable way.

- It presents its results in such a way as to be consistent with a concern to communicate both the 'structures' and 'textures' of the experience. The term 'structure' refers to the 'essences' or 'bare bones' of what makes the phenomenon what it is. In other words, it wishes to articulate the most invariant themes that emerge transferably from one situation or person to another. For example, are there any essential things that can be said about anger that apply to both this individual and that individual and this situation and that situation? This is a scientific emphasis in phenomenology. The term 'texture' refers to the communication of evocative qualities that capture how unique experiences and descriptions can convey the rich and participative nature of 'what the experience is like'. Such presentations require a more elaborate form of writing in which unique experiences are indicated in a way that presents their evocative nature. This is an aesthetic or literary emphasis in phenomenology. How the choice is made to emphasize or combine the presentation of 'structure' and 'texture' depends on the purpose of the research and one's readership. (For a more elaborate discussion of this see Todres (2000).)

- This approach is consistent with a 'knowledge claim' about the primacy of experience – that no matter how much experiences are structurally prefigured by political, cultural and languaged contexts, it is how these contexts are 'gathered' and 'lived out' by people that is an important starting point for qualitative enquiry. The coherence of this 'knowledge claim' is one that is very cautious. It merely says: these seem to be the essential features of this experience as lived through these individuals in these contexts. One can speculate as to why, and offer plausible interpretations in one's discussion but the approach cannot speak of 'causes' or 'explanations' as if such objective 'how-things-are' analyses were possible. The 'knowledge claim' is one that reports 'appearances' in this time and place and offers possible insights that others can relate to in a way that deepens readers' understanding and that can be of use for application. The usefulness of the insights can only be finally validated by interpersonal 'use' and the judgement of that 'use'.

The kind of flexibility that is possible between phenomenology and other approaches may include the following: the use of coherent narratives, presentations of experience that can be linguistically expressed, biographical accounts and texts of experiences, as long as all these accounts have a significant dimension of 'specific occurrences' with all the textures of time, place, sequence and experienced meaning.

Other approaches can use phenomenological analysis (such as those used by Giorgi 1985; van Manen 1990 or Kvale 1996;) for analyzing the meanings of texts or accounts.

In arguing that a phenomenological approach needs coherence and consistency between its goal, research question, data gathering methods, modes of analyses, presentation of results, and modes of 'knowledge claim', we are not primarily interested in preserving the credentials or boundaries of this approach as an ideological commitment for its own sake. Rather, the issue about coherence and consistency refers more simply to a thoughtfulness about whether the empirical claims made by researchers fit with the approach and methods taken.

Grounded theory

The focus of grounded theory research is on developing plausible and useful theories that are closely informed by actual events and interactions of people and their communications with each other. For the researcher this means centring on social and psychological processes such as 'becoming a member of a group', 'learning to live with pain' or 'interaction between patients and professionals'. This entails noting changes in conditions and context. However, the emphasis on these processes also gives grounded theory coherence and consistency:

- Tracing the social/psychological processes that are at the core of people's behaviour and thought is essential. For the researcher it is a journey of discovery where each stage depends on the other. If there is no coherence and consistency within the approach, the processes cannot be followed and theory generation is impossible.

- It is important to formulate a research question or focus on a problem that takes into account the complexity and the process of human action and interaction. This means that the researcher follows the tenets of symbolic interactionism – in particular that human beings are not passive recipients of cues or influences of the social environment to which they merely respond; they must be seen instead as dynamic agents who take an active part in the process, based on the way in which they interpret the situation. In interaction with others they create meaning. This interpretation of social reality and the meaning they attach to action and experience gives consistency to the research. The research aim must be with the original overall intentions of grounded theory.

- The methods of data collection and analysis are consistent with the aim of the research, which is theory development, a notion that should be traceable throughout the research. This means progressive focusing on particular concepts and ideas important for the emerging theory. The collection and analysis of data is therefore interactive. This is a specific feature of grounded theory. It is more developmental than other approaches, and the development is reflected in the interaction between data collection and analysis. Theoretical sampling based on previously occurring concepts ensures coherence and consistency. Initially the focus centres on the phenomenon; then the theoretical ideas are further developed so that the theory can 'emerge'.

- The categories emerging from the analysis can all be linked to each other, and to the developing theory.

Flexibility is possible in a number of ways:

- Aspects of grounded theory are often used in other approaches (see Hammersley and Atkinson 1995); theoretical sampling in particular is seen as a useful tool for many researchers who are able to give direction to their various forms of qualitative research. The description of a culture or of social change may contain elements of a core category and theory development.

- The presentation of findings may also be similar when the focus is on meaning and interpretation of experience. However, the similarities to grounded theory that can be found in a number of approaches do not necessarily mean that grounded theory research has been carried out; it has to have other important elements of grounded theory, the ongoing interaction of data collection and analysis (which gives direction to further data collection), and the generation and construction of theory. However, certain methods of data analysis used by grounded theory such as coding and categorizing can be employed by other approaches at certain phases of analysis.

- The theoretical ideas, which the researcher elicits from the data, are always provisional and may be subject to change depending on further incoming data. For this the approach must be flexible and the researcher open-minded. This emphasis on 'being-on-the-way' is useful for other qualitative approaches as well.

Ethnography

The origins of ethnography lie in cultural anthropology but it is now applied to a range of different fields. During the late 1920s and early 1930s, when the Chicago School of Sociology became active and acquired a reputation, much of the field-work carried out by its members was called ethnography. Ethnography in its early days had as its focus a culture and initially focused its holistic portrayal, the perspective of its members – the informants of the research – on the values and knowledge they share. Through its portrayal in 'thick description' (Geertz 1973), readers obtained an understanding of the workings of the culture and its cultural members, including its rituals, rules and beliefs. However, in more recent times it has been used in a number of different disciplines, and, according to Atkinson *et al.* (2001: 1) 'escapes ready summary definitions'. It has changed from a 'monolithic understanding' of culture, and the approach relates to people's understanding of society and their positions within it; while formerly it focused on the shared elements of culture, it now demonstrates and presents cultural diversity. For instance, ethnographic fieldwork may focus on a hospital setting, the way in which nurses or doctors in the organization are located within it, their situation in the structure, and indeed their relationships with each other which are linked to the cultural context of the organization. Coherence and consistency can be discerned in the following aspects of ethnography:

- The aim of ethnography is to reveal structures and interactions in a society, the contested nature of culture, the meaning that people give to their action and interaction. It also reveals how people are situated within a cultural context. Through this, it demonstrates internal coherence. These elements or building blocks of ethnography are consistent with its foundations but also with recent changes.
- A coherent story is organized around research participants' positions in society and the varied meanings they give to their location, relationships with others and their behaviour.
- One of the main commitments of ethnography is the first hand experience of a social situation or setting on the basis of participant observation and intensive fieldwork.
- Ethnography also relies strongly on naturally occurring language of the participants in the field.

Flexibility is possible through certain procedures which ethnography has in common with other approaches:

- The researchers approach the data collection without strong prior assumptions and do not impose their own views on the words and actions of the research participants. This is difficult, of course, whether researchers are strangers to the setting they observe or, indeed, overfamiliar with it.

- Like grounded theory, ethnography is capable of producing testable theories that might be applied to other settings. As in other approaches, there is a reliance on language and text.

- Data analysis demands certain procedures but the choice and development of taxonomies and typologies depends on the individual researcher who adds the etic (outsider) view to the perspectives of the participants. Researchers are generally aware that, although shared perspectives exist, there is no unified perception and that participants have many voices. This stance is shared with other qualitative approaches, in which there is a movement to represent the multiplicity of voices and perceptions of the participants as well as the researcher's own views and interpretations.

Combining approaches

Some writers claim that different methodological approaches within the qualitative research paradigm can be usefully adopted. For instance, Maggs-Rapport (2000) suggests combining qualitative methodologies through triangulation of data, as this might assist in understanding. However, while one might argue for triangulation 'within-method' for data collection in some approaches – for instance, observation and interviewing – one could also suggest that triangulation between qualitative methods would not only blur the boundaries but also generate confusion about the epistemological and ontological bases that underlie each distinct approach and which give it coherence. Baker *et al.* (1992) describe the way in which the differences in two particular types of inquiry sometimes become blurred, and why data collection procedures must be made explicit and consistent with the chosen approach.

Qualitative research is even more complex than the three approaches on which we have concentrated (for example, nuances of difference between descriptive and hermeneutic phenomenology and the nuances of difference between Glaserian and Straussian versions of grounded theory). This thus suggests that although we have offered some useful general distinctions, qualitative researchers cannot simply use methodological strategies without understanding the intentions and philosophical underpinnings of the different approaches.

It is interesting that even in specific approaches, there is not always consensus about the exact methods, strategies and procedures to adopt. The Glaserian and Straussian versions of grounded theory have developed not only separately over time but also tend to have different purpose, procedures and outcome, or so their defenders believe (Glaser 1992; Strauss and Corbin 1998). Critical ethnography is not only based on assumptions that have their roots in past anthropological ideas, but it also adopts a Marxist stance on power and control (Thomas 1993). This growing complexity of the nuances of qualitative research thus appears to ask for more thoughtfulness about the dimensions used in our diagram, and generates the following questions when engaged in qualitative research practice:

- Is the phenomenon or research question the primary consideration in choosing the approach?
- Do the data collection, sampling and analysis procedures 'fit' the chosen approach?
- Does the study produce the kind of knowledge where the findings and presentation match the goals of the study?
- Has the researcher made explicit that the phases are consistent with the overall parameters of the research design?

Conclusion

Precise definitions of specific qualitative approaches are still not settled and boundaries often blurred. We do not wish to advocate exclusivity or an elitist approach, nor do we see pragmatism as a 'methodological crime'. However, it is argued here that unreflexive and undisciplined eclecticism might be avoided by being specific about the approach adopted.

Unless we say that our insights, as outcomes of qualitative research, are arbitrary, we cannot ignore the issues that are raised by philosophers of science to account for the credibility of whatever claims we make about the truth-value of our qualitative research endeavours. While we may not like the terms 'validity' or 'reliability' we believe that we are accountable to be explicit about the epistemological status of our outcomes, and what we are claiming for these outcomes. Seale (1999), for example, states that the terms 'validity' and 'reliability' are no longer adequate for the issues that are linked to the 'quality' of qualitative research, while Morse et al. (2002) strongly dispute this. Following the dimensions that we have offered in this chapter, we believe that it is possible to be more specific in the write-up of research that begins its methodological section with a claim about the particular status of the chosen research as well as claims about its manner of coherence, consistency and flexibility. This may include references to some of the alternative terms to 'validity' that have been generated such as credibility or trustworthiness and authenticity (Lincoln and Guba 1985; Erlandson et al. 1993; Lincoln 1995; a large list is given by Byrne-Armstrong et al. 2001). Such a section may also include an explicit consideration of whether any methodological procedures or personal disciplines were brought to bear in achieving its claims. It may also include a reflexive account of the intended audiences for which the presentation was written, the kind of knowledge production that was intended, and some of the historical and cultural contexts within which the presentation was written. Such transparency may empower readers to evaluate the range of relevance of the research as well as its possible transferability at different levels or to other situations.

These tentative suggestions are offered as a contribution to emerging challenges of shifting the emphasis away from 'method for method's sake' to a consideration of a more reflective, thoughtful research practitioner who may represent much diversity in approach and practice, but who earns our consideration as a faithful mediator between communities in their quest for understanding.

References

Alvesson, M. and Sköldberg, K. (2000) *Reflexive Methodology: New Vistas for Qualitative Research*. London: Sage.

Atkinson, P., Coffey, A., Delamont, S., Lofland, J. and Lofland, L. (eds) (2001) *Handbook of Ethnography*. London: Sage.

Bailey, P.H. (1997) Finding your way around qualitative methods in nursing research, *Journal of Advanced Nursing*, 25 (1): 18–22.

Baker, C., Wuest, J. and Stern, P.N. (1992) Method slurring: the grounded theory/phenomenology example, *Journal of Advanced Nursing*, 17 (11): 1355–1360.

Brewer, J.D. (2000) *Ethnography*. Buckingham: Open University Press.

Bryman, A. (2001) *Social Research Methods*. Oxford: Oxford University Press.

Byrne-Armstrong, H., Higgs, J. and Horsefall, D. (eds) (2001) *Critical Moments in Qualitative Research*. Oxford: Butterworth Heinemann.

Crabtree, B.F. and Miller, W.L. (eds) (1999) *Doing Qualitative Research*, 2nd edn. Thousand Oaks: Sage.

Creswell, J.W. (1998) *Qualitative Inquiry and Research Design: Choosing Among Five Traditions*. Thousand Oaks: Sage.

Erlandson, D.A., Harris, E.L., Skipper, B.L. and Allen, S.D. (1993) *Doing Naturalistic Inquiry*. Newbury Park: Sage.

Gadamer, H.G. (1975) *Truth and Method*. New York: Seabury Press.

Geertz, C. (1973) *The Interpretation of Cultures*. New York: Basic Books.

Giorgi, A. (1970) *Psychology as a Human Science: A Phenomenologically Based Approach*. London: Harper & Row.

Giorgi, A. (ed.) (1985) *Phenomenology and Psychological Research*. Pittsburgh: Duquesne University Press.

Glaser, B.G. (1992) *Basics of Grounded Theory Analysis*. Mill Valley, CA: Sociology Press.

Hammersley, M. and Atkinson, P. (1995) *Ethnography: Principles in Practice*, 2nd edn. London: Tavistock.

Janesick, V.J. (2000) Choreography of Qualitative Research Design: Minuets, Improvisations, and Crystallization. In Denzin, N.K. and Lincoln, Y.S. (eds) *Handbook of Qualitative Research*, 2nd edn. Thousand Oaks: Sage, 379–399.

Kisiel, T. (1985) The Happening of Tradition: The Hermeneutics of Gadamer and Heidegger. In Hollinger, R. (ed.) *Hermeneutics and Praxis*. Notre Dame, Indiana: University of Notre Dame Press, 3–29.

Knafl, K.A. (1994) In Dialogue: More on Muddling Methods. In Morse, J.M. (ed.) *Critical Issues in Qualitative Methods*. Thousand Oaks: Sage, 210.

Kvale, S. (1996) *InterViews*. Thousand Oaks: Sage.

Lincoln, Y.S. (1995) Emerging criteria for quality in qualitative and interpretive research, *Qualitative Inquiry*, 1 (3): 275–289.

Lincoln, Y.S. and Guba, E.G. (1985) *Naturalistic Inquiry*. Beverly Hills: Sage.

Maggs-Rapport, F. (2000) Combining methodological approaches in research: ethnography and interpretive phenomenology, *Journal of Advanced Nursing*, 31: 219–225.

Morse, J.M., Barett, M., Mayan, M., Olson, K. and Spiers, J. (2002) Verification Strategies for establishing reliability and validity in qualitative research, *International Journal of Qualitative Methods*, 1 (2): Article 2, from http://www.ualberta.ca/~ijqm/.

Potter, J.W. (1996) *An Analysis of Thinking and Research about Qualitative Methods*. Mahwah, NJ: Lawrence Erlbaum.

Seale, C. (1999) *The Quality of Qualitative Research*. London: Sage.

Strauss, A.L. (1987) *Qualitative Analysis for Social Scientists*. New York: Cambridge University Press.

Strauss, A. and Corbin, J. (1998) *Basics of Qualitative Research: Techniques and Procedures for Developing Grounded Theory*, 2nd edn. Thousand Oaks: Sage.

Thomas, J. (1993) *Doing Critical Ethnography*. Newbury Park, CA: Sage.

Todres, L. (2000) Writing phenomenological–psychological descriptions: an illustration attempting to balance texture and structure, *Auto/Biography*, 8 (1 and 2): 41–48.

van Manen, M. (1990) *Researching Lived Experience: Human Science for an Action Sensitive Pedagogy*. London, Ontario: The Althouse Press.

Note

[1] We would like to acknowledge and thank Sage Publications for permission to use and modify this chapter which first appeared as: Holloway, I. and Todres, L. (2003) The status of method: flexibility consistency and coherence, *Qualitative Research*, 3 (3): 345–357.

7

LES TODRES
Clarifying the life-world: descriptive phenomenology

Introduction

Phenomenology has a strong philosophical and epistemological heritage (Spiegelberg 1994) and has been an important source of reference for the development of qualitative research in general. This is because it provides a philosophical rationale for approaching the intelligibility of human experience on its own terms as a source of study. This chapter proceeds by placing descriptive phenomenology within its philosophical context, and then moves to demonstrate in some detail one approach to translating the philosophical insights into the practice of human science research.

Descriptive phenomenology as philosophy

Edmund Husserl (1859–1938) was a philosopher and mathematician whose life work focused on some of the fundamental problems of epistemology (Kockelmans 1967). Such a concern examines the foundation and status of knowledge and includes questions such as: what is 'real' and 'valid', what constitutes 'evidence', and what is the relationship between the 'knower' and the 'known'? His contributions heralded a substantial philosophical tradition that has gone through a number of twists and turns. I cannot do justice to the core philosophical ideas of this tradition within the scope of this chapter (see Spiegelberg (1994) for a historical introduction), but would like to consider briefly two concepts that are important when considering the practice of descriptive phenomenology as an empirical qualitative research approach: the terms, 'life-world' and 'essences'.

- *Life-world.* Husserl used the term, 'life-world' to indicate the flow of experiential happenings which provide the 'thereness' of what appears prior to categorizing it into 'packages'. It is the life-world that is the source of all experiential qualities. Distinctions such as hot, far and the number three all refer to a life-world of happenings without which any thought or construct would have no 'about'. Husserl wished to *intuit and describe* what was given to consciousness by the life-world. The term '*intuition*' was used by Husserl in preference to terms like 'sense', 'think', 'feel', to indicate the presence or appearance of a phenomenon that is then open to faithful description. By sampling phenomena in this way Husserl was able to reflect on the nature of what appeared.

• *Essences.* Plato hypothesized a realm of ideal essences of which this world was an imperfect modification. Such essences constituted ideal archetypes that defined the possibilities and patterns for the phenomena of this world. Husserl used the word 'essence' to indicate something different. In this conception, essences do not exist apart from or prior to the everyday world. Essences refer to invariant structures that can be intuited within an experienced world of meaning. Such essences are neither objective nor subjective but refer to an intelligible order that is intuited in the way things are given to consciousness. So, for example, there are some invariant features that make 'anger' what it is, and some invariant features that make the experience of 'red' what it is. Such experiential phenomena are recognized again and again in spite of their unique variations and contexts. Essences thus refer to the qualities that give an experiential phenomenon its distinctiveness and coherence; the qualities that make something what it is as it appears relationally to consciousness. The meanings of an essential structure can be clarified and expressed in different ways depending on the purpose of one's inquiries. Essences have sometimes been referred to as the relational structure of an experiential phenomenon or the general thematic structure. Husserl was interested in these orders and unities of experiential life and believed that this could be articulated with the help of a method he called *imaginative variation*. The 'whatness' (or essence or structure) of an experience such as 'anger' or an 'experience of an imaginary friend' or 'back-pain' could be arrived at by imaginatively varying the constituents of the experience in order to consider its boundaries and internal relationships. At what stage does it imaginatively stop being what it is and become something else? In such a way Husserl comes to describe the invariant features of something (its bare bones) and how these essential features interrelate to constitute the order of the experience as a phenomenon. Some essences may be valid within a planetary context and are very general such as the experience of gravity whereas others may be very specific and highly context-bound such as the experience of receiving a medical diagnosis within a particular culture or social group. To pursue the articulation of essences does not necessarily mean that one has an essentialist philosophy in which essences precede existence: it leaves open the question as to whether any essences are universal and ahistorical.

Since Husserl, there have been a number of philosophers who have modified his philosophical project in different ways, taken it in different directions, and disagreed with some of his core ideas. These continuities and discontinuities are complex and sometimes overstated. For example, Husserl's student, Heidegger adopted what he believed was a phenomenological attitude in his famous work,

Being and Time, and often used the term 'essence' in his writings. But he focused more and more on what he believed were undeveloped themes in Husserl, notably on the role of language and the problems of ontology – the question of being, as a more primary consideration than the question of knowing. It is not difficult to understand how Husserl's thought, with its invitation to describe the life-world and to find essential qualities inspired a whole generation of existential philosophers such as Sartre, Marcel, Buber and Levinas as well as literary figures and artists.

In conclusion, it could be said that Husserlian descriptive phenomenology is based on the intuition that when one is open to phenomena as relationships there is an intrinsic intelligibility to what appears and that this intelligibility can 'come to language' and be described in productive ways. Experience is restored as a valid focus for inquiry on its own terms without reducing it to biology, behaviour, or sociology.

Descriptive phenomenology: a methodological approach in qualitative research

There have been various attempts to consider the implications of Husserlian phenomenology for the human sciences, for example Alfred Schutz (1972) in sociology, Harold Garfinkel (1967) in ethnomethodology and Maurice Merleau-Ponty (1962) in child psychology. At the philosophical level, Husserl has been at least pivotal in helping to articulate the differences between a natural science and a human science (Merleau-Ponty 1963; Giorgi 1970). But more than this, Husserl's thought has been used in productive ways to go beyond these debates in the philosophy of science and to be used as a template for the practice of human science research. In this chapter I will present the broad approach taken by Amedeo Giorgi (1975, 1985, 1997, 2000) and more recently Giorgi and Giorgi (2003a, 2003b) as it is an example of how to take forward all the core concepts discussed above into the practice of a phenomenologically-oriented qualitative research. To date, many phenomenological research projects have been conducted based on this approach or on some modification of its guiding principles (see, for example, Fischer and Wertz 1979; Aanstoos 1985; Fow 1996; Fischer 1998).

Giorgi's descriptive phenomenology: the practice of a human science approach

Giorgi has made an important distinction between phenomenology as a philosophical project and as a scientific practice:

> Phenomenological philosophy is a foundation for scientific work; it is not the model for scientific practice. The insights of the philosophy have to be mediated so that scientific practices can be performed.
>
> (Giorgi 2000: 4)

In order for it to become a scientific practice, Giorgi (1997) retains the essential spirit of Husserl's philosophy as well as a number of core concepts as articulated by Husserl. The major change that is made is to use descriptions of experiences from others and not just from oneself as in philosophical reflection on experience. The central features of a descriptive phenomenological research approach are then characterized by the following components:

1. The researcher gathers detailed concrete *descriptions* of specific experience from others.
2. The researcher adopts the attitude of the *phenomenological reduction* in order to intuit the intelligibility of what is given in the experience.
3. The researcher seeks the most *invariant meanings* for a context.

These central features have been carried out in a number of different ways in practice. Although Giorgi has offered specific detailed suggestions on how these steps may be achieved, he is keen to point out that these steps may be pursued in different ways. For example, concrete experiential descriptions may be obtained by interviews, by written accounts or even by drawings or experiential exercises on which the respondent comments. Seeking invariant meanings may be aided by various strategies that help the phenomenological researcher to slow down, to intuit invariant meanings, and to express these meanings in a helpful and com-municative manner (see Wertz 1983; Polkinghorne 1989; Moustakas 1994; Von Eckartsberg 1998; Churchill and Wertz 2001; Dahlberg *et al.* 2001; Giorgi and Giorgi 2003a, 2003b for different strategies of articulating meanings in a faithful and rigorous way). The method that follows is thus by necessity indicative, and phenomenological researchers are invited to find new creative ways of expressing the spirit and goals of descriptive phenomenological research. Methods can ensure rigour but cannot replace phenomenological presence and insight. Descriptive phenomenology is essentially the use of self in relation to the discipline outlined previously, and one offers both one's procedures and findings to others for scrutiny.

1. Formulating a research question that has a phenomenological character

Formulating a research question that has a phenomenological character involves two steps: finding a phenomenological focus of interest and formulating a life-world-evoking question that could be addressed to respondents.

1.1 Finding a phenomenon of interest

The phenomenologically oriented researcher wishes to see what the experiences of people can tell us about a phenomenon of interest. The phenomenon of interest is clarified by how it occurs in the concrete life-worlds of people who have gone through the relevant experience. One could start with a very broad phenomenon of interest such as: What are the essential features of the experience of anxiety? (Fischer 1982). One could also focus on a more specific but still fairly general question such as: What are the essential differences between the experience of shame and the experience of guilt? Or one could have a highly specific focus such as: What are the essential attractions of a particular computer game for a particular twelve-year-old? One can see from these examples that the phenomenological character of an interest focuses on the *meaning* of lived experiences, *what* they are and *how* they are lived in concrete ways. The initial question for the researcher is then how to find a phenomenon for focus that is relevant and interesting. This interest may have arisen out of a combination of contextual factors such as previous literature, research, practical or personal interests or some combination of these. This is the stage where the researcher acknowledges his or her embeddedness within a historical community of scholars. A literature search can thus be very helpful at this stage for the purpose of understanding the current issues, theories and questions in the area. One interrogates this literature in order to see where a phenomenological approach may be needed with its benefit of bracketing preconceptions and going back to the life-world in an open-minded way. So, for example, Hartley *et al.* (2002), when reviewing the literature on post-natal depression noticed that there were many assumptions about what was 'normal' for women going through the birth experience. The nature of the experience of the transition to motherhood was not appreciated as a context within which depression could occur. The literature provided little understanding of the complexity of this experience as a whole. This gave the researcher a phenomenological question that was interesting, topical and relevant in relation to current issues and practices. In practice, asking oneself the question 'what is the phenomenon I wish to study' is often a process of refining one's focus through reading, reflection and even by doing pilot studies to see whether the focus reveals discoveries that are relevant and interesting. For example, in my own research into the meaning of self-insight for clients in psychotherapy which is used as an illustration later in this chapter (Todres 2000, 2002a, 2002b), a pilot study revealed two kinds of phenomena: insights that led to a greater sense of freedom and insights that did not lead to a greater sense of freedom. I then became interested in studying a more refined phenomenon: the kind of therapeutic self-insight that carries a greater sense of freedom. In my experience, not enough time is spent on this early phase of reading and reflection in which the phenomenon of interest is specified. Context, purpose and ethical considerations are all central to this refining process.

1.2 Formulating an initial life-world-evoking question

At this phase the phenomenological researcher wishes to have access to descriptions of life-world experiences that are relevant to the phenomenon that he or she is studying. These life-world experiences are of other people who have lived through such experiences and who are able to describe such happenings in context, and as richly as possible. One could perhaps find such faithful experiences existing already in autobiographies or other diaries of experience. However, it is more usual that such exemplars of experiential phenomena need to be generated on the basis of a researcher's question. One would like the question to be open enough so that it gives the respondent enough freedom to describe the relevant experiences (whether in writing or verbally) in his or her own terms. The initial life-world-evoking question does, however, focus the respondent on two concerns:

1. A request to *describe* the experience or experiences as fully as possible as he or she personally lived them. This could take a number of forms such as: 'please describe a situation in which you experienced ...', or 'a time within the last three months when ... happened'. Notice that the request is formulated in such a way as to elicit concrete events and experiences that naturally have a narrative form full of happenings that include descriptions of personal time and space, things, interpersonal relationships, thoughts, feelings and actions. Also notice that the initial life-world-evoking question avoids more abstract requests such as 'what do you think of ...?' or 'what is your view of ...?' Descriptions of lived experience are usually found to be much richer than the conclusions and generalizations that respondents make of them. So views, feelings and attitudes form only a part of the whole experience as lived through by the respondent.

2. A specification of the *kind of experience or experiences* to be focused on by the respondent. Here one needs to indicate the phenomenon in such a way that the respondent can recognize the relevant experience indicated. The researcher needs to be careful not to use jargon in the question but to find experience-near terms that occur in everyday language. For example, in my own research I found that the term 'self-insight' was too technical to include within the life-world-evoking question. More respondents could relate to the terms 'seeing or understanding something about oneself or one's life in a new or different way'. It is the experiential term that one uses that becomes the focus of the study and one suspends one's views about whether this is the same thing as the technical term that one initially started off with. It is part of the phenomenological analysis that comes later that considers the extent to which the technical terms or other disciplinary terms from the literature are adequate to the lived phenomenon as studied. What is sometimes found is that the technical term (like self-insight) is too general for the phenomenon studied and the study serves to differentiate more than one kind of phenomenon that is usually encompassed by a single technical term.

So the general logic of the initial life-world-evoking question is: 'Have you had this kind of experience, and if so, how did it occur for you and what was it like for you?'

2. Data collection

In descriptive phenomenological research the researcher wishes to sample expressions of life-world experiences relevant to the phenomenon of interest. The question often arises: what is an adequate 'sampling' of experience for the sake of the aims of phenomenological analysis. 'Sampling' within this framework is not about size but about quality. The aim is not to count how many people have had a particular experience or to make quantitative comparisons between different populations of people. Rather, the aim is to understand a phenomenon more deeply through adequate exposure to the qualities of the phenomena that are given by the living of the phenomenon. This phenomenon could be highly unique and specific, like the 'experience of discovering a new uninhabited country' or could be a shared experience such as 'learning and understanding a mathematical formula'. The nature of human experience is such that there are always unique as well as shared features to experience. Even studying one case of an experience can be highly instructive. Sartre (1956), for example, has been skilful in communicating essential features of a particular kind of alienation from one's own body by describing, in one case, the concrete details of a woman who came to regard her own hand as 'a stranger' in an uncomfortable interpersonal situation of physical contact. The essence of this experience could be understood by many readers. But it is helpful to have a number of variations or exemplars of an experience for two reasons, a scientific one and a communicative one. The scientific reason is that the phenomenological researcher may better intuit and see essential structures by finding them in a number of variations of the experience. How many variations are enough for this purpose? There is no technical answer to this as it is not the method that ensures the intuition and understanding of an essence. Rather, it is the quality of the expression of the presence of the phenomenon in combination with the insight of the researcher. The communicative reason for using more than one life-world description is that it provides rich and thick 'material' with which to communicate the sense and logic of the phenomenon to others (Todres 1998, 1999; Halling 2002). So, the researcher may then be able to present his or her findings in the following form: 'this is the essential structure of the phenomenon that can be formulated on the basis of these cases, and here are some indications of how this structure lives for Jane, Mary and Peter in different and unique ways.' Indicating both the essence and some of its variations help to communicate a richer and deeper understanding of that essence within the studied context. The above considerations thus result in the following sampling strategy:

(a) A purposive sampling strategy is designed to gather a depth and richness of the experience. Three good descriptions can be better than twelve poor ones.

(b) A full description is articulated of the context of the participants and their experience. So, for example, if one were studying the experience of receiving bad news, it would be important to understand which respondents received this information by post and which respondents received this in an interpersonal situation. Such differing contexts may define two different kinds of experience rather than one, and this is central to defining the kind of phenomenon one is studying.

(c) Apart from ethical procedures common to other qualitative research projects, the phenomenological researcher is also explicit to the respondents about the nature of phenomenological analysis and that, at a certain stage, the researcher will express his or her own understanding of encountering the different descriptions. The researcher is nevertheless accountable to the respondent to the extent that the original interviews or accounts are accurate and faithful. At the 'understanding and analysis' stage, the researcher is accountable to the broader aims and rigours of phenomenological analysis.

There are particular guidelines for conducting phenomenologically oriented interviews as one variation of sampling life-world experiences (Kvale 1996). In essence, the interview needs to be conducted in a way that clarifies rather than directs, while making sensitive decisions about keeping the interview focused on the phenomenon of the study. It is thus an open-ended interview that begins with the initial life-world-evoking question in all cases and then sensitively and facilitatively follows the descriptions and narratives as they unfold.

As an example of an instruction to elicit a written narrative, Sundstrom in Dahlberg *et al.* (2001) asked nursing students to write one detailed account of a concrete situation in their education when they had felt confirmed, and one account when they had felt excluded rather than confirmed. The narratives that were elicited in this way were able to illuminate these two phenomena in a variety of contexts.

3. Data analysis

Descriptive phenomenological analysis involves a disciplined procedure designed to ensure that the details of experiences intimately contribute to an articulation of a level of generality that is helpful to one's interests. The products of such a level of generality has been called a 'general structure' or 'an essential structure'. The concept of generalization within this framework is different to the idea of generalizability within the context of quantitative research. In phenomenological research, generality refers to expressions of patterns or 'wholes' that coherently make sense of the examples on which they are based. These expressions of patterns are able to conceptually describe and qualitatively organize the 'whatness' of a phenomenon and how its elements inter-relate and function together. Such 'generalities' are insights that may be transferable in useful ways. The general structure may be derived from one person's experience or more than one person's experience. This procedure is usually carried out by an analysis of the texts generated through sampling experiences. If the source were interviews, the interviews are transcribed. The phenomenological researcher then enters the attitude of the phenomenological reduction in order to become as faithfully present to the intrinsic intelligibility of the meaning of the narratives. In the process of understanding, one is present not to words in themselves, but to the meanings given through the words. Such understanding and insight can be aided by steps of procedural discipline that help to focus on the meaningful sense of the text as a whole as well as the details within the text. One is trying to engage with the text in such a way as to achieve descriptive adequacy (Ashworth 2000). This means that there is a 'goodness of fit' between one's general formulations and the specific details of the text and how they interrelate. Different steps have been suggested (Wertz 1983; Fischer 1985; Hycner 1985) but essentially involve one or more of the following ideas described in the next five sub-sections.

LIBRARY
EDUCATION CENTRE
PRINCESS ROYAL HOSPITAL

3.1 Obtaining a sense of each protocol as a whole experience

Each complete protocol is read as many times as necessary in order to understand it as a whole experience. This involves the adoption of an empathic attitude that is attuned to the linguistic content, not merely in itself, but as revelatory of the lived experience that the description intends.

Such a reading is already active in two ways:

1. One immerses oneself in the world of the description by disciplining oneself to become open to such world. Such discipline requires the suspension of one's preconceptions as much as possible. This constitutes the kind of phenomenological reduction that brackets theory and jargon from outside of the phenomenon as explanatory concepts.

2. One, nevertheless, maintains an understanding that the description does not just reveal a world-in-general, but an experience of a specific phenomenon in its context. One tries to 'see the phenomenon there' as this is what the description is about. This sense of the whole then provides an intuitive reference within which the specific details can become intelligible.

3.2 Discrimination of meaning units

This step refines the contextual understanding achieved in the previous step by focusing on discrete changes of meaning within the larger context of each individual protocol.

Each protocol is re-read noticing and marking each time a change of meaning occurs with reference to the phenomenon studied. This is a way to ensure that one is accounting for all relevant nuances and details in one's further analysis, and that one will spend some time to consider all meanings when moving to a greater degree of generalization later.

At this stage the protocol is left intact: both the order of the units as well as the language of the respondent remain the same; the meaning units are marked or perhaps numbered for further consideration.

3.3 Formulation of transformed meaning units

Here the respondent's everyday expressions and language are transformed into expressions of meaning for the phenomenon of study that carry more general and transferable insights. Each meaning unit is read by the phenomenological researcher with the following questions in mind: 'Within the total context of this protocol, what does this change of meaning tell me about the experience of the phenomenon in a more general way? How can I express this specific quality in such a way that it does justice to the concrete situation, yet indicates its more general meanings?' Here the researcher may go beyond the language used by the respondent to formulate the sense and meaning of the particular expression for what it can tell us further about the phenomenon under study. For example, in a study of the experience of the transition to motherhood, Hartley (personal communication), considered a number of examples where 'planning' entered life in a much more insistent way.

Here is an example of an actual detail from the description of a respondent:

Normally if I wanted to go anywhere I'd get up, get dressed and go out whereas now it's get up, get 'A' fed, bathed, get the car-seat out, get his change bag out, check his nappy, then by the time you've done all that you think, I'll just change his nappy one more time before we go out. Then you've got to sort of get him down to the car, it's just a lot of hassle as opposed to literally getting up, getting yourself ready and going out.

There are particular qualities to this experience that can be named in a more general and transferable way, and were expressed as follows:

Prior to motherhood, going out was a spontaneous activity involving minimal preparation. However, with a baby to organize, outings have to be planned in advance and the logistics are time-consuming and complicated.

3.4 Formulation of essential general structure or structures

This step involves a synthesis of transformed meaning units into a consistent statement of the invariant themes that run through the different experiences and concrete occasions. The aim is to establish what is typical of the phenomenon and to express such typicality in an insightful and integrated manner. Phenomenological researchers use their intuition of the whole sense of the different accounts of the experiences as well as the transformed insights contained in the discrete meaning units to articulate a formulation that synthesizes the typical themes that arise from the life-world descriptions. How do we express such typicality? Such phenomenological sensitivity is complex but draws on capacities we all use when we try to put experience into language in a communicative way. In this pursuit there is both a scientific concern and a communicative concern. The scientific concern is to achieve descriptive adequacy (Ashworth 2000), that is, to arrive at a linguistic synthesis which can account for the specific meaning units. This process usually means that the researcher has gone back and forth between the emerging formulation of the general structure of the phenomenon-as-a-whole and the individual experiences (parts) to see how the formulations better make sense of the parts, and to see whether the emerging formulation may need to be refined in some way in order to better account for some part. The communicative concern is to find ways of expressing the general structure in a narrative form that facilitates understanding in readers. The phenomenological researcher has by now achieved his or her own digested understanding of the essential structure of the phenomenon. He or she has gone through quite a long and complex process to achieve this. The communicative task is then to express this understanding in a narratively accessible form. Guidance for addressing both the scientific and communicative concerns can be taken from Reed (1987: 102):

... to describe the structure is to describe how the elements of a phenomenon function constitutively, how they interrelate to form the unity of the experience.

Although a single coherent phenomenon often emerges in this phase, it is possible that more than one coherent phenomenon emerges. The researcher does not force this, and one of the values of such discovery-oriented research is that more than one type and kind of phenomenon may be discovered.

3.5 Indicating the value of the essential structure/s for understanding the variations of lived experience

In this step one goes back to the respondents' initial experiences to see how their various specific experiences are understood in the light of the constituents of the general structure. The general structure is made up of constituent parts that relate to one another in a coherent way. For example, in a study on a patient's experience of going through intensive care in hospital (Todres *et al.* 2000) the general structure was made up of a number of phases such as 'entering a twilight world', 'the frightening nature of breathing problems', and 'ambivalent feelings during the weaning process'. Each of these constituents can be 'fleshed out' with reference to different quotations from the patients' narrative. This not only serves the communicative concern to demonstrate how the structure lives in people's lives, but also shows the kinds of variations that can empirically occur within a structure. A structure gives a coherent range of possibilities, but is open enough to allow empirical variations within those possibilities. Thus for one person going through intensive care, 'entering a twilight world' may be welcome whereas for another, it may be fought against. The 'results' of essential structures thus have the character of possibilities that make sense of unique variations. It is this indication of both commonality and uniqueness that is crucial to a human science approach that wishes to avoid both deterministic lawfulness on the one hand, and relativistic solipsism on the other.

Like other forms of qualitative research the findings of the study are finally considered in dialogue with the literature and current research in order to offer critique, possible applications, and further directions for research.

Critique and evaluation of the approach

The value of a descriptive phenomenological approach may be summarized as follows:

- It is based on an epistemological position that can be examined with reference to a long history of philosophical debate. This philosophical framework offers a way to differentiate between the goals and methods of natural science and the goals and methods of human science. As such, a phenomenologically based human science focuses on meaning rather than measurement and articulates the rationale and method relevant to such a concern (Giorgi 1970).

- Although it acknowledges that no method can take the place of insight with regard to qualitative matters, it offers methodological guidelines and procedural steps of discipline that can aid phenomenological presence and the articulation of meaning.

- By wishing to study experience on its own terms without reduction to 'outside' perspectives and theories, it tries to find a language that cares for the human order. This is a language that is full of human participation and one that allows human beings to intuitively share in the phenomenon described; a language that finds the 'I in the thou'.

- It champions the value of the human individual as a starting point in human science. This includes a return to concrete experiences and the attempt to address the balance between articulating unique variations of experience with the 'ground' that we share. The approach moves from the particular to the general, attempting to honour both levels of understanding and their complementarity.

- It remembers the freedom of the unique human occasion by expressing essences and themes, not as final and conclusive law-like absolutes, but rather as possibilities about which unique variations and actualities can occur. Truth in this perspective is thus an ongoing conversation which is not arbitrary but which is never finished and depends on questions and context.

Criticism of descriptive phenomenology as a qualitative research approach may be summarized as follows:

- On epistemological grounds. Relativists would argue that looking for order in experience and between experiences is arbitrary. The most one can do is offer multiple perspectives from multiple positions and contexts and sometimes argue for the relative benefits of some position over another. Objectivists on the other hand would argue that discovering order in experience needs recourse for validity to measures outside of experience such as brain states or behavioural observation. Valid intelligibility cannot be asserted with reference to qualitative meanings for actors: some form of objective measurement is needed in order to make valid assertions that are empirically general and gives scholars a sense of statistically informed confidence.

- On methodological grounds. Some critics have argued that phenomenological philosophy loses its essential character when translated into a qualitative research method (Hoeller 1982/1983; Crotty 1996; Paley 1997). On the other side of this debate, respondents (Giorgi 2000; Davidson and Cosgrove 2002) reply with some variation of the argument that Husserl's philosophical project changed over time and that its insights can be fruitfully used in modified form for qualitative research with productive results.

- Another criticism on methodological grounds occurs in a more specific debate, those phenomenologists informed by Husserl (descriptive phenomenology), and those informed by Heidegger and Gadamer (hermeneutic phenomenology). The extreme form of the criticism by hermeneutic phe-nomenologists is that there is no such thing as description of meaning; it is all interpretation. This philosophical debate is far from settled. Giorgi's (1997) position is that both description and interpretation in human science are legitimate endeavours and that researchers should be clear about such dif-ferences in emphasis and approach.

Claims and limitations

It may be important to understand the claims and limitations of descriptive phe-nomenology as a research approach based on its epistemology. It does not claim to answer questions of measurement or to define phenomena in ways that can be quantitatively measurable. It does not even claim a subtle variation of this, such as 'counting meanings' as indications of their prevalence, importance or power. The limitation of descriptive phenomenology is bound by its concern to study experiential qualities on their own terms. Its 'findings' are experientially intelligible insights about the life-world that are transferable as ways of seeing other life-world experiences of similar type, or even as ways of understanding different life-world phenomena in relation to the phenomenon studied. Its findings are not necessarily final ways or best ways of articulating these insights. The validity of such insights is in their ability to facilitate better or deeper understanding of the phenomenon for readers. Whether this is the same phenomenon studied as that of another study is always to be examined as an open question, and the transferability of insights is always a reflectively critical process. Lawfulness and closure are seldom achieved in studies of the human realm. In science it is possible to have many new 'facts' with very little understanding. In the study of the intelligibility of human experi-ence, the goal is to approach further coherence of understanding about life-world phenomena and this may be evaluated by different audiences in terms of whether it takes understanding forward in meaningful ways. In this regard, phenomenological findings have found to be enlightening for audiences beyond the academic and professional arenas such as informed lay-people who may have a particular interest in the phenomenon studied.

Given these comments about the claims and limitations of descriptive phe-nomenology, a few things may be said about its differences and possible overlaps with other qualitative approaches (these are explored in greater detail in Chapter 6).

Implications for professional practice

In common with other approaches to qualitative research, descriptive phenom-enology is becoming increasingly relevant to a health- and social-care arena that has highlighted the importance of understanding the experiences, stories and 'journeys' of patients and users of services (Heyman 1995; Bray et al. 2000; Rose 2001).

An indication that a life-world methodology is entering mainstream health- and social-care services is evidenced by the United Kingdom's National Health

Service Modernization Agency, which is adopting a methodology of 'discovery interviews' where detailed guidance is given to health- and social-care practitioners of how to elicit experiential descriptions from users in order that services may be improved (Wilcock *et al.* 2003).

This approach is consistent with both the philosophy and data collection phase of descriptive phenomenology, and elicits concrete descriptions of patients' experiences that are far richer than just expressions of attitudes and opinions. The value of such life-world descriptions is that they provide sources of information that may have been unanticipated by both the respondent and researcher. It does not depend on the ability of the respondent to come up with already formulated views or well-articulated generalizations. It provides descriptions of the lived experience on which the views may be based, and as such, provides important references for what the views *mean* in specific terms, and how the experience was lived. The most interesting, surprising and useful insights are often in the detail. Respondents have said that such an approach makes them feel more 'heard' than if they were required to come up with ready-made answers and conclusions. The concerns that arise are often more nuanced and help to form transferable meanings that are more novel and helpful than the reification of an already formulated opinion. So, for example, one respondent may have expressed the view that the doctor did not tell her the truth. We could imagine this theme becoming a reified category and find a number of cases in which the doctor 'did not tell the truth'. But, what is the experience that this view refers to? This is a life-world question. And we may find that when the respondent describes the situation, we begin to understand what 'not telling the truth' means. We may find, for example, that a story emerges of confusions and missed opportunities in very specific places rather than a simple 'not telling the truth'. Such detailed descriptions then have the benefit of informing insightful and nuanced directions such as 'confusion of the patient occurred most when provided with a report of a special investigation which came out as normal'. How to deal with the communication of the complexity of special investigations then becomes a much more 'lively' and informative issue than the earlier reified view.

In this way, studies using a descriptive phenomenological approach may 'humanize' health- and social-care, not just by representing the 'voices' and views of patients, users and professionals, but by accessing descriptions of experiences that carry the intelligible meanings and textures of what it is like to be there.

Illustration: an example of one way of presenting an essential structure

Phenomenon: the kind of therapeutic self-insight that carries a greater sense of freedom

In this chapter I have already referred to my own research on the 'kind of therapeutic self-insight that carries a greater sense of freedom'. This research was used as an illustration in the sections on 'finding a phenomenon of interest', 'formulating a research question', and in the data collection phase of 'formulating transformed meaning units'.

In this section I wish to provide an example of formulating and expressing an 'essential general structure' with reference to this research. The manner of doing this depends partly on the purpose of one's presentation, the nature of one's audience, and the kind of questions one is trying to address. In this particular example I am paying attention to narrative coherence. That is, I wish to show how the various meanings and phases of the phenomenon interact and make sense as a structure that is faithful to the cases I studied. If one is to adequately communicate such narrative coherence, the presentation of the essential structure may need to be quite lengthy, as the sequence, meanings, interrelationships and complexities of the phenomena are laid out. I thus present most of my findings without summary as I have previously expressed them (Todres 2002b). In this presentation, I combine aspects of the final two phases of data analysis, that is, I formulate an essential general structure and combine this in places with an elaboration that refers to particular individual experiences and variations of the structure.

The study resulted in an essential structure that included the following constituents:

(a) the enabling factors of the therapeutic situation and the person of the therapist;
(b) the quality and nature of the kind of therapeutic self-insight that leads to a greater sense of freedom;
(c) the kind of freedom that occurs.

Context of study

Ten people (six men and four women) who had been in psychotherapy for a minimum of four months were asked to describe a situation in psychotherapy in which they saw or understood something which carried with it a greater sense of freedom. All respondents had been in an open-ended conversational therapy with therapists who would describe their practice as being broadly informed by one of the following orientations: psychodynamic, analytic, integrative, phenomeno-logical or existential. The respondents did not necessarily know the orientation of their therapist. For the purpose of this chapter, all identifying features of the participants have been changed.

Enabling factors of the therapeutic situation and the person of the therapist

The first thing that the analysis revealed concerned the enabling situation of psychotherapy.

A structured freedom

Both the therapist and the situation provide a kind of human space that has an ambiguous quality. This ambiguity expresses how there are certain dimensions of the situation that provide clear structures and other dimensions that emphasize a lack of structure. The ambiguity of such a situation articulates a certain 'shape' to psychotherapy, one that is expressed in the phrase 'a structured freedom'.

On the one hand a sense of structure is constituted by experiences of continuity of time, place and person, a growing sense of familiarity with the focus on the client's life, a growing sense of comfort and safety to explore within this context. Such a safe structure is a shape that does not emerge complete, all at once, but one which is realized and tested for over time.

Sometimes an informant would speak more about how the person of the therapist provided the sense of a safe structure and shape. Other informants would speak more of how the situation of therapy, the room and the timing were important in facilitating this sense of safe structure. But in all this, a certain experience of familiarity and continuity were important – a settling down, a gathering together, an interpersonal 'home-coming'.

On the other hand, there was a certain freedom, a lack of structure, in the happenings within the session and the interpersonal space of client and therapist.

This freedom essentially involved an unknown dimension: neither client nor therapist knew much in advance about the direction that the specific content of the conversation would take. No matter how theoretically sophisticated the therapist was or how much the client rehearsed in advance what would be talked about, both came to accept that surprising directions were always possible. For some clients this was scary, for others, this was exciting, and usually clients had both these experiences at different times in response to the open freedom of the potential content of the sessions.

The second thing that the analysis revealed was about the quality and nature of the therapeutic self-insight that occurs.

The quality and nature of this kind of therapeutic self-insight

We now move on to the nature of the kind of therapeutic self-insight that carries a greater sense of freedom. What is the nature of this phenomenon that has been enabled by the structured freedom given by the situation and person of the therapist? There are a number of dimensions and sub-components of this phenomenon:

1. *It is not the self-insight on its own that has power: rather it is its 'before' and 'after', the entire narrative that is understood and experienced, that has freeing power*

   Firstly, although there were often particular self-insights that were important, their credibility were only meaningful because of the personal narrative that had been forged as their context. Here are some examples of specific self-insights that occurred:

   • I have been living as if I always expect to be rejected.

   • There were some important and valid reasons why I needed to hide and protect myself which often no longer apply.

   • Although trying to be like my sister has been restrictive for me, it has given me a sense of security.

   • If I am more assertive towards women, I am afraid that I will lose the relationship.

These were important moments of self-insight, but they were only given freeing power by the narrative that came both before and after these moments. It appears that it is the whole quality of the meaningful personal narrative that is crucial to the value of the therapeutic self-insight. This becomes clearer as we consider the qualities of the narratives that came 'before' and 'after'.

2. *A meaningful personal narrative is a linguistic and emotional work of under-standing patterns and linkages over time: particular self-insights imply the work of 'patterning' that has preceded it, and the implied directions that can come after it*

Over time, descriptions of personal behaviours, feelings, and interactions are seen in a way that form a pattern. For example, for Mary, the theme of wanting to be a 'good girl' first became vividly articulated in terms of the therapist–client relationship. She became aware that she was trying very hard to 'produce the goods' in therapy in order to please her therapist. She then became aware of this theme occurring in other interpersonal situations as well. She also began to remember situations that took place earlier in her life, particularly with her mother, where this was an important concern. This personal narrative of pattern-making/discovery is linguistic and emotional work which links parts into wholes. It both feels and sees this relationship. As such the client is both a participant as well as an observer and develops a rhythm of closeness and distance to her own experience in which seeing patterns gives distance, whereas the experiencing of details gives closeness and emotional authenticity. The insightful quality of this pattern discovery/creation is in its 'sense-making', and such 'sense-making' is emotionally healing in a number of ways. This becomes clearer as we consider the emotional impli-cations of such a 'sense-making' narrative activity.

3. *There is an emotional healing to 'sense-making'*

There were three interrelated ways in which the narrative linguistic work was emotionally healing:

(a) **The felt credibility of 'sense-making'**
   The 'sense-making' process of the personal narrative in which part and whole, or particular events and their themes, come together, produces a sense of felt credibility and personal truth. This is not just a freely im-aginative process – it is much more rigorous than that if the sense of felt credibility is going to occur. It is as if there are certain intuitive standards and questions in the process for the client: 'is this theme supported by the details of my life? Does this way of saying things, say it better than an alternative phrase or word?' There appears to be an aesthetic quality that satisfies a client emotionally when words fit experiences. For example, when a therapist used the phrase: 'you seem to be saying that you want to develop further in this way', the client paused and said: 'not so much *develop* but rather *moving on*'.
   This is a kind of 'sense-making' that is credible to the client. And here we

move to two related qualities of therapeutic self-insight that brings past, present and future into a workable relationship.

(b) *Self-forgiveness*

In the personal narratives that were forged, there was usually an understanding in which repetitive patterns were seen as understandable within a human story.

Thus early on in Bill's therapy he saw himself in a judgemental way as 'pathetic' and 'weak' about his lack of assertiveness. As the narrative evolved, he found credible details about his present and past interactions in which his lack of assertion took on a more complex meaning. He saw how he was afraid of being more powerful in a number of present interactions and also remembered how, as a boy, he wanted to show his little sister that he was not scary like their abusive father – he remembers how much he wanted to protect her. His protective wishes towards others could be seen not just as a weakness but as a strength and even an admirable quality. So the emerging narrative recovers a more complex, human story and this can constitute a sense of self-forgiveness about being the way one is. This does not necessarily condone one's behaviour, but at least makes one less worthy of simple rejection. The healing factor of such self-forgiveness or self-accepting-understanding is that it empowers the kind of self-care that is needed to 'unhook' one from premature, conclusive self-definitions and judgements. And here we come to hope.

(c) *Hope*

This dimension involves a component of self-insight in which:

- A present restrictive, repetitive pattern that has been articulated, is seen as *not inevitable.*
- Also, the client sees more about where *personal agency* is possible and where it is not. As such, the client sees a different path forward from a mere repetition of the pattern and this constitutes an experience of *hope.*

Here is an illustration of these components taken from the study:

Jane came into therapy because she felt that her anger could destroy people she cared about. In therapy, a narrative emerged in which she came to realize that a pervasive angry attitude towards her ex-husband obscured a 'huge grief' about what had happened to her and her children. As the narrative progressed, a de-centring of her anger as a central determinant of her existence occurred and was expressed by her in the following way: 'Behind the walls is not an overwhelming anger that is going to make me kill someone.' This was a great relief and a 'hope' that she needed. The sense of increased personal agency came with a dream that made her realize that significant relationships do not have to end painfully or threateningly. This helped her to feel that she could tolerate her youngest child leaving home. Subsequently their relationship improved. The healing factor of such increased personal agency is that it recovers the sense in which one is not merely a victim of circumstance and that the future does not have to be determined by the past.

All in all, the quality and nature of this kind of therapeutic self-insight describes a 'sense-making' personal narrative with moments of liberating self-insight that are credible and that 'unfreezes' personal time so that one can move into the future in a more active and hopeful way. Going one step beyond this, however, all this is able to tell us something more essential about the kind of freedom that occurs.

4   *The sense of freedom that occurs is essentially an experience of 'being more than...'*

Here, the question that is addressed is: What is the essential nature of the kind of *freedom* that occurs in a self-insightful narrative process?

Now we move to a more philosophical level of phenomenological analysis, one which was approached in the transcendental phenomenological tradition. Here I am interested in the phenomenology of freedom. Such a question focuses on the implicit preconditions that underlie the kind of freedoms expressed by the informants. Within this task, the essential meaning that I intuited from the whole structure of the experience was that the phenomenology of this kind of freedom is revealed by articulating the phenomenology of experiencing personal identity as 'being more than'. What is *in* this experience of *being more than*?

- Being more than what I had previously thought and felt.
- Being more than what I had said up till now.
- Being more than any premature judgement of myself – good or bad.
- Being more than any 'thing' or self-enclosed entity that reacts to forces and causes.

Conclusion

At the end of this analysis, I was prompted to say that therapeutic self-insight is not the fundamental point of psychotherapy: it is more a means to an end, and points to an experience of 'more'. It is this experience of 'being more than' or of 'being as possibility' that is the essential power of psychotherapy (Todres 2002a, 2002b).

References

Aanstoos, C.M. (1985) The structure of thinking in chess. In Giorgi, A. (ed.) *Phenomenology and Psychological Research*. Pittsburgh, PA: Duquesne University Press, 86–117.

Ashworth, P. (2000) The descriptive adequacy of qualitative findings, *The Humanistic Psychologist*, 28, 1–3: 138–152.

Bray, J.N., Lee, J., Smith, L.L. and Yorks, L. (2000) *Collaborative Inquiry in Practice: Action, Reflection and Meaning Making*. Thousand Oaks: Sage.

Churchill, S.D. and Wertz, F.J. (2001) An introduction to phenomenological research in psychology. In Schneider, K.J., Bugental, F.T. and Pierson, J.F. (eds) *The Handbook of*

Humanistic Psychology: Leading Edges in Theory, Research and Practice. London: Sage, 231–262.

Crotty, M. (1996) *Phenomenology and Nursing Research.* Melbourne: Churchill Livingstone.

Dahlberg, K., Drew, N. and Nystrom, M. (2001) *Reflective Lifeworld Research.* Lund, Sweden: Studentlitteratur.

Davidson, L. and Cosgrove, L. (2002) Psychologism and Phenomenological Psychology Revisited, Part II: The Return to Positivity, *Journal of Phenomenological Psychology*, 33 (2): 141–177.

Fischer, C.T. (1998) 'Being angry revealed as self-deceptive protest: an empirical phenomenological analysis'. In Valle, R. (ed.) *Phenomenological Inquiry in Psychology: Existential and Transpersonal Dimensions.* New York: Plenum Press, 111–122.

Fischer, C.T. and Wertz, F.J. (1979) Empirical phenomenological analysis of being criminally victimized. In Giorgi, A., Smith, D. and Knowles, R. (eds) *Duquesne Studies in Phenomenological Psychology*, Vol. 3. Pittsburgh, PA: Duquesne University Press, 135–158.

Fischer, W.F. (1982) An empirical–phenomenological approach to the psychology of anxiety. In de Koning, A.J.J. and Jenner, F.A. (eds) *Phenomenology and Psychiatry.* London: Academic Press, 63–84.

Fischer, W.F. (1985) Self-deception: an existential–phenomenological investigation into its essential meanings. In Giorgi, A. (ed.) *Phenomenology and Psychological Research.* Pittsburgh, PA: Duquesne University Press, 118–154.

Fow, N.R. (1996) The phenomenology of forgiveness and reconciliation, *Journal of Phenomenological Psychology*, 27 (2): 219–233.

Garfinkel, H. (1967) *Studies in Ethnomethodology.* Englewood Cliffs: Prentice Hall.

Giorgi, A. (1970) *Psychology as a Human Science: A Phenomenologically Based Approach.* New York: Harper and Row.

Giorgi, A. (1975) An application of phenomenological method in psychology. In Giorgi, A., Fischer, C. and Murray, E. (eds) *Duquesne Studies in Phenomenological Psychology*, Vol. 2. Pittsburgh, PA: Duquesne University Press, 82–103.

Giorgi, A. (1985) *Phenomenology and Psychological Research*, Vol. 2. Pittsburgh, PA: Duquesne University Press, 82–103.

Giorgi, A. (1997) The theory, practice and evaluation of the phenomenological method as a qualitative research procedure, *Journal of Phenomenological Psychology*, 28 (2): 235–260.

Giorgi, A. (2000) The status of Husserlian phenomenology in caring research, *Scandinavian Journal of Caring Science*, 14: 3–10.

Giorgi, A. and Giorgi, B. (2003a) Phenomenology. In Smith, J.A. (ed.) *Qualitative Psychology: A Practical Guide to Research Methods.* London: Sage, 25–50.

Giorgi, A. and Giorgi, B. (2003b) The descriptive phenomenological psychological method. In Camic, P.M., Rhodes, J.E. and Yardley, L. (eds) *Qualitative Research in Psychology: Expanding Perspectives in Methodology & Design.* Washington, DC: American Psychological Association, 243–273.

Halling, S. (2002) Making phenomenology accessible to a wider audience, *Journal of Phenomenological Psychology*, 33 (1): 19–38.

Hartley, J., Todres, L. and Alexander, J. (2002) The Journey to Motherhood: a phenomenological approach to understanding how women experience becoming mothers. Unpublished Conference Paper: *Qualitative Research Conference*, September 2002, Bournemouth.

Heyman, B. (1995) *Researching User Perspectives on Community Health Care.* London: Chapman and Hall.

Hoeller, K. (1982/1983) Phenomenology, Psychology and Science: II, *Review of Existential Psychology and Psychiatry*, 18 (1–3): 143–154.

Hycner, R.H. (1985) Some guidelines for the phenomenological analysis of interview data, *Human Studies*, 8: 279–303.

Kockelmans, J.J. (ed.) (1967) *Phenomenology: The Philosophy of Edmund Husserl and its Interpretation*. New York: Doubleday and Co.

Kvale, S. (1996) *InterViews: An Introduction to Qualitative Research Interviewing*. London: Sage.

Merleau-Ponty, M. (1962) *The Phenomenology of Perception*. Trans.: Smith, C. London: Routledge and Kegan Paul.

Merleau-Ponty, M. (1963) *The Structure of Behaviour*. Trans.: Fischer, A. Boston: Beacon.

Moustakas, C. (1994) *Phenomenological Research Methods*. London: Sage.

Paley, J. (1997) Husserl, phenomenology and nursing, *Journal of Advanced Nursing*, 26: 187–193.

Polkinghorne, D.E. (1989) Phenomenological research methods. In Valle, R.S. and Halling, S. (eds) *Existential Phenomenological Perspectives in Psychology*. New York: Plenum Press, 41–60.

Reed, D.L. (1987) An empirical phenomenological approach to dream research. In Van Zuuren, F., Wertz, F.J. and Mook, B. (eds) *Advances in Qualitative Psychology*. Swets, North America: Berwyn, 101–113.

Rose, D. (2001) *Users' Voices: The Perspectives of Health Service Users*. London: The Sainsbury Centre for Mental Health.

Sartre, J.P. (1956) *Being and Nothingness*. Trans.: Barnes, H. New York: Philosophical Library.

Schutz, A. (1972) *The Phenomenology of the Social World*. Trans.: Walsh, G. and Lehnert, F. London: Heinemann.

Spiegelberg, H. (1994) *The Phenomenological Movement: A Historical Introduction*, 3rd and rev. edn. Dordrecht: Kluwer Academic Publishers.

Todres, L. (1998) The qualitative description of human experience: the aesthetic dimension, *Qualitative Health Research*, 8 (1): 121–127.

Todres, L. (1999) The bodily complexity of truth-telling in qualitative research: some implication of Gendlin's philosophy, *Humanistic Psychologist*, 23 (3): 283–300.

Todres, L. (2000) Writing phenomenological–psychological descriptions: an illustration attempting to balance texture and structure, *Auto/Biography*, 3: 1 and 2: 41–48.

Todres, L. (2002a) Globalisation and the Complexity of Self: the relevance of psychotherapy, *Existential Analysis*, 13(1): 98–105.

Todres, L. (2002b) Humanising forces: phenomenology in science; psychotherapy in technological culture, *Indo-Pacific Journal of Phenomenology*, 3: 1–16.

Todres, L., Fulbrook, P. and Albarrran, J. (2000) On the receiving end: a hermeneutic–phenomenological analysis of a patient's struggle to cope while going through intensive care, *Nursing in Critical Care*, 5 (6): 277–287.

Von Eckartsberg, R. (1998) Existential–phenomenological research. In Valle, R. (ed.) *Phenomenological Inquiry in Psychology: Existential and Transpersonal Dimensions*. New York: Plenum Press, 21–61.

Wertz, F.J. (1983) From everyday to psychological description: analyzing the moments of a qualitative data analysis. *Journal of Phenomenological Psychology*, 14 (2): 197–241.

Wilcock, P.M., Brown, G.C.S., Bateson, J., Carver, J. and Machin, S. (2003) Using patient stories to inspire quality improvement within the modernisation agency collaborative programmes, *Journal of Clinical Nursing*, 12: 1–9.

8

FRANCES RAPPORT
Hermeneutic phenomenology: the science of interpretation of texts

Introduction

Interpretive phenomenology, hermeneutic phenomenology or 'hermeneutics', as it is more commonly known, is the science of interpretation of texts, whereby language, in its written or spoken form, is scrutinized to reveal meaning in phenomena. The hermeneutic phenomenologist emphasizes the 'ordinary language' of everyday experience, the words we use on a day-to-day basis, to describe and explain cultural mores, behaviours, events and actions and the relationship between 'ordinary language' and daily social life. Hermeneutic phenomenologists strive to understand the nature of human beings and the meanings they bestow upon the world by examining language in its cultural context; the way language is given meaning and is interpreted. By attempting to clarify meaning and offer plausible explanations for human experience, the hermeneutic phenomenologist illuminates what it is to be human in the 'life-world' – the world as we immediately experience it – in order to offer a deeper meaning to experience (van Manen 1990).

Underlying philosophical and historical developments

To clarify the main features of hermeneutic phenomenology in its methodological form, this chapter begins by placing hermeneutics in the context of a phenomenological history.

In the eighteenth century, phenomenology was first practised as the examination of religious texts. Explorations of understanding (*Verstehen*) restricted to 'religious exegesis' (Mueller-Vollmer 1986) were extended to include broader linguistic understanding through the writings of Droysen and Dilthey, Simmel, Weber, and later by Garfinkel and other ethnomethodologists (Outhwaite 1987; Thompson 1987). In the nineteenth century Dilthey's work was particularly influential, emphasizing the need to see text as just one element of understanding within the broader framework of historical knowledge. Dilthey viewed historical knowledge as an interrelationship between experience, expression and understanding (Thompson 1987), arguing that it was the human spirit that drove human studies, and that all experience was contextualized in terms of past and future possibilities.

Husserl, Heidegger and interpretive phenomenology

Edmund Husserl (1859–1938) is considered the founding father of phenomenology. Starting his career as a mathematician under Franz Brentano, he gained a reputation as a post-Cartesian philosopher, abandoning plans to teach mathematics and science, to dedicate his life to a thesis of 'transcendental' or 'Husserlian' phenomenology (Laverty 2003). Husserl concentrated on the subject–object divide and in defiance of Cartesian thought, which suggested that mind and body were distinct substances with determinate essences (MacDonald 2001), described the relationship between subject and object as inextricably linked through conscious knowing. Objects were considered to be 'objects of consciousness for us' (Dreyfus 1987: 254), understood through their range of forms using transcendental phenomenological processes such as 'intuition' and 'free imaginative variation' (Husserl 1931). Husserl argued that by suspending or rendering non-influential the outer world, it was possible to clarify how objects appear to consciousness. In order to do this, Husserl recommended putting reality on hold, 'bracketing out' all extraneous thoughts using 'the phenomenological reduction', or *epoché* as it is also known. Husserl argued that all objects could be described exactly as 'intuited'. However, his exploration extended well beyond an understanding of the relationship between consciousness and 'real objects' such as tables and chairs, to a plethora of objects or 'phenomena of experience' such as feelings, concepts, dreams, hallucinations, emotions, sensations, fantasies, referential objects and thoughts. Indeed, anything that presented itself to consciousness and that could be 'intuited' phenomenologically became an object of consciousness and the basis for Husserl's 'science of consciousness' (Husserl 1931). Here the boundaries of understanding could be extended to encompass a complete, existential contemplation of the world.

Husserl's ideas had a profound effect on his protégé, Martin Heidegger (1889–1976), who at the University of Freiburg, moved from studying theology to studying phenomenological philosophy under Husserl's guidance (Laverty 2003). Once established to succeed Husserl's professorship, Heidegger reacted against Husserl's ideas of intimate subject–object relationships and concentrated on modes of being. Heidegger wrote his famous book *Being and Time* in 1927 (Heidegger 1927/1962) to stimulate a movement away from transcendental phenomenology towards a more interpretive approach to understanding.

Heidegger's writing had a profound effect on continental European thought, especially the existential philosophers such as Jean-Paul Sartre, who wrote *Being and Nothingness* (Sartre 1992) in deference to his work.

Heidegger questioned the ability of transcendental phenomenology to elucidate objects of consciousness for us. He described human experience as 'already within the world', saying that we relate to the world in integral ways, not as subjects related to objects, but as beings inseparable from a world of being. We live in and among the world as an essential part of our own reality (Heidegger 1927/1962). As Todres comments, 'the body has experiential access and is always already there as part of our everyday lives' (Todres 2004: 14). We know the world, not as 'the pure ego and pure consciousness', but in ways '*a priori* to conscious knowing' (Walsh 1996: 232). Heidegger described this situation as 'Being-in-the-world', the fundamental ontology – the meaning of being in general and the ground upon which the human sciences could be constructed (Heidegger 1927/1962).

In order to explore 'Being-in-the-world' in more detail, let us consider the example of hanging a painting on a wall. To hang a painting we must first hammer a nail into the wall. We may, however, be unaware that we are hammering until such time as our activity changes, a break in our concentration, for example, would enable us to consider the action and its range of outcomes. Yet, while hammering, we work automatically, 'beyond conscious knowing'. The action does not need to enter consciousness to be successfully completed and though the experience may be interpreted in a number of ways, for Heidegger this was evidence of a world in which experience and history are shared. We 'know' the world and our everyday practices within it intimately, and knowing gives meaning to our 'existent state'. We make sense of experience through our existence within the world and by sharing knowledge and history with others, we confirm our being. According to Dreyfus, this is what Heidegger meant when he said '*Dasein* is its world existingly'. *Dasein*, which in translation means 'being there', conveys the idea that our activity is one of 'being the situation in which coping can go on and things can be encountered' (Dreyfus 1987: 263).

Unlike his predecessor Husserl, Heidegger concentrated on understanding and our interpretation of phenomena, believing that it was through language and speech that our 'Being-in-the-world' was both manifest and understood. Researchers following a Heideggerian tradition emphasize the interpretive approach to understanding phenomena. They attempt to develop notions of the way human beings give meaning to experience, behaviour and action, while making sense of the world through understanding and the clarification of speech and language.

In his latter work Heidegger moved on from *Dasein* to explore our place in historical thinking, but it is for his work on *Dasein* that he will best be remembered.

Hans Georg Gadamer and hermeneutic phenomenology

Before considering the impact of Hans Georg Gadamer's writing on the hierarchy of phenomenological history, it might be worth re-iterating the major differences between Husserl and Heidegger. Husserl emphasized that we as 'subjects' know 'objects' through a state of pure consciousness. He questioned the possibility that objects can have a separate existence from us and recommended we use the 'phenomenological reduction' to explore the way in which objects are 'intuited'. Heidegger argued that we are always already in the world and that our experience or our 'knowing', is '*a priori* to conscious knowing' (Heidegger 1927/1962; Husserl 1931).

Hans Georg Gadamer (1900–2002) was deeply influenced by the works of

both Husserl and Heidegger and as Heidegger's pupil, 'moved to extend Heidegger's work into practical application' (Laverty 2003: 9). Gadamer developed
interpretive phenomenological thought into a philosophy of Gadamerian hermeneutics. Considered as one of the most critical thinkers of the twentieth century, he
concentrated on how language reveals *being*, building on the idea that all understanding is phenomenological and that understanding can only come about
through language. For Gadamer, language, understanding and interpretation were
inextricably linked.

Following in the tradition of his mentor, Gadamer questioned the meaning of
being by selecting specific aspects of Heidegger's phenomenology to utilize within
his own philosophical writings, namely: *historicity* and *language and its ontological
connections* (Heckman 1986) (see Table 8.1 on page 131 for key terminology).
According to Honey (1987: 75), Gadamer was thus able to identify that:

> It is language that preserves, transmits, and carries tradition along. Language
> is not only an object in our hands, it is the reservoir of tradition and the
> medium in and through which we exist and perceive our world. One's
> belonging to a tradition is only uncovered through the interpretation of signs,
> words and texts that embody cultural heritage.

The main features and key terms of hermeneutic phenomenology

Art aesthetic as a kind of play

Although Gadamer saw understanding as phenomenological in nature, he was
concerned that the human sciences were evolving within the natural science tradition with its emphasis on the discovery of general laws, rather than the
uniqueness of phenomena (Gadamer 1975/1996). In order for the human sciences
to rediscover their humanist culture, Gadamer proposed an analysis of the aesthetic experience of art, to reveal the limitations of the natural science's concept of
'truth'. Understanding the art aesthetic is an experience of self-understanding in
relation to something else that is already understood. It removes us from our life
context to a context that embodies the whole of existence (Heckman 1986).
Gadamer described the art aesthetic as a kind of play (Gadamer 1975/1996), with
him as a player absorbed in neither a subjective nor objective way in the game.
Objectivity for both Heidegger and Gadamer was anathema, suggesting the
individual, as a self-conscious being with a superior position on 'truth' (Weinsheimer 1991). Subjectivity was also unacceptable, with its emphasis on the individual over and above the phenomenon. Instead, the notion of play dispelled the
subject–object divide through its suggestion of constant movement – movement
between player and ball, movement between player and game. In the notion of
movement neither player nor that which is played with has the upper hand; they
are in constant flux. This state can be found in the words we chose to depict
movement such as: 'play of the breeze, play of colours' (Walsh 1996: 236) and
even 'play on words'.

Language and its ontological connections

'We possess the world through language', said Anderson *et al.* (Anderson *et al.* 1986: 74), in response to Gadamer's suggestion that language is the precondition for understanding. But language does two things. Not only does it transpose concepts into a form we can understand; in the written text it also becomes an object of interpretation. In order for this to happen there must be a reciprocal question–answer relationship between text and interpreter (Gadamer 1975/1996). That is to say, meanings that come to us through interpretation are given to pose further questions and further puzzles to be understood and interpreted in different ways. Understanding text takes place within the historical context that permeates all understanding and through which understanding becomes meaningful.

Gadamer (1975/1996: 401) argued that language is not independent of the world:

> Not only is the world 'world' only insofar as it comes into language, but language, too, has its real being only in the fact that the world is re-presented within it. Thus the original humanity of language means at the same time the fundamental linguistic quality of man's being-in-the-world.

Through this statement, Gadamer connected language with ontology and following Heidegger's lead, focused on a mode of being rather than the epistemological mode of knowing that characterized much of nineteenth- and twentieth-century philosophy.

Personal prejudice and horizon

Gadamer strongly believed that it was counter-productive to consider 'ordinary language' while removing oneself from the situation of discovery – putting aside personal opinion and presupposition. He dismissed the negative connotations given to personal opinion by Husserl and incorporated the concept into his own writings. Gadamer saw prejudice (or *fore-knowledge*) in positive terms, as affirmative of all presupposition that underlies judgement. In order to understand or interpret a phenomenon, he suggested, the interpreter must both overcome the phenomenon's strangeness and transform it into something familiar, thus uniting the horizon of the historical phenomenon with the interpreter's horizon. For Gadamer, prejudice not only gives the hermeneutic problem its real thrust, but is the means by which the truth about a phenomenon is established (Gadamer 1975/ 1996). Thus the association between truth and prejudice is integral to understanding.

'Historicity', fusing horizons and the hermeneutic phenomenologistic circle

It has been argued that the relationship between interpreter and interpreted is wholly dependent on historical time, with both interpreter and interpreted caught up in a continuing cultural tradition known as 'effective history' (Mueller-Vollmer

1986: 39). In order to lay bare our own beliefs, we must first be aware of the *historicity* of understanding that governs all our prejudices. Events have an influence on our study of them. By ignoring historical understanding, we are distorting our knowledge base, but by allowing historical understanding to speak to us, we are making clear its true meaning. However, we can only understand the historical horizon through our own contemporary comprehension, so we need to meld horizons in order to complete the act successfully. This notion is called the 'fusing of horizons' – horizon being a metaphor for our range of vision, which includes the historical perspective. It is important that the notion of history is not confused with the lapsing of time, but rather our ability to be aware of our own past, incorporating that awareness into our history (Giddens 1982). The process of fusing horizons is circular and following Schleiermacher, who coined the term, Gadamer went on to describe it as a *hermeneutic circle* (Schleiermacher 1833/1977; Gadamer 1975/1996). With no beginning nor end, top nor bottom, interpretation is revealed as a process of circular movement – a continuum.

Distinctions between interpretive and descriptive phenomenology

In this section, differences in the theoretical and practical positions of descriptive and interpretive phenomenology are explored and the way phenomenology is transposed into scientific method discussed alongside an exposé of data collection and analysis techniques.

Paley argues that the very nature of phenomenological philosophy, be it Husserlian, Heideggerian or Gadamerian, disclaims the existence of a workable method (Paley 1997). Paley suggests that the transcendental idealism espoused by Husserl, by which we explore pre-reflective experience, removes us from the social world making judgements about 'lived experience' totally inaccessible. This line of thought has fuelled a divide between Husserlian (descriptivist) and Heideggerian/ Gadamerian (interpretivist/hermeneutic) camps and as philosophical phenomenology becomes the ground for scientific practice, the divide is further widened. Though there are phenomenologists wishing to draw our attention to the complementarity of different phenomenological perspectives (Todres and Wheeler 2001), we are more frequently reminded of differences between them, with the interpretivist upholding that:

- Meaning is unique and cannot be described.
- Interpretation is vital if we are to move beyond the data.

While descriptivists argue:

- 'Unified meaning can be teased out and described precisely as it presents itself' (Giorgi 1992: 123).
- Description is vital to account for variety in phenomena.

The interpretivist argument currently holds most sway among phenomenologists

Table 8.1. Key terminology in hermeneutic phenomenology

Terminology	Description
Heideggerian phenomenology	We are beings in and among the world and inseparable from a world of being
Hermeneutic phenomenology	Description of experience mediated by interpretation
Life-world	Our sense of lived life
Being-in-the-world	Beings in, among and inseparable from a world of being, existences in an existing world
Lived experience	Immediate, pre-reflective consciousness. The reality of lived experience that belongs to any one individual
Unready-to-hand	The way things show up for us when there is a problem
Interpretation	Pointing out the meaning of something
'Dasein'	People's everyday existence, 'being-there', being part of the situation where things are encountered
Attunement	A basic characteristic of *Dasein*, a basic way of being where our situation always already matters to us
Discourse	The world as always already articulated
Phenomenological description	One interpretation, non-exhaustive
'Verstehen'	Concept of understanding (including linguistic understanding)
Personal prejudice	Understanding others through language, history and tradition
Horizon	Range of vision
Fusing horizons	Melding positions that are in themselves forever changing
Hermeneutic phenomenologistic circle	Circular process of understanding, explication and interpretation. Circle defined by our personal horizon of understanding
Play	A losing of the subject–object distinction as in one's conduct within the hermeneutic circle
Historicity	An awareness of the cultural tradition of understanding that governs all our prejudices

today, but descriptivists nevertheless claim to have the upper hand on exclusivity of data, saying that although one may present an interpretive account of a phenomenon, it is with the understanding that there could be other interpretations. Thus according to Giorgi, 'the motive for interpretation is usually a situation of doubt, ignorance, or lack of clarity' (Giorgi 1992: 122).

However, the authenticity of phenomenological description has not escaped criticism:

> It is difficult to understand how a 'description of meaning' can be a description of something which 'patterns the specific experience uniquely' and, *at the same time*, a description that is 'essential to the experience no matter which specific individual has that experience'. The logical relationship between structure and experience must be either one-one or one-many; it cannot, presumably, be both. A structure which determines the individual uniqueness of an experience cannot, by definition, be a structure which defines all experiences of the same kind.
>
> (Paley 1997: 192)

Though both descriptivist and interpretivist approaches are concerned with meaning, the interpretivist is involved with the clarification of meaning in terms of plausible hypotheses or theoretical models while the descriptivist defines how meanings are presented to consciousness, precisely as they are presented. Other differences between the two include:

- The descriptivist suggestion that the researcher is the expert in judging the validity of a subject through the reduction using imaginative variation, contrary to the interpretivist recommendation for the use of external judges to test the validity of findings.
- The descriptivist suggestion that all interpretation can be described and that if data are coherent, coherent descriptions can be made, contrary to the interpretivist suggestion that data can only be interpreted because humans are self-interpretive.

Hermeneutic phenomenological method

This section considers hermeneutic method, concentrating in particular on the work of the educational theorist Max van Manen to explore data collection and analysis techniques.

For the hermeneutic phenomenologist working in health services research today, there is a marked concentration on the transposition of philosophical hermeneutics into a workable method for data collection and analysis. Hermeneutic phenomenologists consider philosophical hermeneutics as the foundation stone for their scientific method, not a model for scientific practice. By separating out theory and practice, they avoid the methodological impasse suggested by Paley (above), setting aside the purist view that hermeneutic philosophy is counter to a workable method and looking instead at method development.

A number of suggestions have been made for a hermeneutic approach to method development. First, it is advised that researchers using hermeneutic phenomenology should work closely with others during data collection and analysis with formal/informal group analysis techniques recommended (van Manen 1990). Second, that others' experiences and reflections are valid and should be considered alongside the experiences and reflections of the researcher (Jones 2004). Third, that researchers should be open to practical and theoretical challenges during the course of a research study (Dahlberg and Halling 2001). Considered together, these recommendations encourage the hermeneutic researcher to concentrate on workable methods underpinned by rigorous research design and internal validation processes.

Various hermeneutic methods have been developed with these considerations in mind, in the field of nursing, predominantly through the work of nurse researchers such as Diekelmann and Allan (Diekelmann *et al.* 1989) (see also Diekelmann 1992), while in the field of education, through the work of educational theorists such as van Manen (1989; 1997). Van Manen describes our understanding actions through verbal or visual expression as challenging us to return to the pre-reflective state. Pre-reflection demands that data are collected immediately following the events being described, before research participants have had time to reflect on their experiences. According to van Manen, it is only through a sense of immediacy that we will really get to 'know' the *life-world* of the research participant.

Van Manen's (1990: 30–31) method progresses through six basic steps:

1. turning to a phenomenon which seriously interests us and commits us to the world;
2. investigating experience as we live it rather than as we conceptualize it;
3. reflecting on the essential themes which characterize the phenomenon;
4. describing the phenomenon through the art of writing and rewriting;
5. maintaining a strong and oriented . . . relation to the phenomenon;
6. balancing the research context by considering parts and whole.

This method enables researchers to:

- explore meanings people give to their lives;
- concentrate on 'ordinary language' (descriptions in the participants' own words);
- examine phenomena immediately and directly, using first-hand experience;
- develop 'conversational relationships' with research participants;
- develop trust between researcher and participant;

- understand the links between meaning, language and the world in which meaning exists;
- recognize personal prejudice;
- search for hidden meanings embedded in the words of research participants.

Data collection

Van Manen describes twelve different aspects of investigating 'lived experience'. The majority of these have their basis in the act of writing, including: 'diaries and journals as sources of lived experience'; 'lived experience descriptions through protocol writing' and 'experiential descriptions in literature'.

Writing is said to fix thought on paper, externalizing what in some senses is internal or inter-subjective. It 'distances us from our immediate lived involvements with the things of our world' (van Manen 1989). It is clear that deciding on how best to address a research question will have impact upon the methods adopted. One of the data collection techniques proposed, 'interviewing to gather personal stories' has been described as a vehicle for gathering rich, in-depth data that are dependent on the interviewees description of events as an example of the original. Hermeneutic interviews encourage the development of 'conversational relation-ships' between interviewer and interviewee through in-depth discovery and inti-macy and intend to build trust within the relationship by offering interviewees 'space' to translate knowing into telling (van Manen 1990). The building of trust is further encouraged through the interviewer's judicious use of prompts and interjection and through the employment of 'active listening' techniques. However, according to Walters (Walters 1995) interviewers must feel confident to add their own perspective to the process when necessary in order to signify their own 'being-in-the-world'. Multiple perspectives, including the researcher's own, help the researcher prepare for data analysis where it will be important to respond to the participant's story through personal interaction with the data.

When conducting a hermeneutic study, Gadamer recommends the researcher keep a study diary. Other phenomenologists agree with this, commenting that diaries focus the mind not only on the story being told, the semantic expression, but also on the emotive qualities of data collection, the mantic expression, which together offer a more holistic view of experience. Where interviews are concerned, diary entries follow immediately after the interview is finished while the experience is still uppermost in the interviewer's mind (Thompson 1990; Koch 1998).

Data analysis

In a hermeneutic study, data analysis enables the researcher to objectify and interpret accounts in order to understand more clearly the world of the research participant. Interpretation depends heavily on the use of personal historical background, concentrating on one's own response to the language used by the participant, which carries along with it history and tradition. Explanation must be correlated with understanding to 'know' the phenomenon in all its forms and to develop an interpretive account. If interviewing is the method of choice, when a number of interviews are analyzed together, the variety of constructions that exist around the phenomenon may be brought into consensus to reveal the 'essential' quality of that phenomenon. This process includes 'fusing horizons', to compare and contrast a variety of ideas expressed and to arrive at a definitive understanding of the text. Koch (1998), citing Grenz (1996), describes this as an undertaking whereby the researcher has a 'dialogue' with the text – a hermeneutic conversation – to build on and reveal new understanding. The relationship is dynamic with a constant rhythm and has been linked to the 'hermeneutic circle' (understanding, explication, interpretation). Geertz (1975) adds to this, remarking that parts of texts and whole texts are independent of each other, but by moving between them, the researcher seeks to turn them into explications of each other.

Again we turn to van Manen to consider a thematic analysis approach to interview transcripts. The technique in question, one of three analytic approaches that van Manen proposes, has been described as 'the selective or highlighting approach' (1990: 79) and it consists of four stages:

1. Searching for 'structures of experience' (van Manen 1990: 79).
2. Describing how structures are thematic of the phenomenon.
3. Searching for essential and incidental themes.
4. Explaining and interpreting essential and incidental themes.

Each stage is rigorously selective and it is important to move slowly through the data so as not to overlook essential detail. Structures of experience, or sentences of great relevance to the research question, that stand out for the manner in which they are thematic of the phenomenon, are selected to help throw light on recurring themes, incongruities or puzzles within the data. Structures of experience also serve as useful quotations to illustrate study findings. Once revealed, they are described in the order in which they were discovered to show not only how each one is thematic of the phenomenon, but to present a decision trail through the data that illustrates the process of revelation. Analysis leads to a focusing-in on essential and incidental themes. Essential themes are those which, should they be absent from the final description of the phenomenon, would render the phenomenon incomplete. They help give shape to the data, and as a cognitive process, searching for essential themes, encourages a thoughtful and controlled response to participant stories. The researcher melds personal knowledge with emergent understanding, in effect, taking part in a 'hermeneutic conversation' with the text, to reveal new understanding underlying the words. Individual analysis is enhanced by collaborative analysis, through either formal or informal group sessions. Collaborative analysis leads to 'a common orientation to the notion of the phenomenon that one is studying' (van Manen 1990: 100), offering new insights or corroboration with researcher perspectives. Once analysis is complete, the researcher turns to the activities of report writing and publication, thus completing van Manen's six-step approach.

Critical issues

Differences from other qualitative approaches

The main difference between hermeneutic phenomenology and other qualitative approaches lies in the fact that hermeneutic phenomenologists believe that humans are self-determining beings. Furthermore, self-determination merits in-depth examination of how we shape the world through shared history and understanding. This is apparent, for example, in the contrast between hermeneutic phenomenology and ethnography. Ethnographers concentrate on cultural knowledge and how cultural knowledge is presented through participants' day-to-day routines, use of artefacts and cultural understanding. In ethnography, meaning is predominantly cultural, considered in terms of the descriptions people give to their own and others' cultural positioning. Hermeneutic phenomenologists, in keeping with an examination of self-determination, consider how meaning (be it cultural or otherwise) is revealed through 'ordinary language'. The hermeneutic phenomenologist tries to move towards an essential understanding of our 'being-in-the-world' through 'embodied understanding' and interest lies in how we develop awareness of new meanings in 'lived experience'.

Another example of an approach that compares dramatically differently to hermeneutic phenomenology is critical social theory. Here the theorist emphasizes the political, moral and social junctures between communities, societies and individuals, to understand the effects of action and communication on the way we constitute the social world. The critical social theorist, unlike the hermeneutic phenomenologist, will use an action research approach to data collection that enables the researcher to become part of that which is being studied. By so doing s/he attempts to 'equal out' political and social agendas and offer resolution to difference through social cohesion. The critical social theorist is particularly interested in issues surrounding the co-ownership of data, hoping to engender personal and societal change towards a sense of 'inclusivity'. The hermeneutic phenomenologist concentrates on 'lived experience', rather than power relationships and prompting activities towards change. In hermeneutic phenomenology what is important is how meanings are given to the *life-world*, not whether situations are appropriate or effective. The hermeneutic phenomenologist attempts to uncover reality as it is experienced, rather than indicate unanticipated conditions and unintended consequences.

Hermeneutic interviews

These differences are clearly reflected in the data collection techniques different researchers employ. Again if we look at interviewing, the hermeneutic researcher uses interviews to uncover meaning by:

- Gathering experiential narrative material.
- Conducting face-to-face interaction that captures mantic and semantic levels of understanding.

- Engaging in conversational development.
- Gathering experience as immediately lived.
- Incorporating the views of the participant with those of the researcher.
- Concentrating on the immediacy of data collection.

While other qualitative interviewers are likely to:

- Gather information, sometimes cultural, about actions, behaviours, conversations, beliefs and artefacts.
- Not necessarily conduct face-to-face interviews (they may also be telephone interviews).
- Emphasize information elicitation.
- Distance themselves from their own experience as immediately lived.
- Dissociate from personal prejudice, pre-supposition and individual assumption.
- Not necessarily concentrate on the immediacy of data collection.

Implications for professional practice

The implications for professional practice are manifold. If we can understand the potential for using hermeneutic phenomenology to explore people's 'lived experiences' through in-depth learning, sound critique and methodological evaluation, we can gather rich data to influence service delivery, treatment of patients and policy agendas. Methodological rigour is necessary in this pursuit. Researchers should be encouraged to publish in peer-reviewed journals that highlight best research 'evidence' and impact on professional practice. By raising standards of good practice through recognition of the value of sound qualitative studies, qualitative researchers can encourage others to broaden their horizons to different ways of collecting and analyzing data that most appropriately answer health-care questions.

The National Health Service Executive (NHSE) is one of a host of professional bodies continuing to support models of best practice based on 'evidence-based' health care (httpp.//www.dh.gov.uk). In spite of the fact that the 'evidence' such bodies refer to continues to predominate within a positivistic paradigm, the value of humanistic research is beginning to be recognized and frameworks developed for assessing the 'quality' of qualitative research. (See, for example, the 2003 document for the Cabinet Office written by the National Centre for Social Research httpp.//www.strategy.gov.uk/files/pdf/quality_framework.pdf. Also, see the ESRC Teaching and Learning Research Programme Research Capacity Building Network 2004.) It has been suggested that such frameworks may still be based on inappropriate evaluation criteria and as a consequence, remain ineffective in developing health-care policies and programmes (Torrance 2004). However, as the development of any assessment criteria of this nature is well overdue, such attempts should perhaps be welcomed.

Nevertheless, hermeneutic studies continue to be present in the nursing and psychological literature (see, for example, Van Kaam 1959; Colaizzi 1978; Giorgi 1985; Draucker 1999; Dahlberg and Halling 2001; Todres and Wheeler 2001). When these are rigorously conducted and underpinned by sound methodological frameworks, they have the potential to reinforce an evidence-based agenda and can develop sound professional knowledge, particularly when supported by evaluation structures. As an integral element of 'good evidence', the ability to highlight how the science behind the method is appropriate to a research study and transferable to others is of paramount importance. Moreover, there is value in informing researchers of the significance of the relationship between methodology and method, as this will impact significantly on their understanding of study findings (Maggs-Rapport 2001).

Hermeneutic phenomenology: an extended example

This section presents an example of a hermeneutic phenomenological study that took place between 1999 and 2001, the data of which have been recently re-analyzed; to explore 'decision-making' in egg donation. The original study examined women's motivation to donate eggs as well as their experiences of being potential 'egg share' donors. (For more in-depth information, please refer to Rapport (2003).)

Background

Original forays into explorations of gifting of body parts and different donation types was stimulated by the writings of Richard Titmuss, who was Professor of Social Administration at the LSE from 1950 until his death in 1973. In 1970 Titmuss wrote a seminal book on blood donation. *The Gift Relationship: From Human Blood to Social Policy*, in which he developed a social welfare model of blood donation based on a comparison of voluntary donor motives in the UK with those of paid donors in the USA. In his thesis, Titmuss described the creative act of giving as 'altruistic', saying inequality sets in when systems determine acts of giving according to economic criteria. For Titmuss, the voluntary donation system allows the self to be realized with the help of anonymous others and this 'allow[s] the biological need to help to express itself' (Titmuss 1970: 212). The work of the anthropologists Levi-Strauss (1969) and Malinowski (1922), writing on the act of gifting, was also taken into consideration though these writers presented the act of giving quite differently. For them it was one of expectant reciprocity – the expectation of a counter-gift that binds giver and receiver in complicit relationships far outreaching the act upon which the gift is based. Gifts were said to be about self-interest, acting as pledges of repayment or 'mandates of trust' to be taken forward at a later date.

In view of these very different interpretations, it was clear that a study exploring women's motivation to donate eggs would develop within the context of two premises. First, the premise that donation is based on an altruistic desire to help others. Second, the premise that donation is about assumed reciprocal agreements.

Egg sharing

Egg sharing is a self-help scheme, pioneered in the UK in 1993 by Ahuja and Simons of the Cromwell Hospital, London. The scheme encourages a woman, the donor, who can produce eggs of her own but needs fertility treatment to achieve a pregnancy, to enter into a private treatment programme of her choice. The donor is asked to donate approximately half of her eggs to another woman, the recipient, who cannot produce eggs of her own and by so doing will side-step lengthy NHS waiting lists of around five years. The donor's treatment will be heavily subsidized while the recipient pays in full. Donor and recipient remain anonymous to each other, though the donor may write a pen portrait for the recipient to receive with unidentifiable information included.

Recruitment procedures

Women were recruited opportunistically into this study from a single fertility centre in the UK between October 1999 and June 2000. The sampling strategy was time-based, as the number of people entering the scheme was very small. Consequently, all women were approached to take part over an eight-month period and this was the potential study cohort. An information sheet and consent form was sent out to all women expressing an interest in the scheme by the fertility nurse before their first appointment. Thus women gave consent before taking part in their first consultation, unsure of their suitability for egg sharing. It was evident that potential donors were in an extremely fragile and emotive state, often changing their minds about consent on a number of occasions.

Results of recruitment

Out of thirty-two women who applied for an initial consultation for egg sharing over an eight-month period, sixteen consented to take part in the study. However, only eleven of the sixteen were interviewed, as five withdrew after they were told in their first consultation that they were unsuitable for the scheme. Interestingly, the intention had been to interview all women who applied, irrespective of actual participation, although the outliers in this case declined.

Hermeneutic interviews

Following on from the description of hermeneutic method in this chapter, this study chose hermeneutic interviews as its data collection method. Interviews were chosen to encourage women to express their views immediately after the initial consultation as well as to endorse face-to-face data collection. In keeping with van Manen's views on the need for pre-reflective data, all interviews were conducted directly following the initial consultation, before women had had time to fully consider their reactions to the first consultation. As a result, all interviews were at the fertility clinic in a room close to the fertility specialist's consulting room. All interviews were taped, were extensive and open-ended in style, depending on the interviewees' descriptions of their experiences and their ability to put those across using 'ordinary language'. I was intent on developing trust between the interviewer and interviewee and this was facilitated through empathic listening which involved little interjection but encouragement nevertheless, through active listening techniques. At the analysis stage not only the interviewees', but my own personal 'horizons' were taken into account. However, during data collection, it was important to 'actively listen' to the stories being told and the meanings being put across.

Data analysis

Data were transcribed and transcripts analyzed using van Manen's 'selective or highlighting technique'. While data were being honed down to explore the 'structures of experience' displayed within the texts, I was orientating myself to the way in which women described egg sharing at both mantic and semantic levels. The emotive nature of the language used helped determine the strength of feeling expressed, while the semantic storyline helped uncover the linguistic meaning which makes social understanding possible (Van der Zalm and Bergum 2000). Mantic expression was noted during and directly following all interviews. Consideration of layers of meaning led to a progressive focusing in on emergent textual themes and these, alongside notes taking in reference to structures of experience exposed during analysis, helped me arrive at four essential and no incidental themes. As an example of the analysis process, Figure 8.1 shows the first sentence, the verbatim quotation from one of the interviewee transcripts. This is followed by my own interpretation of how the 'structure' was thematic of egg sharing. This should not be seen as a reiteration of the quotation, but an understanding of how it 'spoke' to me and thus to the phenomenon. The final sentence is the note I wrote to myself about my own response to this 'structure of experience'. This process was repeated throughout each and every transcript. Every sentence labelled a 'structure of experience' was removed from the text in the order in which it was presented and treated in this fashion.

Figure 8.1 Example of analysis

1   *'Tried everything ourselves first, because we really wanted to do it on our own.'*
2   The optimal situation is not egg sharing but natural reproduction.
3   Egg sharing is not something couples set out to do, but something they arrive at after alternative treatments.

In the search for meaning, as I continued to explore the data, I experienced the cognitive process of slowing down that seemed necessary to the experience of continuously reviewing the text. The passage of time during which analysis took place was also important, acting as a sort of 'rites of passage' through which I needed to pass in order to 'know' the data and thus make sense of the interviews. Such engagement has been described as dynamic. It suggests a constant rhythm as 'interpretation reveals understanding and understanding, in turn rewrites interpretation' (Allen and Jensen 1990), and it is in the sense of constant movement that defines the 'hermeneutic circle' of understanding, explication and interpretation.

Following individual analysis, three academic colleagues took part in two group analysis sessions. Colleagues were given a small number of transcripts to read and were asked to list major issues arising from each transcript to develop a common orientation towards the data. Colleagues wrote summaries of their own interpretive understanding, which were compared with my own and discussed through group meetings. Collaborative analysis helped ensure the 'trustworthiness of data' and encouraged an examination of the degree of similarity between views.

The four essential themes of egg sharing

Four essential themes and no incidental themes emerged from the data, encapsulating the decision-making process. It is worth noting that the dominant theme 'egg sharing as motherhood' subsumed all other themes as women expressed an overwhelming desire to conceive.

Egg sharing as context

Women's decisions to 'egg share' should be considered in the context of fertility treatment. Women consider their decision to take part in the scheme in relation to NHS treatment rationing, NHS waiting lists and the length of time they feel they have left before their body clock stops 'ticking'. Women also take into account their physical and emotional capacity to continue with alternative treatment options and this becomes integral to decision-making. Financial considerations, such as paying a reduced fee, also play a crucial role in the decisions made. While discussing the available treatment options, women revealed the options already exhausted, weighed up the ethical implications of one treatment option over another and explored the degree to which they were prepared to adapt to changing personal, emotional or physical circumstances. Women frequently changed their minds about the acceptability of one treatment option over another, with those treatments demanding the fewest personal compromises the first to be accepted.

Egg sharing as exchange

Women described egg sharing as a kind of exchange that was mutually but not necessarily equally beneficial. Recipients were likely to gain more than they were, as they were giving away their eggs to allow someone else to have a baby. Nevertheless, donors saw themselves as being in the stronger position, as they could keep trying for a baby and thus their reproductive potential was not in jeopardy. Donors expressed a strong sense of pleasure in being able to help another woman conceive, however, when pressed, donors suggested it was their own needs that were paramount.

Egg sharing as empathy

There was a strong sense that donors were doing recipients a favour resulting in empathetic concern for another's need. Donors described themselves as 'special', fulfilling an act of charity or a unique role and the decision to continue with egg sharing was strongly associated with not wishing to 'let the recipient down'.

Egg sharing as motherhood

The desire to experience motherhood was described as the driving force behind egg sharing. The goal of motherhood was expressed passionately and in great detail and there were a number of reasons for this. Women talked about how they wanted someone to depend on them, someone to keep them young and happy, company in old age and the opportunity to watch a child grow up.

Decision-making in ART

The findings indicate that participants were donating not out of an altruistic desire to give but were intent on helping another woman conceive. Though ambivalent about giving away half their eggs, women were desperate to be afforded the opportunity to try for a baby and while agreeing to participate in the scheme, discussed the need for more structured information giving and more discussion around personal need. They wanted to be brought in line with process and outcome through clearer channels of information giving and information sharing and expressed doubts about being in control of their fates and the fate of their offspring. Women were most concerned about giving away genetic material, the parental abilities of recipient couples and chance meetings between donor, recipient and offspring. However, in spite of these doubts, they continued to donate. While such extreme rationing for NHS treatment occurs, despite the implications of success for the recipient, donors will pursue donation.

How decisions were made

During thematic analysis, secondary analysis of the decision-making process was undertaken to reveal women's clear frustration and bewilderment at the lack of information available and the apparently inconsequential manner in which information was passed between professionals and patients. These findings confirm those of previous studies, which have highlighted a lack of satisfaction with information giving around possible causes of infertility, drugs and the time scale for investigation and treatment (Monarch 1993; Souter et al. 1998; Kerr et al. 1999). There is a lack of structure to information giving, leading to a sense of anxiety and abandonment while women are left to fend for themselves to acquire the information necessary to make decisions about treatment and care. This seeming lack of structure emphasizes a continual hierarchy in the relationship between patients and professionals. Surprisingly perhaps, women continued to express their deep felt gratitude to the health professionals for helping them try to conceive.

Study conclusions

Decisions about donating eggs are being taken within a context of rationing of treatment, a desperate desire to achieve a pregnancy, doubts about process and outcome and a lack of clear information leading to uninformed decisions. Women continue to enter a scheme with concerns about the future for their potential offspring. Though fully aware of the emotional, physical and mental toll that treatment takes on their lives and the limited success rates for different fertility treatments (the majority of women interviewed had been attempting to conceive for between six to twelve years) women are keen to pursue motherhood through egg sharing as this is one of the only avenues left to them. This study brings into question the premise that donation is borne out of an altruistic intent. For these women, taking the private treatment route through the egg sharing scheme offers a rare opportunity for motherhood. It is this that draws women into what I describe as 'the fertility syndrome' and keeps them on the treadmill well past their first donation attempt.

The hermeneutic study: enhancing dependability and validity

Researchers working in hermeneutic phenomenology regard the study as a complete process. It must be holistic and integrated, with no one part of study design more important than another. In addition, the researcher must be able to account for the data while displaying process, procedure and outcome. Consequently, the decision trail must be highly visible so that the researcher can illustrate the study's dependability, by showing how decisions were arrived at about data collection and analysis and how methodology relates to method (Maggs-Rapport 2001). By so doing, decisions are made visible for others' scrutiny with publications and other documentation considered in terms of internal validity, data evidence and 'trustworthiness' of data. As Koch comments, emphasizing the study's dependability through the researcher's ability to leave a decision trail, 'entails discussing explicitly decisions taken about the theoretical, methodological and analytical choices throughout the study' (Koch 1998). To encourage study dependability, it is recommended that the researcher keeps a study diary (Gadamer 1975/1996). The diary helps the researcher note aspects of the research design integral to findings and conclusions and additional information about the participants themselves, such as their reactions to events and comments made. The diary really comes into its own at the writing-up stage, the moment when the researcher makes public the private workings of the research, further contextualizing personal actions and behaviours. Validity is not only apparent through the smooth progression from data collection to data analysis and study findings but, as already mentioned, through group analysis, note taking and self-reflection. The reflexive mode is particularly pertinent to the hermeneutic study, where data collection will be dependent on the recognition of 'historical connections' linking researcher interpretation to the participant story (van Manen 1989).

Writing and re-writing reinforces the inbuilt veracity of the study and the researcher's ability to show the workings of the text, the 're-thinking, re-flecting, re-cognizing' (van Manen 1989: 32). This is the stage where in-depth analysis is clarified, lived experience displayed and complex choices illustrated. Anecdotes and stories can be incorporated at this point too, to add to participant stories with examples offering rich description using verbatim quotation.

Conclusion

This chapter has presented a phenomenological history alongside a presentation of the major theoretical premise upon which a hermeneutic study can be built. It has indicated how hermeneutics differs from other qualitative research frameworks and has displayed the unique attributes of hermeneutics through an extended example within a health services research context. I would contend that if hermeneutic in nature and of good scientific quality it is not enough to have an interesting and novel research question. The academic pursuit must be built on a firm foundation predicated by sound judgement and critical analysis. Workings should be displayed wherever possible and decisions accounted for through in-depth critique and the leaving of a decision trail. This will illustrate how 'evidences' are both employed and produced. Hermeneutic phenomenological studies have the potential to open up pathways towards best research and practice. Consequently the strengths of a well-thought-out, accountable and practical study, justified by clear methodological underpinnings should not be underestimated.

References

Allen, M.N. and Jensen, L. (1990) Hermeneutic inquiry: meaning and scope, *Western Journal of Nursing Research*, 12: 241–253.

Anderson, R.J., Hughes, J.A. and Sharrock, W. (1986) *Philosophy and the Human Sciences*. Kent, England: Croom Helm.

Colaizzi, P. (1978) Psychological research as the phenomenologist views it. In Valle, S.R. and King, M. (eds) *Existential Phenomenological Alternatives for Psychology*. New York: Oxford University Press, 48–71.

Dahlberg, K. and Halling, S. (2001) Human science research as the embodiment of openness: swimming upstream in a technological culture, *Journal of Phenomenological Psychology*, 32 (1): 12–21.

Diekelmann, N.L. (1992) Learning as testing: a Heideggerian hermeneutical analysis of the lived experiences of students and teachers in nursing, *Advanced Nursing Science*, 14 (3): 72–83.

Diekelmann, N.L., Allen, D. and Tanner, C. (1989) *The NLN Criteria for Appraisal of Baccalaureate Programs: A Critical Hermeneutic Analysis*. New York: National League for Nursing Press.

Draucker, B.C. (1999) The critique of Heideggerian hermeneutical nursing research, *Journal of Advanced Nursing*, 30 (2): 360–373.

Dreyfus, H.H. (1987) Heidegger, Modern Existentialism. In Magee, B. (ed.) *The Great Philosophers: An Introduction to Western Philosophy*. Oxford: Oxford University Press, 254–277.

ESRC Teaching and Learning Research Programme Research Capacity Building Network (2004). *Building Research Capacity*. Cardiff University.

Gadamer, H.G. (1975/1996) *Truth and Method.* Trans.: Barden, G. and Cumming, J. London: Sheed and Ward.

Geertz, C. (1975) On the nature of anthropological understanding, *American Scientist*, 63: 47–53.

Giddens, A. (1982) *Profiles and Critiques in Social Theory.* London: Macmillan Press.

Giorgi, A. (1985) *A Sketch of a Psychological Phenomenological Method.* Pittsburgh: Duquesne University Press.

Giorgi, A. (1992) Description versus interpretation: competing alternative strategies for qualitative research, *Journal of Phenomenological Psychology*, 23 (2): 119–135.

Grenz, S.J. (1996) *A Primer in Postmodernism.* Grand Rapids: William B. Eerdmans.

Heckman, S.J. (1986) *Hermeneutics and the Sociology of Knowledge.* Cambridge: Polity Press.

Heidegger, M. (1927/1962) *Being and Time.* Oxford: Blackwell.

Honey, M.A. (1987) The interview as text: hermeneutics considered as a model for analysing the clinically informed research interview, *Human Development*, 30: 69–82.

Husserl, E. (1931) *Ideas: General Introduction to Pure Phenomenology.* London: Allen and Unwin.

Jones, K. (2004) The turn to a narrative knowing of persons: minimalist passive interviewing technique and team analysis of narrative qualitative data. In Rapport, F. (ed.) *New Qualitative Methodologies in Health and Social Care Research.* London: Routledge, 35–54.

Kerr, J., Brown, C. and Balen, A.H. (1999) The experiences of couples who have infertility treatment in the United Kingdom: results of a survey performed in 1997, *Human Reproduction*, 14 (4): 934–938.

Koch, T. (1998) Story telling: is it really research? *Journal of Advanced Nursing*, 28 (6): 1182–1190.

Laverty, S.M. (2003) Hermeneutic phenomenology and phenomenology: a comparison of historical and methodological considerations, *International Journal for Qualitative Methods*, 2 (3): Article 3.

Levi-Strauss, C. (1969) *The Elementary Structures of Kinship.* London: Eyre and Spottiswoode.

MacDonald, P. (2001) Husserl's preemptive responses to existentialist critiques, *The Indo-Pacific Journal of Phenomenology*, 1: 1–22.

Maggs-Rapport, F. (2001) Best research practice: in pursuit of methodological rigour, *Journal of Advanced Nursing*, 35 (3): 373–383.

Malinowski, B. (1922) *Argonauts of the Western Pacific.* London: Routledge.

Monarch, J.H. (1993) *Childless: No choice: The Experience of Involuntary Childlessness.* London: Routledge.

Mueller-Vollmer, K. (1986) *The Hermeneutics Reader.* Oxford: Blackwell.

Outhwaite, W. (1987) *New Philosophies of Social Science: Realism, Hermeneutics and Critical Theory.* London: Macmillan.

Paley, J. (1997) Husserl, phenomenology and nursing, *Journal of Advanced Nursing*, 26: 187–193.

Rapport, F. (2003) Exploring the beliefs and experiences of potential egg share donors, *Journal of Advanced Nursing*, 43 (1): 28–42.

Sartre, J.P. (1992 [1943]) *Being and Nothingness: A Phenomenological Essay on Ontology.* New York: Washington Square.

Schleiermacher, F.D.E. (1833/1977) *Hermeneutics: The Handwritten Manuscripts.* Atlanta, Georgia: Scholar's Press.

Souter, V.L., Penney, G, Hopton, J.L. and Templeton, A.A. (1998) Patient satisfaction with the management of infertility, *Human Reproduction*, 13 (7): 1831–1836.

Thompson, J.B. (1987) Hermeneutics. In Kuper, J. (ed.) *Methods, Ethics and Models*. New York: Routledge and Kegan Paul.

Thompson, J.L. (1990) Hermeneutic inquiry. In Moody, L.E. (ed.) *Advancing Nursing Science Through Research*, Vol. 2. Newbury Park, CA: Sage.

Titmuss, R.M. (1970) *The Gift Relationship: From Human Blood to Social Policy*. London: Allen and Unwin.

Todres, L. (2004) The meaning of understanding and the open body: some implications for qualitative research, *Existential Analysis*, 15 (1): 38–54.

Todres, L. and Wheeler, S. (2001) The complementarity of phenomenology, hermeneutics and existentialism as a philosophical perspective for nursing research, *International Journal of Nursing Studies*, 38: 1–8.

Torrance, H. (2004) Quality in qualitative evaluation – a (very) critical response, *Journal of the ESRC Teaching and Learning Research Programme Research Capacity Building Network*, May 2004 (8): 8–10.

Van der Zalm, J.E. and Bergum, V. (2000) Hermeneutic-phenomenology: providing living knowledge for nursing practice, *Advanced Nursing Science*, 31 (1): 211–218.

Van Kaam, A. (1959) Phenomenological analysis: exemplified by a study of the experience of being really understood, *Individual Psychology*, 15: 66–72.

van Manen, M. (1989) Pedagogical text as method: Phenomenological research as writing, *Saybrook Review*, 7 (2): 23–45.

van Manen, M. (1990) *Researching Lived Experience: Human Science for an Action Sensitive Pedagogy*. London, Ontario: Althouse Press.

van Manen, M. (1997) From meaning to method, *Qualitative Health Research*, 7 (3): 345–369.

Walsh, K. (1996) Philosophical hermeneutics and the project of Hans Georg Gadamer: Implications for nursing research, *Nursing Inquiry*, 3: 231–237.

Walters, A.J. (1995) The phenomenological movement: implications for nursing research, *Journal of Advanced Nursing*, 22: 791–799.

Weinsheimer, J. (1991) *Philosophical Hermeneutics and Literary Theory*. New Haven: Yale.

LIBRARY
EDUCATION CENTRE
PRINCESS ROYAL HOSPITAL

9

ROSALIND BLUFF
Grounded theory: the methodology

Introduction

The purpose of this chapter is to explore the main features and nature of grounded theory. The origins and history of grounded theory will be considered and the research process examined, with particular emphasis on the characteristics that make it different from other qualitative research approaches. Critical issues such as the erosion or evolution of the methodology and its relevance to health-care practitioners will also be explored.

The nature of grounded theory

Grounded theory is one of the main approaches to qualitative research (although it was not initially intended as a purely qualitative method). A number of key features, however, ensure it maintains its own unique identity. Of these the development of theory is particularly important (Glaser and Strauss 1967; Strauss 1987; Glaser 1998; Strauss and Corbin 1998). Theory explains and provides insight into the phenomenon under study. Grounded theory is therefore a creative process that is appropriate to use when there is a lack of knowledge or theory of a topic (Glaser and Strauss 1967; Schreiber and Stern 2001), where existing theory offers no solutions to problems (Chenitz and Swanson 1986) or for modifying existing theory. Glacken *et al.* (2003), for instance, chose grounded theory for their study of the experience of fatigue in individuals living with hepatitis C because this phenomenon had not previously been explored in patients with liver disease. Grounded theory also identifies a series of events and how these change over time which is appropriate when patients have to live with a medical condition. It will be shown that the development of theory is facilitated through an interactive process of collecting and analyzing data.

Origins and history

Grounded theory was first developed by two American sociologists, Glaser and Strauss, in the 1960s when they explored the experience of patients dying in hospital (Glaser and Strauss 1965, 1968). Glaser with a background in quantitative research and Strauss with a grounding in qualitative research sought to understand human beings and their behaviour by developing systematic and detailed procedures which would be viewed as scientific.

Their original text (Glaser and Strauss 1967) provided some insight into how to undertake a grounded theory study, but over the years the method has been refined and become more transparent with the publication of *Theoretical Sensitivity* (Glaser 1978), *Qualitative Analysis for Social Scientists* (Strauss 1987) and *Basics of Qualitative Research* (Strauss and Corbin 1990, 1998). The real essence of grounded theory has, however, become an issue for debate. Glaser (1992) strongly believes that his approach is grounded theory, and that Strauss has developed a new method which should be called 'full conceptual description'. Other well-known researchers such as Stern (1994) debate the question whether the methodology has evolved or been eroded. Glaser has since written a number of texts that he sees as being in the spirit of the original grounded theory approach (for instance, 1998 and 2001).

Glaserian and Straussian perspectives of grounded theory

Over the years two perspectives of grounded theory have emerged (Strauss and Corbin 1990; Glaser 1992) although Stern (1994) and Schreiber (2001) suggest these differences have always existed and evolved over time. This may be a reflection of the different background of Glaser and Strauss. Their differences became a public issue with the publication of Glaser's (1992) book in response to the collaborative work by Strauss and one of his former students (Strauss and Corbin 1990). Glaser verbally attacks Strauss for deviating from what he regards to be grounded theory and requests him to withdraw *Basics of Qualitative Research* (Strauss and Corbin 1990) because it 'distorts and misconceives grounded theory'. Strauss and Corbin (1990, 1998) adopt a detailed, systematic and more prescriptive approach, which, according to Glaser (1992), forces the development of theory. Glaser (1992) believes that more flexibility allows the theory to emerge. The differences between these two approaches will be considered as each component of the research process is explored.

Glaser (1992) believes that Strauss and Corbin (1990) eroded the method by omitting some of the original procedures (his subsequent work, mainly in 1998 and 2001 develops his recent ideas on the debate). Strauss and Corbin assert that their approach has evolved (Strauss and Corbin 1994), and that over time they have adapted grounded theory to meet the needs of the phenomenon under study. However, Strauss and Corbin (1994) also express concern that the increasing popularity of grounded theory has resulted in researchers who lack understanding of some of its components. Thus the latter do not always set out to develop theory, fail to develop a dense theory or believe they are using grounded theory because they are using an inductive process. Strauss and Corbin (1994) acknowledge that the lack of clarity in the original text (Glaser and Strauss 1967) may to some extent account for this. However, one could argue that all approaches evolve over time, some of the original ideas may be modified and new concepts and procedures added in the process of carrying out the research. Glaser (1998), however, talks about 'rhetorical wrestling' and states that there is no need to rewrite and that everything necessary is already contained in previous texts.

Symbolic interactionism

The assumptions on which grounded theory is based are rooted in symbolic interactionism which, according to Travers (2001), can be viewed from a number of perspectives. Blumer (1971) who articulated the views of Mead (1934) believed that the behaviour of individuals and the roles they adopt are determined by how they interpret and give meaning to symbols. The meaning of symbols such as language, dress and actions is shared by individuals within a culture and is learnt through a process of socialization. Behaviour is therefore influenced by the context in which it takes place. It is the meaning given to these symbols, which enables the behaviour of others to be predicted. Individuals respond to these predictions by adapting their behaviour towards others. Human behaviour and the roles that individuals fulfil are therefore negotiated and renegotiated in a process of inter-action and consequently change over a period of time rather than remaining static. Feedback from these interactions enables individuals to recognize how others perceive them and hence develop a perception of 'self'. The self is therefore influenced by the expectations of others and by the example that they set. Individuals can respond to others without thought, but interpretation of symbols implies a cognitive analysis. People thus have active control of the way they present themselves rather than passively allowing themselves to be moulded by the environment. Reality of the self and the environment is therefore socially constructed. The social processes within these interactions are explored. In doing so, grounded theory makes explicit the reality of how individuals perceive their world and the way they interact with others.

Glaser and Strauss (1967) accepted the fundamental principles of Mead's perspective of symbolic interactionism. Although an inductive process, like all approaches to qualitative research, grounded theory – particularly Straussian grounded theory – seeks to make theoretical assertions that can subsequently be tested and verified and is hence deductive as well as inductive. The systematic approach to data collection and analysis and the use of terminology such as working hypotheses, variables and precision emphasize its link with the quantitative paradigm. Pidgeon (1996) comments that in saying theory is 'discovered from data' Glaser and Strauss (1967) imply an objective relationship between psychological and social events. When placed on a continuum with other qualitative approaches grounded theory can be sited closest to the quantitative paradigm (Cluett and Bluff 2000) when compared with other qualitative approaches.

The research question and the use of literature

The research question identifies the phenomenon to be studied. The area of the study needs to be broad, at least initially. Glaser (1992) believes that if the focus is too narrow there may be insufficient data to formulate a theory. Strauss and Corbin (1998) emphasize that the focus narrows as the study progresses and the important issues emerge, 'progressive focusing' occurs. Although there is still openness to discovery the focus is on the evolving theory. Some studies begin with a question while others may state an aim. Specific objectives are avoided as these determine the focus of the study from the beginning and inhibit the process of discovery.

A literature review is an overview of the literature on issues relevant to the phenomenon to be studied. There is a debate about the timing of the literature review. It is recognized that preconceived ideas can inhibit the process of discovery; they can provide a framework for data collection that results in confirmation of what is already known about a phenomenon (Glaser and Strauss 1967; Glaser 1992; Strauss and Corbin 1998). Theory is generated from and grounded in the data. For this reason Glaser (1978, 1992, 1998) does not believe an initial review is appropriate. However, avoiding a literature review prior to commencing a study will not necessarily eliminate any preconceived ideas. If the phenomenon under study is related to the researcher's own practice setting then knowledge and experience of the phenomenon is inevitable. Morse (2001a) believes that an initial literature review combined with bracketing prior assumptions provides novices with knowledge that they can then use to compare with their categories as they emerge. In this way they are less likely to become swamped in data. This comparison can therefore help to initiate the creative process of analysis. Whether bracketing can really be achieved is, however, questionable. Clegg (2003) argues that if there is a dearth of literature related to the phenomenon being studied then the initial literature review is likely to have little influence on the outcome.

Strauss and Corbin (1998) suggest it is not necessary to review all the literature prior to a grounded theory study but this raises a question about how much literature should be reviewed at the very beginning. Inevitably researchers have to make sure that they do not study an area which has been researched many times before in a similar way, so that their study adds something new. For this they need an overview of the literature. Ultimately researchers have to be pragmatic. Justification for the methodology and rationale for studying the chosen phenomenon requires some form of literature review. The decision to adopt grounded theory is based on the amount of knowledge known about the phenomenon.

The ongoing use of the literature has a number of purposes (Glaser 1978, 1992). It can enhance theoretical sensitivity to the data, that is the ability to determine what is or is not important to the emerging theory (Glaser 1978; Strauss and Corbin 1998). The literature is also incorporated into the study confirming or refuting ideas emerging from the data. Questions or ideas from the literature are also sought in the data to extend the theory. Literature accessed at this stage tends to be different from that used in the initial review because the focus is now on developing the emerging theory. Glaser as well as Strauss and Corbin acknowledge that reading literature related to other disciplines is necessary as this can enhance conceptualization of the data as well as theoretical sensitivity.

Whether to undertake an initial review, how much literature to access at this time and when to commence the subsequent review will be a matter for professional judgement. Cutcliffe (2000) argues that the decision about when to access the literature may depend on which version of grounded theory the researcher has chosen.

Sampling

Like many other types of qualitative studies sample size in grounded theory research can vary but tends to be small. For example, Clegg (2003) chose four patients and three relatives to participate in her study, while Glacken *et al.* (2003) included twenty-eight individuals. Sample size may, however, be larger. Fifty-five first-time mothers took part in a study by Rogan *et al.* (1997) that explored the experiences of becoming a mother.

Purposive or purposeful sampling is used in the beginning. This means participants have knowledge of the phenomenon being studied. Initially *open sampling* takes place. Selection means acquiring participants who will provide data relevant to the study. As a theory begins to emerge, *theoretical sampling* is included. This means that analysis of the data informs sample selection (Glaser and Strauss 1967) which is based on further development of the emerging theory. This selection may be based on participants or emerging concepts.

Purposive sampling may also be one of convenience such as a cohort of students rather than a number of students from several cohorts. Alternatively participants may select themselves. These types of sample are atypical of a population and therefore might be called biased (Smith and Biley 1997), but the purpose is to provide insight into a phenomenon that only those with specific knowledge have. The inclusion of negative (deviant) cases or the views of participants that differ from others provide a balanced perspective. When researchers are dependent on others, such as health-care workers, for selecting their sample, lack of sufficient variation in the data may be a limitation of a study (Landmark and Wahl 2002).

An additional type of purposeful sampling is snowballing or chain referral sampling whereby one participant informs the researcher of someone else who might be willing to participate in the study. This may be necessary if the phenomenon under study is uncommon such as, for instance, the experience of caring for a baby with phenylketonuria.

Data collection

Qualitative data in GT are derived from the same sources as those of other qualitative approaches. This involves collecting data by means of interviews and/or observation of the phenomenon that is being researched. In addition, health-care practitioners may collect data in the form of records such as medical or maternity notes, off duty rotas and minutes of meetings. Strauss and Corbin (1998) suggest diaries; autobiographies, letters and historical accounts, but many other sources can be used.

Interviews may be unstructured or semi-structured. Unstructured interviews generally consist of one or two open-ended questions. Participants are then free to say as much or as little as they wish and the researcher does not impose their own ideas. Questions that prompt or encourage participants to elaborate can be posed (Patton 2002). It is at this stage of the research process that having knowledge and experience of the topic can facilitate data collection (Strauss 1987). Indeed, Pidgeon (1996) believes that without some prior knowledge sense cannot be made of any research data. Smith and Biley (1997) acknowledge the tension that exists between putting aside any preconceived ideas and using knowledge and experience to facilitate the development of theory. The use of a reflective diary can raise researchers' awareness of their preconceived ideas and the influence of these on data collection and analysis. This awareness is also important if the perspective of another is to be understood (Hutchinson and Wilson 2001). Obtaining the insider perspective and interpret it requires empathy or the ability to place oneself in the shoes of another. This process of looking back on the self (Mead 1934) continues throughout the research. The researcher is an integral part of the research process. The desirability of being able to suspend knowledge is likely to be difficult or even impossible to achieve.

The study may begin with semi-structured interviews (indeed Strauss himself prefers these). There are no guidelines to stipulate the number of questions this involves. It is, however, important to remember that the more questions that are asked the more structured the interview becomes. Too many questions, and the researcher determines the agenda. The process of discovery is then inhibited, and what is important to participants may never be revealed. Morse and Bottorff (1992) in a study that explored the emotional experience of breast expression following the birth of a baby posed three questions. Landmark and Wahl (2002) sought to explore the experiences of women who had recently been diagnosed with breast cancer. They identified six key issues which included *reactions to the diagnosis, every day living patterns* and *thoughts about the future*. Although these were stated to be guidelines their purpose was to provide structure to the interview.

In reality most grounded theory interviews become semi-structured because, as the key issues emerge, there is a need to focus on these to facilitate development of the theory. Issues that lack relevance to the emerging theory are not pursued. An interview guide can be used to record questions that highlight these key issues (Holloway 1997). If these issues do not arise spontaneously the researcher can then address them; such questions will be important in developing the emerging theory. An alternative to the individual interview is the focus group, an approach adopted for instance, by Rogan *et al.* (1997). Interactions of a small group of individuals generate ideas and facilitate exploration of the phenomenon (Holloway 1997). It might, however, be more difficult to carry out theoretical sampling with focus groups.

Holloway (1997: 94) suggests that the interview is a 'conversation with a purpose', a phrase used by the Webbs in the nineteenth century. Conversations are verbal interactions between two or more individuals who ideally all have an equal opportunity to express their viewpoint. If, however, researchers say too much, there is a real possibility that they will introduce their own ideas and thus influence the incoming data. Interviews are often referred to as 'in-depth', implying a considerable amount of detailed data are collected. Although they can vary in length for example 50–180 minutes (Glacken *et al.* 2003), this is a short timespan in the trajectory of an experience such as permanent fatigue. To regard such interviews as in-depth may therefore be inappropriate. The sensitive nature of a phenomenon studied may result in distress to participants. For this reason it is important to ensure participants have some form of support following the interview. Landmark and Wahl (2002) offered their participants the opportunity to talk with a medical consultant or nurse according to their needs.

Observation provides an opportunity to witness the interactions that take place between individuals in a social setting. The researcher provides the interpretation of events. Combining observation with interviewing clarifies the meaning of those events from the perspective of the participants. This can be useful in discovering whether what is said corresponds to what is done in practice and can provide opportunities to clarify any discrepancies. Researchers need to be aware of the ethical issues that can arise when observing others. These include the Hawthorne effect, when the presence of the researcher alters the behaviour that is being observed, and what action to take if practice that is witnessed causes concern.

Fieldnotes

Fieldnotes are the written account of the researcher's thoughts and observations and therefore enhance data collection. When interviewing they might include aspects of the context of the study, facial expressions and gestures that cannot be recorded on a tape. Descriptions of participants and the researcher's perceptions of what is happening in the setting will also be important. For this reason Holloway (1997) believes they are a combination of the researcher's personal reflections as well as detailed descriptions that enhance remembrance of events in the setting. When observation is the mode of data collection, fieldnotes are vital as they provide the only means of data collection (Morse and Field 1996) unless videotapes are used.

Data analysis

The process of analysis can begin as the data are being collected and fairly soon after the interview or observations have been undertaken and transcribed. The transcription includes coughs, pauses, laughs and so on, while in observations actions and interactions are described in the fieldnotes. All of these have meanings and may influence interpretation of the data.

A key feature of grounded theory is the constant comparative method of analysis (Glaser and Strauss 1967) in which data collection and analysis is a simultaneous and interactive process. The process also involves constant comparison between words, sentences, paragraphs, codes and categories. The purpose of this is to identify similarities and differences in the data. Each interview and observation is also compared. This process continues until the final write up of the report has been completed. It is a detailed and thorough process involving repeated reading or listening to the tape recordings. The interaction with the data enables the researcher to understand the phenomenon that is being researched.

Coding

Open coding (Strauss and Corbin 1998) or *Level 1 coding* (Hutchinson and Wilson 2001) is initially employed to name and give meaning to the data. This may involve use of 'in vivo' codes that are the participants own words. Codes with similar meaning are linked together and renamed as categories to provide more abstract meaning. In addition, each property or characteristic of the category can be located along a continuum (Strauss and Corbin 1998). For example, in a study that analyzed women's initial experiences of motherhood, Barclay *et al.* (1997) developed a category that they entitled 'unready'. At one end of the continuum women were totally unready for motherhood while at the other extreme were those who were completely ready. This process is known as dimensionalization.

Glaser (1992) and Strauss and Corbin (1998) adopt a different, though similar, approach to coding. While the naming of categories and identification of properties and dimensions appears to be the same whichever method is used, the approach to initial coding adopted by Strauss and Corbin is a very detailed one.

During open coding and the subsequent analytic process, questions are generated and answers sought in the data. Future participants can be asked these questions if they are likely to facilitate the development of a theory. These questions can also generate working hypotheses or propositions that can be validated in subsequent data collection. Unlike other qualitative approaches, grounded theory is therefore an inductive and deductive process. According to Glaser (1992: 51) neutral questions should be asked such as 'what is actually happening in the data?' This permits the data to tell their own story. In contrast, Strauss (Strauss and Corbin 1998) asks 'what if?' (Stern 1994), and considers all possibilities whether they are in the data or not. This involves asking questions such as *who?, what?, where?, how?* and *when?* According to Glaser (1992) his approach permits the theory to emerge while Strauss forces the data. Strauss and Corbin (1998) dispute this, saying that the data are allowed to speak for themselves.

Axial or *Level 2 coding* (Hutchinson and Wilson 2001) follows open coding. This process is used to make connections between categories and sub-categories and allows a conceptual framework to emerge. Using a paradigm model, relationships are established by determining causes, contexts, contingencies, consequences, covariances and conditions (Glaser 1978). At this stage some open codes may be discarded because there are no connections. The relationship between concepts is verified by constant comparison and enables the theory to be developed. The link between conditions, consequences and interaction can be expressed in the form of a conditional matrix (Strauss and Corbin 1998). Lugina *et al.* (2002) provide a good example of this, while Rogan *et al.* (1997) acknowledge that their theory was not fully developed. The data are therefore put back together in new ways. According to Glaser (1992) the paradigm model forces the data into a predetermined structure hence his use of the term 'full conceptual description' for the work of Strauss.

Selective coding for Strauss and Corbin (1998) is the process that links all categories and sub-categories to the core category thus facilitating the emergence of the 'storyline' or theory. Perhaps unsurprisingly Glaser (1992) disagrees and clearly states that selective coding is about confining coding to those categories that relate to the core category. Keddy *et al.* (1996) in a discussion of how grounded theory can be used for feminist research acknowledge that more than one story might emerge from the data. A decision therefore has to be made about choosing which story to develop.

The core category is central to and links the data; it accounts for the variations in the data (Strauss and Corbin 1998). It therefore provides a theory to explain the social processes surrounding the phenomenon. Integrating ideas from the literature and undertaking further sampling can expand this theory (Stern 1980). Subsequent interviews can verify this theory and enhance its development. Concepts and codes that lack relevance to the developing theory are discarded, but negative cases are retained. Rogan *et al.* (1997) identified six categories: 'realizing', 'unready', 'loss', 'aloneness', 'drained' and 'working it out'. Linking these together was the core category 'becoming a mother'. Their theory explains how women move through a trajectory of recognizing life changes, something that they were not ready for, to making the adjustment to motherhood. The ability to give meaning to the data, in other words to recognize what is relevant and important, and what lacks relevance for the emerging theory requires theoretical sensitivity (Glaser and Strauss 1967; Glaser 1978). It is this that also helps to determine theoretical sampling. Pidgeon (1996) believes that novices may be unable to theorize beyond the context in which their own study took place, and grounded theory therefore may become little more than content analysis.

It has been acknowledged that the Straussian version of grounded theory is very structured, and concerns have been expressed that some researchers may follow it as a prescription (Pidgeon 1996). This implies 'linear thinking' (Keddy *et al.* 1996: 450), which is contrary to the intention of constant comparison. In contrast, the Glaserian approach could be perceived as being rather vague.

When each category is conceptually dense, variations in the category have been identified and explained, and no further data pertinent to the categories emerge during data collection, saturation is said to occur (Strauss and Corbin 1998). At this point in the study all participants are expressing the same ideas relevant to the developing theory, and nothing new is emerging from observations in the field. No further data collection is necessary, and the final sample size is known. Some codes and categories will be saturated before others, hence some data collection appears to become irrelevant but confirms what has already been said. It is interesting to note that the issue of saturation was originally discussed by Glaser and Strauss in *The Discovery of Grounded Theory* (1967) and is now included in *The Basics of Qualitative Research* (Strauss and Corbin 1998) although it was not mentioned in their 1990 edition. Glacken *et al.* (2003) maintain that they did achieve saturation while Clegg (2003) admits her small sample size may not have permitted this. There is then the potential for the theory to be incomplete

(Hutchinson and Wilson 2001). It is, however, difficult to state categorically that saturation has been achieved.

Memos and diagrams

Memos are the written records of abstract thinking about the data. They are therefore a record of the data analysis (Strauss 1987) which can include questions that are generated and directions for future data collection. Diagrams provide a visual form of the data that is clear and concise. The relationship between codes and categories is clearly visible. Areas for further data collection will be evident as will gaps in knowledge (Strauss and Corbin 1998). Strauss and Corbin place great emphasis on the use of memos. They provide a record of the research process and its progress, hence memos become increasingly complex as comparisons are made with the data; links between codes and categories establish the variations which all contribute to the development of the theory.

Evaluating a grounded theory study

Evaluation of a study is about making judgements of its worth. In this case it is about judging the theory, the research process used in developing it and deciding if the methodology was appropriate. Any criteria used to evaluate a grounded theory study should take into consideration whether a Glaserian or Straussian approach was adopted (Smith and Biley 1997).

Trustworthiness and credibility of the data needs to be established to ensure rigour. Reasons for choosing the grounded theory approach and provision of an audit trail therefore need to be made explicit. A detailed description of the context in which the study took place is essential, yet Morse (2001b) acknowledges that many studies she receives for publication fail to elaborate on this important component.

The research question or aim needs to be sufficiently broad, and data collection and analysis should demonstrate how the important issues emerged and the study became more focused. Evidence of initial and subsequent sample selection should therefore be apparent. How concepts were derived from the data should be shown as well as how categories were formed and categories and sub-categories linked together. Examples should be provided. Also, examples of questions and working hypotheses should be explained, and whether these were proven or not. There also needs to be evidence of any discrepancies, and how these were accounted for.

The core category or storyline needs to be evident and demonstrate how it links all the data. In the absence of a core category (Hutchinson and Wilson 2001) the study may be merely descriptive. A good theory is 'conceptually dense' (Strauss and Corbin 1998) and comprehensive if it accounts for all variations in behaviour. Peer review of the analytic process can enhance trustworthiness.

Theory is constructed from the data and should represent the social reality as perceived by participants. In other words it 'fits' (Glaser and Strauss 1967). These will not only be recognizable to the participants when they review the findings but also to others who are familiar with the social setting (Glaser and Strauss 1967; Strauss and Corbin 1998). Quotes from the data will demonstrate how the theory was constructed. Understanding of the theory is also important if it is to be effectively used (Glaser and Strauss 1967). Glaser and Strauss suggest that a grounded theory should have 'relevance' or 'grab' and 'work'. It explains what is actually happening in the setting and can predict what will happen under certain conditions. Lugina *et al.* (2002) believe they achieve these criteria. They provide a framework that expresses midwives' views about their role in postnatal care and what they can do to enhance the quality of care they give. The theory therefore provides guidelines for action. These criteria imply the theory is useful, and this is very important in health research.

Findings cannot be generalized to a total population but may have meaning for others in a similar social setting (Strauss and Corbin 1998). Likewise a grounded theory study cannot be replicated, but if another researcher follows the audit trail, the theoretical explanation for the phenomenon should be similar (Strauss and Corbin 1998). Glaser (1992) questions why any one would want to do this!

Application of grounded theory

Grounded theory is now a very popular approach to doing qualitative research in health care. Schreiber and Stern (2001) state that this is true for nursing and the same could be said for midwifery. Despite this, its impact on practice and education has been minimal (Hall and May 2001).

The environment in which health care is provided is dynamic. Practitioners' perspectives of giving care are important and so is the impact of policies on the provision of care. Using grounded theory to make these explicit can provide others with knowledge to change or enhance their own practice for the benefit of clients.

The delivery of health care involves interaction between practitioners, clients, managers, educationalists, and members of the multi-professional team including students. Emphasis is now placed on inter-professional education to facilitate understanding of each others' roles, remove inter-professional rivalries and thus enhance the quality of care clients and patients receive (DOH 2001a, 2001b). Implementation of this new style of education is being piloted with the support of funding from the Department of Health. Evaluation of these and other programmes from student and teacher perspectives may lead to modifications in structure and content as well as enhance student and teacher performance. There is also the potential to gain insights into how students from a number of professions relate to each other and work together. What follows is an example of an educational study that uses grounded theory and aims to illustrate some of the features included in this chapter.

An example of grounded theory research

Learning and teaching in the context of clinical practice: the midwife as role model

Introduction and justification for methodology

The aim of this study was to develop a theory to provide insight and understanding into how student midwives learned the role of midwife from their midwifery role models. Emphasis was therefore placed on eliciting the influence of midwifery role models on students and the impact of this on their practice. An initial literature review was sufficient to identify a lack of literature related to role modelling in midwifery although aspects of the phenomenon had been explored in nursing and medicine (Dotan *et al.* 1986; Lublin 1992; Davies 1993; Nelms *et al.* 1993; Wiseman 1994). These studies were, however, undertaken in Australia, America and Israel where culture and practice differs from that in England. Emphasis in these studies tends to be placed on positive role models with limited attention paid to poor role models and their impact on those who observe and interact with them (exceptions are the study by Davies and that by Nelms *et al.*). Gaps in knowledge and how the study might contribute to what is already known about the phenomenon were therefore made transparent. According to Stern (1980) grounded theory is a suitable means for exploring phenomena that have been investigated by others but not by one's own discipline.

Well-known studies that have explored the concept of socialization such as those by Becker *et al.* (1961), Dingwall (1977), Fretwell (1982) and Melia (1987) revealed that learning a role is a process of interaction that participants actively engage in. Roles are negotiated and renegotiated and are dynamic changing over time. It therefore seemed logical to suppose that students would interpret the actions of their role models and allow these to influence their own behaviour. Students are also likely to have shared meanings as they practise in the same social settings. These notions of interaction support the underlying belief on which grounded theory is based. The methodology was therefore appropriate for making this process of interaction explicit.

Background to the study

Prior to 1993 the medical model of care was the accepted form of practice. Interventions associated with this model of care were devised mainly by doctors and expressed in written policies (Garcia and Garforth 1989). Following these policies lead to adoption of the role of 'handmaiden' to the doctor (Robinson *et al.* 1983; Askham and Barbour 1996; Begley 1997), a role that some midwives continue to fulfil (Coggins 2002; Richens 2002). Historically the culture of midwifery and indeed the National Health Service (NHS) in Britain was associated with an expectation that practitioners would do as they were told (Hadikin and O'Driscoll 2000). Kirkham (1999) defines midwives as an oppressed group subordinated by doctors. She uses the writings of Freire (1993) on domination and control to explain how midwives came to accept the values and beliefs of the medical profession and in doing so undermined their own profession and practice hence the perpetuation of this model of care.

When data collection began in December 1993 the midwifery culture was beginning to change. Project 2000 (UKCC 1986) emphasized the preparation of a new practitioner through education. There was now an expectation that midwives would be autonomous and reflective practitioners, critical thinkers and knowledgeable doers who could use evidence to inform their practice. The *Changing Childbirth Report* (DOH 1993) also advocated midwifery care that focused on the women, giving them choice of care, control in the care they received and continuity of carer. Students were therefore exposed to two versions of midwifery which raised issues about which role they learned and how they learnt it.

Using grounded theory

The Straussian approach to grounded theory was adopted with detailed, practical advice obtained from Strauss and Corbin (1990). Twenty students and seventeen midwives participated in the study. Students were located in one of two universities in the south of England. Those with no nursing experience were undertaking either a three- or four-year programme while students who were qualified nurses were participating in the seventy-eight-week shortened programme. The midwives practised in the hospital, a midwifery-led unit or in the community setting. The sample was one of convenience. This is contrary to the grounded theory approach, but certain concepts such as 'bullying' were followed up and sampled as they emerged and became important to the developing theory.

Data were collected over a period of three years through unstructured tape-recorded interviews. One open-ended question was posed to students: 'how do you learn the role of the midwife in the clinical setting?' Midwives were asked 'how do you think students learn the role of the midwife when they work with you in the clinical setting?' As important issues emerged, these were listed on an interview guide. If not spontaneously included in the conversation by participants in subsequent interviews questions were raised relating to these issues. Topics were excluded from the interview when it became apparent during the research that they lacked relevance to the emerging theory.

The data were analyzed by the constant comparative method. Open coding enabled the data to be conceptualized. Codes that reflected my own interpretation of the data were identified. These included 'sticking to the rules', 'keeping quiet', and 'being innovative'. 'In vivo' codes (Strauss and Corbin 1998) included 'bending the rules' and 'the way it's always been'. 'Sussing and sizing' was a code initially chosen to reflect how students sought information about the midwives with whom they worked. This corresponded to a category adopted by Davies (1988) in an ethnographic study that explored students' experiences of the first eighteen weeks of their eighteen-month midwifery programme. 'Sussing and sizing' is something all individuals do when encountering new situations. Morse (2001a) emphasizes the importance of labelling concepts with the same name as those in other studies when they share the same meaning. This can enhance the richness of the developing theory. It could also be argued that they confirm what is in the literature and enhance trustworthiness of the data. To invent a new code has the potential to create confusion for readers. 'Sussing and sizing' was initially chosen to reflect how students sought information about the midwives with whom they worked. Ultimately this code was renamed 'seeking information' and reflected the broader perspective of gaining information not only from midwives but also peers. It was also a means of avoiding idiomatic expressions.

A higher level of abstraction was achieved by comparing codes and linking these together to form categories when similarities were found to exist. 'Cheating' and then 'being evasive' became a category that incorporated codes such as 'telling lies', 'withholding information' and 'practising behind closed doors'. These reflected the strategies that some midwives adopted to enable them to avoid criticism while practising midwifery based on a philosophy which did not correspond to that of the other midwives with whom they worked. Categorizing the data in this way reduces the data and thus makes them more manageable (Coffey and Atkinson 1996).

Working propositions were generated in response to questions that emerged from the data. These were subsequently verified by means of 'theoretical sampling'. Junior students, for example, had a need to learn the rules of practice to enable them to fit in and meet the expectations of their role models. The proposition that students would no longer need to fit in with their role models once they had learned the rules of practice was not verified. Properties and dimensions were also identified. The philosophy on which midwives based their practice was a property of a category entitled 'role modelling'. This was dimensionalized by placing a philosophy of childbirth 'only normal in retrospect' and hence requiring routine interventions at one end of a continuum and childbirth as a normal physiological process at the opposing end.

Axial coding took place when categories and sub-categories were linked together by using the paradigm model. This was established by determining their relationship to each other, using the 'six cs' (Glaser 1978): causes, context, contingencies, consequences, covariances and conditions. A sub-category of role modelling for example was labelled 'fitting in'. Making such connections was not always easy. For example, 'keeping quiet' was a passive reaction and consequence of being criticized. It was also a strategy students adopted for fitting in with prescriptive midwives. Similarly 'keeping quiet' was an expectation of prescriptive midwives and a characteristic or condition of submission to authority to those above them in the midwifery hierarchy. 'Cheating' was a strategy for 'fitting in' but it was also a way of practising in the hospital environment.

The process of 'selective coding' identified the core category entitled 'interpreting and using the rules'. It was this category that linked all the data together and helped to provide an explanation of how students learned the role of midwife from their role models. In retrospect this sequential coding was too prescriptive. Relationships between codes were often identified, but these sometimes changed as the core category emerged. It was only at this point in the analytic process that clarity was achieved and axial coding completed. In addition questions posed to participants facilitated the development of the core category rather than establishing the relationship between categories and sub-categories as Strauss and

Corbin (1990, 1998) suggest. Examples of questions, properties and dimensions provided by Strauss and Corbin (1990) were beneficial in offering an initial understanding of the grounded theory process. These were, however, too obvious and simplistic. Attempts to use these questions were ultimately abandoned as it meant forcing the data and inhibiting the process of discovery.

The core category

Analysis of data revealed that central to the data was the issue of how midwives interpreted and used rules to inform their practice. The way in which midwives practised, the care they gave to women, their approach to learning and teaching, the way in which students learned, and the role they learned, was determined by how their role models interpreted and used the rules. This core category was developed from 'in vivo' codes (Strauss and Corbin 1998) such as 'bending the rules' and 'the way it's always been'. The former related to how midwives adapted what they perceived to be rules when giving care, while the latter was an indication that some midwives continued to adhere to rules even when they were outdated. Hence some midwives' practice was based on traditional knowledge. In addition some open codes were formulated from my own interpretation, for example, 'sticking to the rules'. Relationships between codes were identified to form the category while properties such as following written rules, following unwritten rules, bending and breaking the rules became sub-categories.

A conditional matrix

A conditional matrix shown in Figure 9.1 illustrates how the conditions under which interactions take place when students' role models use the rules of practice influence the consequences of their actions. The way in which the rules were used defined the type of midwife, the way in which they practised and the impact of this on maternity care.

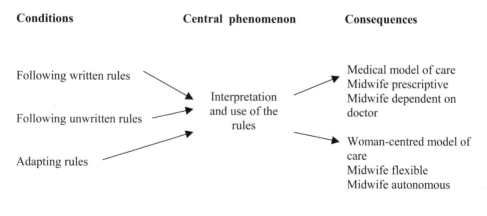

Conditions   **Central phenomenon**   **Consequences**

Following written rules

Following unwritten rules → Interpretation and use of the rules

Adapting rules →

Medical model of care
Midwife prescriptive
Midwife dependent on doctor

Woman-centred model of care
Midwife flexible
Midwife autonomous

Figure 9.1 Conditional matrix

All midwives are unique in the way they practise. What emerged from the data were two 'ideal types' that could be placed at either end of a continuum. Placement on the continuum is based on the degree of autonomy that midwives exert. The literature tends to suggest that midwives have lacked autonomy (Robinson *et al.* 1983; Askham and Barbour 1996; Begley 2001). However, even if midwives rigidly follow rules, an initial decision has to be made about which rule to follow. All midwives are therefore autonomous, but the midwives whom I labelled 'prescriptive' restricted their own practice and in doing so limited the degree of autonomy they exerted. Midwives whom I categorized as 'flexible' adjusted their practice to meet the needs of clients.

It is important to acknowledge that there are more than two types of midwife. For example, McCrea *et al.* (1998) in a qualitative study that explored midwives' approaches to the relief of pain in labour also placed midwives on a continuum. These researchers placed midwives whom they called 'cold professionals' at one end of the continuum and 'disorganized carers' at the opposite end. Midway between each end were midwives classified as 'warm professionals'. Likewise, Emmons (1993) labelled some midwives crusaders, survivors and nurse-midwives. While differences exist, all of these midwives share some similarities with prescriptive and flexible midwives.

Emerging theoretical ideas

What emerged from the data were eight theoretical ideas rather than a single theory (Bluff 2001: 218–219). The core category integrated the data and provided the basis on which these theoretical ideas were formulated.

1. When midwives rigidly follow written and unwritten rules they prescribe midwifery care which corresponds to the medical model. In doing so they act as obstetric nurses or 'handmaidens' to the doctor.
2. When everything is interpreted as rules to be followed, prescriptive midwives appear to be uncaring and detached from the experience of childbirth. The individual needs of women are not met and the relationship between midwife and client is superficial.
3. Midwives who rigidly follow the rules inhibit the growth and development of students providing them with few opportunities to achieve beyond the level of their role model.
4. Midwives are flexible when they interpret the rules for the benefit of women and provide a woman-centred model of care. These midwives therefore act as autonomous practitioners.
5. When rules are interpreted and adapted to meet the needs of women, flexible midwives demonstrate involvement in women's experiences and are empathic, supportive and caring.
6. Midwives who use their professional judgement to interpret the rules provide an environment in which senior students can become autonomous practitioners.

7. When midwives demonstrate the role of autonomous practitioner, practise a woman-centred model of care and meet the learning needs of students, they are appropriate role models and teachers.

8. When practitioners who hold opposing attitudes, values and beliefs practice together there is conflict in the clinical setting. Conflict can be avoided when flexible midwives adopt strategies that involve becoming prescriptive or practising by subterfuge.

The conditional matrix illustrates the first two of these theoretical ideas. When students work in the clinical setting they observe the way in which their role models practise. These role models also act as their teachers. By making explicit the process of how students learn the role of midwife from their midwifery role models the influence of these role models on students was uncovered. These ideas are now presented in a visual form to demonstrate the value of a diagram or theoretical framework for providing both researcher and readers with an overview and clarity of the relationship between the eight ideas and the other perspectives of students and midwives (Bluff 2001: 238). In this instance 80,000 words are condensed to a single page!

The conditional matrix and Figure 9.2 reveal the impact of how the rules are used on the way in which midwives practise and the maternity care they give to women. Figure 9.2 provides more detail and in addition reveals the conflict experienced by flexible midwives when they practise in the same setting as prescriptive midwives, and the impact these role models have on student learning and the role they adopt. It does not identify the nature of the conflict between midwives and the impact of this on morale. It is also does not make explicit students' expectations of adopting the prescriptive strategies or subterfuge to enable them to practise flexibly when they qualify hence the reality of maintaining a culture that promotes lying and subterfuge.

Since data collection was completed a number of years have passed and it is important to remember that the pace of change in the maternity services has been unremitting. Hence when applying findings to practice there is a need to take into account the results of any studies subsequent to this one.

Conclusion

Grounded theory has developed mainly as a qualitative approach in which data collection and analysis are a simultaneous process. It aims to illuminate the social processes of interaction. Interviews and observation are the preferred means of data collection. Data are coded and categorized using the constant comparative method of analysis. The emergence of a core category links the categories and sub-categories together to provide a storyline or conceptually dense theory that explains what is happening in the social setting; theory is therefore generated from the data. Theoretical sampling facilitates development of this theory and memos provide a record of the analytic process. The literature is incorporated into the data

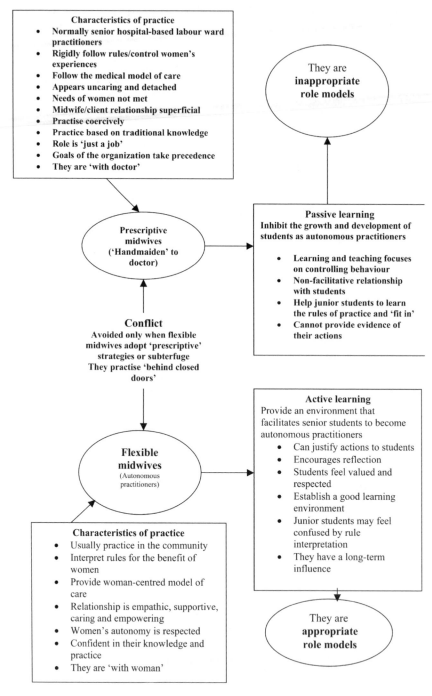

Characteristics of practice
- Normally senior hospital-based labour ward practitioners
- Rigidly follow rules/control women's experiences
- Follow the medical model of care
- Appears uncaring and detached
- Needs of women not met
- Midwife/client relationship superficial
- Practise coercively
- Practice based on traditional knowledge
- Role is 'just a job'
- Goals of the organization take precedence
- They are 'with doctor'

They are **inappropriate role models**

Prescriptive midwives ('Handmaiden' to doctor)

Passive learning
Inhibit the growth and development of students as autonomous practitioners
- Learning and teaching focuses on controlling behaviour
- Non-facilitative relationship with students
- Help junior students to learn the rules of practice and 'fit in'
- Cannot provide evidence of their actions

Conflict
Avoided only when flexible midwives adopt 'prescriptive' strategies or subterfuge
They practise 'behind closed doors'

Active learning
Provide an environment that facilitates senior students to become autonomous practitioners
- Can justify actions to students
- Encourages reflection
- Students feel valued and respected
- Establish a good learning environment
- Junior students may feel confused by rule interpretation
- They have a long-term influence

Flexible midwives (Autonomous practitioners)

Characteristics of practice
- Usually practice in the community
- Interpret rules for the benefit of women
- Provide woman-centred model of care
- Relationship is empathic, supportive, caring and empowering
- Women's autonomy is respected
- Confident in their knowledge and practice
- They are 'with woman'

They are **appropriate role models**

Figure 9.2

to confirm or refute the findings. An extended example of grounded theory has been used to illustrate many of its features.

There is debate about whether the method has been eroded or evolved. Glaser and Strauss view grounded theory from different perspectives. When undertaking a grounded theory study researchers need to make explicit the approach they have adopted. Appropriate criteria can then be used to evaluate the study.

References

Askham, J. and Barbour, R. (1996) The negotiated role of the midwife in Scotland. In Robinson, S. and Thomson, A.M. (eds) *Midwives, Research and Childbirth*. Volume 4. London: Chapman & Hall, 33–59.

Barclay, L., Everitt, L., Rogan, F., Schmied, V. and Wyllie, A. (1997) Becoming a mother – an analysis of women's experience of early motherhood, *Journal of Advanced Nursing*, 25: 719–728.

Becker, H.S., Geer, B., Hughes, E.C. and Strauss, A.L. (1961) *Boys in White: Student Culture in Medical School*. Chicago: University of Chicago Press.

Begley, C.M. (1997) Midwives in the Making: A Longitudinal Study of the Experiences of Student Midwives during their Two-Year Training in Ireland. Unpublished PhD thesis, King's College, Dublin.

Begley, C.M. (2001) Giving midwifery care: student midwives views of their working role, *Midwifery*, 17 (1): 24–34.

Bluff, R. (2001) Learning and Teaching in the Context of Clinical Practice: The Midwife as Role Model. Unpublished PhD thesis, Bournemouth University.

Blumer, H. (1971) *Sociological implications of the thoughts of G.H. Mead*. In Cosin, B.R. (ed.) *School and Society*. Milton Keynes: Open University Press, 11–17.

Chenitz, W.C. and Swanson, J.M. (eds) (1986) *From Practice to Grounded Theory: Qualitative Research in Nursing*. Menlo Park, CA: Addison-Wesley.

Clegg, A. (2003) Older South Asian patient and carer perceptions of culturally sensitive care in a hospital community setting, *Journal of Clinical Nursing*, 12 (2): 283–290.

Cluett, E.R. and Bluff, R. (2000) From practice to research. In Cluett, E.R. and Bluff, R. (eds) *Principles and Practice of Research in Midwifery*. Edinburgh: Balliere Tindall, 11–26.

Coffey, A. and Atkinson, P. (1996) *Making Sense of Qualitative Data: Complementary Research Strategies*. Thousand Oaks: Sage.

Coggins, J. (2002) From student to practitioner: a midwife's view, MIDIRS *Midwifery Digest*, 12 (1): 24–25.

Cutcliffe, J.R. (2000) Methodological issues in grounded theory, *Journal of Advanced Nursing*, 31 (6): 1476–1481.

Davies, E. (1993) Clinical role modelling: uncovering hidden knowledge, *Journal of Advanced Nursing*, 18: 627–636.

Davies, R.M. (1988) The Happy End of Nursing: An Ethnographic Study of Initial Encounters in a Midwifery School. Unpublished MSc dissertation, University of Wales, Cardiff.

Department of Health (1993) *Changing Childbirth: The Report of the Expert Maternity Group*. London: HMSO.

Department of Health (2001a) *Working together, learning together: a framework for lifelong learning for the NHS*. London: DOH.

Department of Health (2001b) *The NHS investment and reform for NHS hospitals: taking forward the NHS Plan*. London: DOH.

Dingwall, R. (1977) *The social organisation of health visitor training*. London: Croom Helm.

Dotan, M., Krulik, T., Bergman, R., Eckerling, S. and Shatzman, H. (1986) Role models in nursing, *Nursing Times*, 82 (3): 55–57, Occasional Paper.

Emmons, E. (1993) A Divided Profession: An Analysis of the Two Cultures in Midwifery Education and Practice. Unpublished PhD thesis, University of Surrey.

Freire, P. (1993) *Pedagogy of the Oppressed*, new rev. edn. New York: Continuum.

Fretwell, J.E. (1982) *Ward Teaching and Learning, Sister and the Learning Environment*. London: The Royal College of Nursing of the United Kingdom, London.

Garcia, J. and Garforth, S. (1989) Labour and delivery routines in English consultant units, *Midwifery*, 5 (4): 155–162.

Glacken, M., Coates, V., Kernohan, G. and Hegarty, J. (2003) The experience of fatigue for people living with hepatitis C, *Journal of Clinical Nursing*, 12 (2): 244–252.

Glaser, B.G. (1978) *Theoretical Sensitivity*. Mill Valley, CA: Sociology Press.

Glaser, B. (1992) *Basics of Grounded Theory Analysis: Emergence versus Forcing*. Mill Valley, CA: Sociology Press.

Glaser, B. (1998) *Doing Grounded Theory: Issues and Discussion*. Mill Valley, CA: Sociology Press.

Glaser, B. (2001) *The Grounded Theory Perspective: Conceptualization Contrasted with Description*. Mill Valley, CA: Sociology Press.

Glaser, B. and Strauss, A.L. (1965) *Awareness of Dying*. Chicago: Aldine.

Glaser, B. and Strauss, A.L. (1967) *The Discovery of Grounded Theory*. Chicago: Aldine.

Glaser, B. G. and Strauss, A. (1968) *Time for Dying*. Chicago: Aldine.

Hadikin, R. and O'Driscoll, M. (2000) *The BULLYING Culture*. Oxford: Books for Midwives, Oxford.

Hall, W. and May, A.L. (2001) The Application of Grounded Theory: Issues of Assessment and Measurement in Practice. In Schreiber, R.S. and Stern, P.N. (eds) *Using Grounded Theory in Nursing*. New York: Springer, 211–225.

Holloway, I. (1997) *Basic Concepts for Qualitative Research*. Oxford: Blackwell Science.

Hutchinson, S.A. and Wilson, H.S. (2001) Grounded Theory: The Method. In Munhall, P. (ed.) *Nursing Research: A Qualitative Perspective*, 3rd edn. Sudbury, MA: Jones and Bartlett.

Keddy, B., Sims, S.L. and Stern, P.N. (1996) Grounded theory as feminist research methodology, *Journal of Advanced Nursing*, 23: 448–453.

Kirkham, M. (1999) The culture of midwifery in the National Health Service in England, *Journal of Advanced Nursing*, 30 (3): 732–739.

Landmark, B.L. and Wahl, A. (2002) Living with newly diagnosed breast cancer: a qualitative study of 10 women with newly diagnosed breast cancer, *Journal of Advanced Nursing*, 40 (1): 112–121.

Lublin, J.R. (1992) Role modelling: a case study in general practice, *Medical Education*, 26 (2): 116–122.

Lugina, H.I., Johansson, E., Lindmark, G. and Christensson, K. (2002) Developing a theoretical framework on postpartum care from Tanzanian midwives' views on their role, *Midwifery*, 18 (1): 12–20.

McCrea, H.B., Wright, M.E. and Murphy-Black, T. (1998) Differences in midwives approaches to pain relief in labour, *Midwifery*, 14 (3): 174–180.

Mead, G.H. (1934) *Mind, Self and Society*. Chicago: University of Chicago Press.

Melia, K. (1987) *Learning and Working: The Occupational Socialization of Nurses*. London: Tavistock Press.

Morse, J.M. (2001a) Situating Grounded Theory Within Qualitative Inquiry. In Schreiber, R.S. and Stern, P.N. (eds) *Qualitative Health Research*. New York: Springer, 1–13.

Morse, J.M. (2001b) The Cultural Sensitivity of Grounded Theory. Editorial, *Qualitative Health Research*, 11 (6): 721–722.

Morse, J.M. and Bottorff, J.L. (1992) The emotional experience of breast expression. In Morse, J.M. (ed.) *Qualitative Health Research*. Newbury Park: Sage, 319–332.

Morse, J.M. and Field, P.A. (1996) *Nursing Research: The Application of Qualitative Approaches*. London: Chapman & Hall.

Nelms, T.P., Jones, J.M. and Gray, D.P. (1993) Role modeling: A method for teaching caring in nursing education, *Journal of Nursing Education*, 32 (1): 18–23.

Patton, M.Q. (2002) *Research and Evaluation Methods*, 3rd edn. Thousand Oaks, CA: Sage.

Pidgeon, N. (1996) Grounded Theory: theoretical background. In Richardson, J.T.E. (ed.) *Handbook of Qualitative Research Methods for Psychology and the Social Sciences*. The British Psychology Society, Biddles Ltd, 75–85.

Richens, Y. (2002) Are midwives using research evidence in practice? *British Journal of Midwifery*, 10 (1): 11–16.

Robinson, S., Golden, J. and Bradley, S. (1983) A study of the role and responsibilities of the midwife. NERU Report no. 1, Nursing Education Research Unit, King's College London University.

Rogan, F., Shmied, V., Barclay, L., Everitt, L. and Wyllie, A. (1997) 'Becoming a mother': developing a new theory of early motherhood, *Journal of Advanced Nursing*, 25: 877–885.

Schreiber, R.S. (2001) The 'how to' of grounded theory: avoiding the pitfalls. In Schreiber, R.S. and Stern, P.N. (eds) *Using Grounded Theory in Nursing*. New York: Springer, 55–83.

Schreiber, R.S. and Stern, P.N. (eds) (2001) *Using Grounded Theory in Nursing*. New York: Springer.

Smith, K. and Biley, F. (1997) Understanding grounded theory: principles and evaluation, *Nurse Researcher*, 4 (3): 17–30.

Stern, P.N. (1980) Grounded theory methodology its uses and processes, *Image*, 12 (1): 20–23.

Stern, P.N. (1994) Eroding Grounded Theory. In Morse, J.M. (ed.) *Critical Issues in Qualitative Research Methods*. Thousand Oaks, CA: Sage, 212–223.

Strauss, A. (1987) *Qualitative Analysis for Social Scientists*. New York: Cambridge University Press.

Strauss, A. and Corbin, J. (1990) *Basics of Qualitative Research: Grounded Theory Procedures and Techniques*. Newbury Park, CA: Sage.

Strauss, A. and Corbin, J. (1994) Grounded theory methodology: an overview. In Denzin, N.K. and Lincoln, Y.S. (eds) *Handbook of Qualitative Research*. Thousand Oaks, CA: Sage, 273–285.

Strauss, A. and Corbin, J. (1998) *Basics of Qualitative Research: Techniques and Procedures for Developing Grounded Theory*. Thousand Oaks, CA: Sage.

Travers, M. (2001) *Qualitative Research through Case Studies*. London: Sage.

United Kingdom Central Council for Nursing, Midwifery and Health Visiting (1986) *Project 2000: A new preparation for practice*. London: UKCC.

Wiseman, R.F. (1994) Role Model behaviors in the Clinical Setting, *Journal of Nursing Education*, 33 (9): 405–410.

10

SIOBHAN SHARKEY AND
JOHN AGGERGAARD LARSEN
Ethnographic exploration: participation and meaning in everyday life

Introduction

Ethnography provides an inside perspective on everyday life through the researcher's engagement with people over time and explores human experience and social interaction as well as the meaning people apply to their experiences, that is, their 'symbolic world'. An ethnographer seeks to explain overt aspects of culture, shared and on the surface, such as language, behaviour, places, actions and relationships, as well as hidden and covert elements, such as humour, silence and irony (Spradley 1980). For some researchers ethnographic pursuit can be a total life commitment to 'a people' or 'a culture', for others ethnography is a strategic approach to data collection for a specific research purpose (Leininger 1985; Morse 1994).

Ethnography can involve different qualitative and quantitative methods and has been described as:

> ... a particular method or set of methods. In its most characteristic form it involves the ethnographer participating, overtly or covertly, in people's daily lives for an extended period of time, watching what happens, listening to what is said, asking questions – in fact, collecting whatever data are available to throw light on the issues that are the focus of the research.
>
> (Hammersley and Atkinson 1995: 1)

This chapter introduces the ethnographic perspective and the evolution of the ethnographic tradition within qualitative research, including description and critique in ethnography. The key methods of data collection: participant observation and interviewing are described along with other methods such as the use of documents and diaries. The importance of writing and the ethnographic text will be discussed as well as the ongoing process of analysis. Issues relating to the utility and role of ethnography in health research and the practitioner/researcher role will also be addressed. Finally, an illustrative case highlights the methods, analysis, ethics and reflexive issues of the approach.

The ethnographic perspective

Deriving from the Greek, ethnography literally means 'writing a people'. The genre of writing ethnography is related to adventurer/merchant texts of the sixteenth century which employed the genre of '*strange adventures*' to document travels for other adventurers (Rose 1990). The account of the Polish–English anthropologist Malinowski about his time in the Trobriand Islands (1922) and his detailed documentation of the everyday life of the islanders, is usually cited as the beginning of formal ethnography. Ethnography has had many influences since the turn of the twentieth century, not least the Chicago School of Sociology (1917–1942) with its 'core ethnographies' of 'the social worlds of every day life' the reality of ordinary people and the influence of symbolic interactionism.

A characteristic of ethnography is the principle of holism aiming to capture an all-inclusive understanding of the social and cultural world of people. Cultural analysis is often presented as the main rationale for the method. Robson (1995: 148) describes the ethnographic approach as seeking to

> provide a written description of the implicit rules and traditions of a group. An ethnographer, through involvement with the group tries to work out these rules. The intention is to provide a rich or 'thick' description which interprets the experiences of people in the group from their own perspective.

Culture

Culture involves belief, ideas, values and knowledge as the shared basis of culture and is often at the centre of definitions of ethnography (Geertz 1973). Spradley and McCurdy (1972: 8) define culture as 'the knowledge people use to generate and interpret social behaviour'. For example, when we greet someone with a handshake or a kiss, we are using our cultural knowledge about behaviour in context but the rules are not always clear or shared by all members of a group. Culture is coded in symbols, the meaning of which have to be learned, be it language or behaviour.

More recently ethnographers are trying to understand (rather than describe) how culture is constructed and negotiated, paying attention to the agency of individuals and interaction between groups. Theoretical perspectives have highlighted a shift away from assumptions about culture as social coherence towards an increased recognition of differences existing within social groups, and indeed, this is reflected in contemporary usage of critical ethnography in illuminating difference in power or access to health services.

Methodology

Ethnography is an unstructured approach to research where the researcher needs to be explorative and flexible to 'follow the data', making decisions throughout the research process about what, where and when data will be collected. As the ethnographer, after the initial phases of fieldwork, develops an insider perspective and becomes more knowledgeable about the field of research, new sources of data may emerge as central and the research questions and strategy have to be adjusted accordingly. Any means for accessing social life and culture can be important to an ethnographer, including the 'bits' that are not there, where even spaces can have meaning. For example, what does it mean when some people are not talked to in certain situations; and why do only some groups of people enter certain buildings?

There is no overall consensus about which type of epistemology underpins ethnography, and different ethnographers apply different paradigms: interpretive, humanist, positivist (Hammersley and Atkinson 1995; Savage 2000). There are some key influences on ethnography which are more fully discussed in other texts (Guba 1990; Oakley 1990; Denzin 1997) and in the chapters of this book. Ethnography focuses on observations of the 'real world' (Hammersley and Atkinson 1995) and on the culture and social world of participants. More recently qualitative researchers have questioned the capacity to portray the 'real' world objectively and highlight the role of research as a means of critique, with increased attention to the role of the researcher in the production of knowledge.

Ethnography has been influenced by various approaches and philosophies such as phenomenology and symbolic interactionism which are more fully discussed elsewhere in this book, and also by naturalism – a perspective which advocates a study of the world in its natural state (opposed to 'artificial' setting of a controlled, experimental setting with its focus on objectivity, standardization and neutrality), with a prime aim being the description of the setting true to its natural form, involving actions, behaviours and contexts through eyes of 'actors' themselves. Symbolic interactionism stressed that human action is based on social meanings. People interpret events and experiences which are constantly under revision and shape action (Blumer 1969; Hammersley and Atkinson 1995). To understand we must *learn the culture* and develop theory from data (Bloor 2001; Rock 2001). Hermeneutics too has significance for the ethnographic principles of holism, context, reflexivity and 'thick description' (Geertz 1973).

Critical ethnography encompasses a model which relies on a view of the relationship between theory and practice derived from Marx and Hegel (who asserted that the goal of practice is to bring reality into line with theory). Research is seen as emancipatory (in feminist models this has largely meant the emancipation of women) – research is part of social transformation, encompassing ideals of freedom, equality and justice (Thomas 1993; Hammersley 1995).

Insider perspective

Traditionally commentators on ethnography suggest that the concept of the insider view is crucial, where ethnographers aim to uncover or 'discover' the point of view of the people or groups of people in the culture of interest. This insider or 'emic' view is in contrast to the outsider or 'etic' view which emphasizes objectivity in data collection. The insider view, on the other hand, focuses on culturally derived meanings – insider terms, meanings, rules and relationships – understanding meaning, an 'actors definition of a situation' (Schwandt 1994: 118). The ethnographer has to consider that insider views may be represented and interpreted in different ways by different people across the timeframe of a piece of research.

Reflexivity

The interpersonal nature of ethnographic research requires a reflexive approach to acknowledge the process and content of the data and knowledge that is generated. Reflexivity is crucial at every stage of the research process and identifies different relationships and perspectives: researcher, researched, readers and funders through careful recording of the processes of decision-making (Fine 1994; Aunger 1995).

Reflexivity in ethnography has three functions (also discussed in Chapter 15) (Meyerhoff and Ruby 1982; Denzin and Lincoln 1994; Aunger 1995):

1. Maintain quality and rigour within research, providing a trail of activity through diary notes, memos and other documentary evidence.
2. Acknowledge and making public the researcher's role in interpreting and producing meaning and representation of 'real world'.
3. Document decision-making around the process and product of generating and analyzing data towards theory development, a weave of the first two functions.

Ethnography is influenced by contemporary economic and socio-political issues, and ethnographers are increasingly aware of the need to reflect on and describe this as part of their research. For example: why is a certain issue studied; who has got the power; who is researching whom? The nature of relationship and interconnections between a researcher and those being researched will strongly influence generated knowledge, and the researcher can therefore be viewed as a research instrument, whose presence has a role in determining fieldwork and data (Savage 2000; Heyl 2001).

Data for ethnography do not exist independently of human intervention as discrete phenomena to be 'collected'. Rather, data are generated in an interpretive effort actively involving the ethnographer. In this sense, 'reality is socially constructed' (Berger and Luckmann 1967). Rather than trying to erase their own presence, ethnographers make sure to describe the nature of their presence through reflection on their relationships with other social actors and their roles in the social field (Adler and Adler 1987).

Goodwin *et al.* (2003: 576), for instance, document a need to manage influx of data and provide good illustration of 'everyday' dilemmas that influence decisions about data generation. Goodwin and her co-authors highlight the 'community being researched' who are not a 'passive component' and have a role in shaping the data – in this case two anaesthetists in a surgical setting who overtly held a confidential conversation within earshot while the researcher was visibly taking notes in her role as a researcher. Goodwin *et al.* also discuss decision-making as it related to dilemmas around whether the researcher should regard herself as an insider or not, and how others would perceive her.

Doing ethnography

Research design

Driven by existing theory, new questions, lack of information or a need for understanding, ethnography generally starts with broadly defined research questions that are likely to change as the research progresses, responding to encounters and experiences in the field. Ethnographers see questions and answers as integrated elements in human thinking, and new questions have the potential to emerge at any stage of the research. Ethnographic design is a trade-off between looseness and selectivity (Robson 2002).

In some research settings a stringent research design can be required to allow access and the use of focused ethnography has increased in health- and social-care research, exploring specific topics or embedded in larger multi-method designs (Morse and Johnson 1991). Focused ethnography emphasizes the importance of having a predetermined research design, providing a detailed rationale for the link between study questions, data collection and conclusions, and in this way could be seen to contradict core values of ethnography, such as the need to be flexible and holistic in order to explore the insider perspective. For example, Hornberger and Kuckelman (1998: 363) undertook a focused ethnography in a rural American state, focusing on a specific question – 'What is your vision of a health community?'; Manias and Street (2000) used a critical ethnographic approach to focus on the use of policy and protocol by nurses as a means of mediating communication between doctors and nurses. This topic-specific approach differs from that which commences with a broad area of interest, where a specific topic emerges and is explored further, for example, in Pols' (2003) study of two psychiatric hospitals in Holland, where the issue of 'modes of doing good' was raised and enabled exploration of the specific tensions between judicial and caring traditions.

Research focus and sampling

In preparing to 'enter the field' the researcher needs to consider how to access data sources in order to address theoretical issues and research aims, dependent on theoretical interests, practical issues and opportunities for participation (Spradley 1980; Hammersley and Atkinson 1995). Settings vary in terms of content and boundaries, and the researcher must make decisions between breadth and depth of investigation as the focus of the work will be shaped by both the researcher's initial interests, and ongoing encounters, influencing specific cases selected. Sometimes research can be opportunistic, driven by a timely or critical issue within a specific setting. For practitioners in health- and social-care settings, opportunities may arise in relation to new interventions or systems of working. Both practitioners and service users are in an ideal position to undertake ethnographic work as 'insiders'; however, to avoid the danger of bias and 'blind spots', a theoretically and methodologically informed 'outsider' perspective is valuable. The ethnographer is constantly balancing insider and outsider perspectives.

A researcher will not be interested in everything, but will select 'cases' across or within settings. These can be theoretically or practically driven, or used in combination. The most important issue in sampling for qualitative research is to cover variation and make sure that different situations and views are represented in the data – also called maximum variation sampling (Patton 2001). In contrast to the statistical generalization allowed by a representative sample, this sampling strategy allows for theoretical generalization in the data analysis (as we will discuss below). Similarly, when taking a grounded theory approach (Glaser and Strauss 1967; Strauss and Corbin 1998) 'theoretical sampling' can be used when the selection of cases is designed to produce categories and identify relationships to each other. Glaser and Strauss undertook research on dying in hospital settings and illuminated issues of awareness, expectation and rates of dying through examining cases in different hospital settings – intensive-care patients; cancer patients; neo-natal babies (Glaser and Strauss 1968). Sampling within cases is also part of the ethnographer's decision trail: when to observe, talk, what to ask, what to record in fieldnotes. Researchers may identify clusters, networks, units or similarities within settings and may identify recurring activities, places, people and times which begin to signify categories of meaning within the group or culture (Spradley 1980; Hammersley and Atkinson 1995; Lofland and Lofland 1995). In this way homogeneity, variation and contextuality are considered.

In health research, especially when the ethnographer is a practitioner, it is important to be aware that informants may approach the researcher for therapeutic reasons, and it may be difficult, and arguably unethical, for the researcher to separate out roles. Research by one of the authors with family carers of people with mental illness living in remote settings in the Highlands of Scotland, raised a dilemma relating to whether to provide information about local services to family carers, when it was obvious that this service would help (Sharkey 2004). Researchers on the other hand may select whom to interview, and choices about sampling within a setting or group may be uncertain. Often decisions about 'who', 'when' and 'how many' are taken repeatedly during the course of the fieldwork and are determined by the researchers aims (initially broad, increasingly selective), previous encounters and practical or access considerations.

Access, role and ethics

Ethnographers who are not already part of the settings they want to study will have to gain access, which is rarely straightforward. Gaining access can be very time consuming depending on issues such as whether it is an open or closed setting; the researchers relationship with the setting and gatekeepers as well as political, ethical and legal issues. Gatekeepers are not neutral to the research setting and gaining access through a gatekeeper is likely to influence not only access to data within the setting, but also how the researcher is perceived by informants. Using a gatekeeper indicates a social alliance and the status and role of the gatekeeper is therefore likely to be 'carried' by the researcher in the research setting, at least initially. In some circumstances a particular study may prove not to be feasible and the setting will have to be abandoned or the researcher may find new research questions which can be studied in the setting. In addition, the dual role as practitioner and researcher can be difficult to manage (Goodwin *et al.* (2003) as highlighted

LIBRARY
EDUCATION CENTRE
PRINCESS ROYAL HOSPITAL

earlier). Preliminary visits and analysis can help both an assessment of the suit-ability of a setting and shaping of the research questions. Who is willing to talk within a setting will also shape the research (Hammersley and Atkinson 1995).

Lofland and Lofland (1995) provide useful guidance on getting into settings, highlighting differences between public or open settings and closed settings. In open settings anyone has the right to be there and might traditionally include places like airports and hospital corridors – but recent terrorist threats and public perceptions of 'safety' have changed the status of these sorts of areas. In closed settings not just anyone is granted access. Health- and social-care settings will vary but are increasingly 'closed' settings. Covert research in public and open settings may have as many ethical issues as research in pre-planned, 'deep-cover' type scenarios (Lofland and Lofland 1995). Even for a researcher negotiating access, whether to go in as an 'outsider' or 'insider' will raise questions about ethics. In health care, stringent ethical application procedures and research governance requirements are adopted from biomedical research to safeguard the rights of research participants and it is highly unlikely that a covert study would be approved.

Overt or covert

Traditionally covert research is viewed as being undertaken without due awareness and consent from 'subjects', where there are ethical questions relating to privacy, confidentiality, autonomy and potentially harmful consequences when an indivi-dual becomes aware of research. However, recently it has been acknowledged that in many research situations it can be difficult to be certain of consent and understanding on the part of those being researched, the participants. There is a sense in which all research is covert to an (unknown) extent, in that a researcher cannot always be certain that their explanations of the reasons for their work are fully understood by those being researched. Does signed consent mean under-standing? It has been observed that '[a]ll research lies on a continuum between overtness and covertness' (Murphy and Dingwall 2001: 342). Particularly in ethnography, with little control over settings and those in them, it is not always practical for the researcher to obtain full consent at the very start from everyone who may ultimately contribute to a study.

Participant observation

A distinction is often made between types of observation – participant and non-participant. However, the notion of non-participant observation is contentious by contradicting knowledge of social interaction, as when standing quietly and observing in a corner the researcher is likely to influence the social dynamic and cultural meaning by being present in the minds of the other actors. Participation suggests some kind of interaction or role on the part of the ethnographer but it is often difficult to determine the exact degree or type. A researcher may go through a spectrum of activity in the course of a piece of research: complete observer; observer as participant; participant as observer and complete participant

(Hammersley and Atkinson 1995). Stressing the researcher's social identity rather than activity in the setting, it can be useful to describe different types of membership roles taken by the researcher: peripheral member, active member or complete member (Adler and Adler 1994). An extreme version of the complete membership role is called 'going native' – in this situation the researcher totally identifies with the people and culture and the critical analytic 'outside' perspective is weakened.

The individual's perception of the researcher will crucially influence access to data. It is important to consider social significance of different groups and individuals and the symbolic and social meaning of particular types and styles of clothing, dialects or mannerisms. Ethnographers have reported how even their body posture can be changed through fieldwork to match that of the people they studied. Cultural knowledge is not only a set of belief systems but is fundamentally embodied (Csordas 2002; Merleau-Ponty 2002 [1945]), as also recognized by the concept of habitus formulated by Bourdieu (1990). As ethnographer you use 'your self' in the widest sense and through the process of fieldwork significant social and cultural knowledge is often embodied in the researcher. This is a key feature of ethnography as it challenges the prevalent rationalist body–mind separation of traditional scientific positivist discourse. Some ethnographers engage in auto-ethnography to explore the experiential aspects of this process of embodiment by using their personal experiences with the engagement in the social and cultural life as the principal data for analysis (Berger 2001; Ellis 2002).

Ethnographic observation takes place in natural settings, among actors in everyday life, aiming to identify meaning to people in that setting, seeking culturally and socially meaningful questions to ask. The researcher has to be able to open up to the newness in surroundings to become 'ethnographically aware' – tuning in, seeing and hearing in a new way. Spradley (1980: 55) talks about the researcher needing to be 'explicitly aware' to overcome years of 'selective inattention'. Observation varies within a setting, initially broad-based but becoming more focused as the researcher spends more time in a setting. This type of funnel structure can help shape theoretical development of the research (see later discussion on analytical process). In everyday life we act subconsciously – 'cultural rules' are implicit. However, as a participant observer, who 'appears' as an ordinary participant, there are differences in terms of thought processes. Spradley (1980) lists six major differences: dual purpose, explicit awareness, wide-angle lens, insider–outsider experiences, introspection and record keeping. The participant observer aims to be both a participant in activities as well as an observer of people, activities and physical aspects of the context – at the same time. Being able to 'do' and observe at the same time requires awareness and attending skills. Researchers use introspection to access embodied knowledge and increase understanding about the process and context of generating data. This means heightened senses which can be tiring for researchers, particularly if they are trying to take in a broad field, and they need to be aware of the potential for stress. The researcher needs to be self-aware about presentation of self, and the dangers of being over-friendly or the 'going native' (as discussed earlier).

Listening to the talk between people in a research setting is a crucial resource for generating data from everyday life. Accepting that there will be some kind of influence from the researcher on the data and trying to understand this in context is part of the reactivity of research. 'Influence' is well illustrated in Leyser's (2003) research in an American psychiatric hospital, where she reflects on the impact of being a woman researching in a predominantly male setting. Trying too hard to minimize influence may indeed be counter-productive in blocking sources of data while merely introducing a different kind of bias into the study (Hammersley and Atkinson 1995). Ethnographers need to be comfortable to use themselves actively to generate data and provide 'thick descriptions' of cultural and social meanings when reflexively describing their involvement in the setting.

Ethnographic interviewing

In combination, participant observation and interviews help illuminate each other. Ethnography utilizes a broad range of interview forms. Informal interviews occur spontaneously in everyday settings, such as talking in the office or ward or at team meetings, and are good opportunities to ask questions relevant to research aims – the dividing line between participant observation and interviews is therefore blurred (Spradley 1979; Hammersley and Atkinson 1995). While taking part in such social interactions an ethnographer is careful to memorize details and, as soon as possible, record them accurately as fieldnotes. Ethnographic interviewing is also associated with formal depth interviews with key informants as a means of eliciting rich material relating to experiences (Lofland and Lofland 1995). Having enough time to explore meaning and perspective is crucial, whether an encounter is spontaneous and informal or pre-arranged, formal and private.

The more formal the interview situation, the more likely that perspective will be removed from actions in natural settings. On the other hand, the formal interview can provide insights into an informant's private experiences and thoughts that would rarely be revealed under other circumstances. The importance of individual interviews is manifest in person-centred ethnography, focusing on the individuals and how their experiences both shape, and are shaped by, social and cultural processes (Hollan 2001). As will be described in more depth later, one of the authors utilized longitudinal in-depth interviews with fifteen users of a mental-health service in order to capture their changed experiences and perceptions over a two-and-a-half-year period (Larsen 2002a).

Issues of power and the researcher–informant relationship will influence what is shared during the interview (both of these may be particularly pertinent if the researcher is also a practitioner or clinician or is perceived as such). The first few minutes of an interview can be crucial in helping to establish a relationship, and how one presents oneself is influential. Building trust and rapport is particularly important where there has been little or no previous participant observation. The researcher needs to take time to provide reassurance relating to anonymity, confidentiality and opportunity to withdraw. Reasons for the study and issues relating to tape-recording and note taking will all help the interviewee understand what is going on. Throughout the interview active listening is crucial where the interviewer responds appropriately, both verbally and non-verbally to what is being said and shows acceptance to the interviewee.

Both the interviewer and informant have roles and responsibilities within the interview and these can shift as the interview or research progresses, especially if the researcher returns time and again to the same interviewee. The setting of an interview may also affect the exchange. How relaxed is it? Whose territory is it? Who is in control? Informants may not wish to be interviewed in their own homes for any number of reasons, and a more neutral setting can be identified. There may be no choice over setting, which might not be physically suited to a long interview process. There may be more than one person and the presence of others will affect and transform the interview. This is illustrated by research of one of the present authors, where a married couple initially asked to be interviewed together. At times what they said and their body language indicated that they were reluctant to go into details in order to 'protect' their partner. This became such an issue for them that they requested that the author return and interview them separately, which she did (Sharkey 2004). Such methodological 'practicalities' are in themselves meaningful events to be recorded, reflected on and analyzed as ethnographic data.

Ethnographic and other qualitative interviewing is characterized by 'open questions' used as prompts. Spradley (1979) talks about 'grand tour' and 'mini-tour' questions the former being broad, open questions, the latter more focused and likely used later in an interview. It is not likely that every informant will be asked exactly the same questions, but the same topics may be covered. While remaining flexible, an interviewer may want to 'nudge' the interview in a particular direction and may use more focused questions or clarifying questions to do so. Is the information detailed enough? Does something said earlier still need clarifying? Has the informant gone off down another (possibly more interesting or relevant and previously unforeseen) route? What to ask and where to go with the interview will be constantly under review and decisions may need to be made 'on the hoof'. This type of flexibility is crucial to the ethnographic approach in order to identify questions which are meaningful for the inside perspective. Focus group interviews have developed as a distinct method that pays attention to group dynamics and how the researcher can utilize these for specific data collecting purposes. (See Chapter 4 on focus groups for more detail.)

Data recording must be managed within the context of an interview about what is said, the context of the interview and about decisions made by the interviewer as to the direction of the interview (discussed later in relation to writing and fieldnotes). Interviewing is an exercise then in multi-tasking, which improves with practice, and is made easier by the process of audio-recording. Audio-recording also needs managing, both in terms of ethics (permissions, etc.) and practicalities – equipment, location, timing and ultimately transcribing and storage as transcribed audio-recordings take on the format of documents and need to be organized and analyzed in this form. Hammersley and Atkinson (1995) suggest that audio-recording has clear advantages over notes of verbal encounters and interviews but may be perceived as intrusive and cause more problems than it solves. If an interviewee is uncomfortable with audio-recording the researcher has to be prepared to rely solely on note-taking.

Additional data sources

Ethnographers can make use of other qualitative (or quantitative) methods available. Plurality of methods is encouraged by the data validation principle of triangulation as well as the holistic perspective of ethnography. Additional data sources enable the researcher to profile the social complexity of research settings. Quantitative methods are not in the 'core tool box' of all contemporary ethnographers, but they can be very useful. For example, a survey can access the views of a large population and allows the researcher to demonstrate how various views relate to socio-economic and other significant variables. Ethnographers increasingly involve their informants in participatory research activities which have the potential to generate different types of data and can help to overcome traditional difficulties related to representation: who has the power to make analysis and present research findings? Research can be emancipatory by involving the informants as active partners. It can also be a means to challenge the 'lone-ranger style' of traditional ethnographies (Sanders 1999; Trujillo 1999) by involving informants in collaborative data generation, analysis and presentation.

Solicited and unsolicited documents and other media may form an additional source of data for a study and can take a wide variety of forms – diaries, poetry, video, photographs and biographies (Harper 2003; Hodder 2003). Data can come from official sources such as (in health settings): case notes, policy documents, meeting notes, manuals and shift schedules. Again, in health research, access and ethical issues will need to be carefully addressed. Hammersley and Atkinson (1995) point out that documentary sources should be viewed as social products, open to bias and should not be relied on uncritically as research resources. Solicited documents such as diaries can also be important sources, particularly relating to aspects of life that are inaccessible or not open to observation. Diaries are a particularly useful source of data in relation to health and illness experiences, for example as observational logs followed by in-depth interviews, as part of a mixed method design or as an exploration of patient or family experiences (Zimmerman and Wieder 1977; Kelleher and Verrinder 2003; Sharkey 2004).

Analyzing data

Ethnographic writing

Writing occurs in different ways throughout the research process in the form of fieldnotes, memos and analytical notes. Fieldnotes form the backbone of participant observation and represent the living evolution of a piece of research in that it is with fieldnotes that the researcher's selections and interpretations are documented and developed. A researcher will identify what he or she regards as 'significant' and hence make selections about how subsequent inquiry is shaped. Fieldnotes are descriptive and cumulative and never form a 'complete picture' and can supplement tape recording. Fieldnote writing should happen as close to interactions and observations as possible without being intrusive. Different types of language and perspectives may need to be reflected within fieldnotes and records of speech should be verbatim where possible, distinguishing between people's own 'emic' terms and observers' 'etic' terms (that is, analytical concepts), ensuring that these differences are 'retrievable'. In this sense fieldnotes are as much about organizing data for retrieval and analysis as a record of fieldwork.

The content of fieldnotes, along with observations, is likely to become more focused as the researcher spends more time in the setting, and pertinent issues and relationships emerge. As analysis progresses with ideas and themes developing, the understanding of what is 'meaningful' will also change, and this will be reflected in the writing. In order to communicate the experiences, values and meanings of people in a setting, the researcher must transform them into the written word and thereby change them. When writing researchers are 'discovering' new things about their field of inquiry, and the choice of language and words helps researchers to bring knowledge and information to the reader. Writing can provide a forum for critical distance, what Jenkins (2002: 12) has also called *epistemological objectivity*. Postmodernist thinking has illuminated how writing is a creative and analytic process – and, as such, a method of inquiry (Richardson 2003) – where experience, knowing and language are intertwined in the personal narrative (Ellis and Bochner 2003). Here it is possible to see how production of the text and analysis in ethnography are interwoven.

Analytical processes

Central to the endeavour of ethnography is the intention to depict the lives and world views of other people and cultures. Analytical aids ensure that the ethnographer's personal experiences and insights have wider validity by integrating different perspectives and data sources in a holistic inquiry. Analysis is ongoing and progressive, interwoven with and shaped by data generation. Analysis cannot be separated from theory or the overall aims of the research and is a process of asking questions of the data and checking how the answers might be interpreted to make sense. Analysis can perhaps best be described in hermeneutic terms as a dialectic movement between data and theory, being shaped and reshaped as knowledge expands and deepens (Gadamer 1989 [1960]). This is why ethnographers, possibly more often than other researchers, can be seen to abandon their initial research aims and, in the middle of their research, formulate radically new questions to investigate. It relates to the point made earlier that ethnographic research is not just seeking answers to questions but, more radically, looking to ask the right questions.

As ethnographic data generally are captured as text, common methods of analysis and data management work with 'free flowing text' in a process of coding, identifying themes and concepts and building conceptual models (Ryan and Russell 2003). Initial organizing or indexing of data can influence subsequent analysis and development of ideas. Spradley (1980) provides a framework for organizing data to identify context by specifying: spaces (physical/places); actors (people); activity (related acts); objects (physical things); acts (single things that people do); events (related activities that people carry out); time (sequences); goals (things people are trying to accomplish) and feeling (emotions felt and expressed). However, not all information can be captured by 'arbitrary' frameworks and the researcher needs to remain open to alternative perspectives (Hammersley and Atkinson 1995). It is important that the ethnographer uses personally experienced insights to guide the analytic process to avoid it developing into a formalistic procedure where the 'sense of life' is lost.

Coding needs to take account of emerging, and potentially changing categories, and data can be allocated to more than one category, which can also change as the analysis proceeds. It is a good idea to keep a 'logbook' on the development of the coding categories and to describe the purpose and content of each code. When codes are either separated into sub-codes or merged, the analytic rationale should be described in the logbook. This procedure provides transparency and enables the researcher to track the development of the coding system.

Analytical notes (sometimes called theoretical notes, see Emerson *et al.* 2001) are important for the next stage of analysis, when 'analytical categories' are identified. The researcher records emerging ideas when reading through data and should regularly 'pull together' analytical notes to make sense of where ideas are going. It can be helpful to make case-specific analytic notes, for example, when analyzing an interview transcript. This allows the researcher to capture insights related to the specific situation in which these data were generated. This process can also be recorded in the logbook as 'analytical memos' which provide reflections on the progress of the ideas in the research. Taking time to reflect on the direction of the analysis is important, although it is often difficult to find sufficient time during parallel fieldwork. Asking questions relating to emerging categories allows the researcher to explore what is theoretically/empirically of interest – a process also called 'funnelling' (Spradley 1980; Hammersley and Atkinson 1995). Whether sorted and stored on computer, using analytical headings (annotated data segments stored as index cards under developing themes) or making physical copies and storing them in different category files, analysis moves on from this initial stage to identifying patterns and relationships within the data.

Hammersley and Atkinson (1995) advise that researchers keep their 'analytical nerve' in tolerating uncertainty and ambiguity in their early readings of text, looking for anything that is interesting or different or reflects a pattern in the data. This is where jotted notes in the field or analytic notes can help the researcher keep the threads of what is interesting and related within the data. The researcher aims to identify common and unexpected experiences that take the data beyond the specific person's experience and says something more about the experience or context. Sometimes observer-identified concepts emerge, where participants provide phrases or words which exactly capture an experience and which can ring true with other participants experiences and stories (Lofland and Lofland 1995). These emerging or 'sensitizing' concepts (Blumer 1954) themselves are altered through the emergence of new codes within new or previous data, until the researcher begins to identify 'stable' sets of categories based on coding of the full range of data (Hammersley and Atkinson 1995).

Identification of relations between categories enables the analysis to move beyond the case to develop models and hypotheses in interpreting the data in a dialogue with existing analytical concepts and theories – that is, theoretical generalization (Patton 2001). The focusing process moves the researcher from descriptions of what is happening towards developing theories or ideas about patterns and relationships. This is illustrated in the example that follows where Larsen's work focused on the concept of 'symbolic healing'. These more analytical categories can themselves then be integrated into a model to be tested and further developed. Ethnography has been used to develop and test theory, but depending on the researcher's epistemological position views differ on the role of theory in data analysis. Arguably, theory testing in itself should not be seen as an end-point of ethnography, but as part of a ongoing process of testing and further development of ideas as indicated by the dialectic back-and-forth movement between data and theory. Constant referral back to the data is essential to enable clarification and to testing of assumptions – allowing the researcher to check the validity of his or her interpretations. Researchers can use a variety of sources to check interpretations and ensure that these are grounded in the data and perceptions of participants. Hammersley and Atkinson (1995) identify social context, time and people as useful dimensions. This means investigating whether the interpretation applies to different social situations and spaces in the field; whether different groups of people have different or similar views and experiences; and whether the interpretation is valid over the entire period of time the research was conducted. Checking with participants or other researchers as to the 'fit' of the concepts is also a useful strategy. However, caution must be exercised as participants' views can change over time or their rationale for being involved may alter, or they might have a specific interest in promoting a particular view or 'finding'. Validatory activities cannot be regarded as achieving 'truth'. Nevertheless, triangulation as such allows the researcher to check interpretations from different perspectives – the participants, the role and impact of the researcher as well as the methods chosen (this will be discussed more fully in Chapter 15).

The management of textual data can be aided by the use of CAQDAS – Computer Assisted Qualitative Data Analysis – where computer programs such as NUD*IST (Fielding 2001) and NVivo (Richards 1999) enable the researcher to code/segment, store and manage data. Such computer programs can be an immense help when trying to oversee huge amounts of data, as are usually generated in ethnography (Hammersley and Atkinson 1995; Fielding 2001). It is, however, important to stress that the use of computer programs to manage data does not eliminate the active interpretive role of the researcher. Safeguards against the dangers of decontextualization when retrieving data according to analytic codes can be secured by making strategic use of the aforementioned case-specific analytic notes. Equally, the researcher has to consider carefully the dangers of becoming absorbed in the alluring technicalities of a potentially endless analytic process, continuously working to improve and refine coding categories. In the analytic process there is a fine balance to be struck between time spent on primary data analysis when reading, coding, organizing, re-coding and re-organizing data and the time spent on secondary data analysis when exploring the meaning of data in relation to existing theoretical frameworks and seeking to develop new theoretical understandings.

Policy and practice

Given its descriptive and model development capacities, how does ethnography feature in relation to practice and policy development in health and social care? Practitioners and service users within health- and social-care settings have most to gain from ethnography, and indeed there is a growing body of writing which reflects this (see Greene's discussion (2003: 610) on the organizational learning potential of involving stakeholders in the process of research). Although Hammersley (1992: 125) suggests that ethnography should be general and not specifically related to policy and practice development, he goes on to list some of the strengths of ethnography in relation to policy development: taking account of diversity and change over time; documenting beliefs and behaviour behind the public front; using multiple sources of evidence and having the potential to discover unanticipated aspects of policy development.

Due to the lack of statistical generalizability of ethnographic findings and the prevalent dominance of a realist and positivist paradigm in the policy field, Bloor (2001) comments that the role of ethnography in contributing to policy development will remain small. Ethnography does, however, have a role in helping to change practice. Bloor's (1997) own work on therapeutic communities led directly to practice change. There appears to be a growing appreciation of the value of ethnographic research in health and social care. By detailing social and cultural processes in treatment and support and by analyzing the involvement of different institutions and professional groups ethnography can improve our understanding of the ways in which complex interventions work. To this end researchers and policy developers are increasingly recognizing the utility of ethnography and other qualitative methods to assist the traditional use of randomized controlled trials (Campbell *et al.* 2000; Savage 2000).

Example of an ethnography: a case study

Experience and identity processes in a mental-health intervention

The field

This case study presents an ethnography of a mental-health service for early intervention in psychosis. The social and the health sectors in the Danish capital, Copenhagen, collaborated to provide community-based intensive treatment and support over a two-year period for people aged 18 to 45 who for the first time had experienced psychosis or other serious mental illness within the 'schizophrenic spectrum' (WHO 1993).

Access and role

I was employed as internal programme evaluator in the social sector of the Municipality of Copenhagen to document the social aspects of the intervention. This position gave me an active membership role in the setting (Adler and Adler 1987). Over the same period I was registered as a PhD student of sociological studies at the University of Sheffield. These two roles strengthened my independence as researcher while at the same time complicating the insider–outsider characteristic of my position. The research was carried out over a four-year period and altogether I spend about two years in the field.

Entering the field

My first day in the job as evaluator was 1 April 1998. It was a Wednesday. I met with my new colleagues at half-past eight in the morning in a Community Mental Health Centre in the outskirts of Copenhagen. I felt slightly overdressed in my shirt and jacket since everybody else around the table dressed more casually. To fit in better I would later leave the jacket in the closet and put on a pullover instead. On my request, to immerse myself in the setting and be directly involved in the day-to-day activities of the intervention, I moved my office from an administrative building in the city centre to share offices with three other staff members. Throughout the fieldwork I engaged on a daily basis with my clinical colleagues and took part in the weekly social 'breakfast meeting' in a team as well as the regular meetings between leaders and staff. In the first months of my employment I sought to gain further understanding of my colleagues' backgrounds and motivations through informal conversations and individual interviews. I also handed out notebooks to all staff members for them to make observations and thoughts on their work to strengthen their reflexivity. I presented the research openly and collaboratively.

Becoming ethnographically aware

Even if the broader cultural context of the fieldwork, Danish society, as well as the location of my hometown Copenhagen, was familiar to me, the institutional context of psychiatry and experiences with mental illness were 'remote areas' to me (Ardener 1987). I was 'a stranger' in the field, and the individual experiences as well as the cultural practices that were revealed to me were unfamiliar and in many instances disturbing. Writing in my fieldwork diary helped me to deal with the experiences and, at the same time, maintain a critical stance towards the psychiatric perspective on mental illness. As I became familiar with the language, meanings and implicit rules of interaction I was able to provide more in-depth and detailed descriptions. I developed an insider perspective. However, I did not attempt to take a role as clinical practitioner in the service. This was primarily because of my research interest in the clients' perspectives and experiences to examine identity processes in the course of the social and health intervention (cf. Csordas 1994; Jenkins 1996).

Person-centred ethnography and methodological flexibility

Using participant observation to study the clients' perspectives was problematic. First, I had already been identified as evaluator and my credibility as 'client' would therefore be dubious. Second, the interventions were largely based on individual treatment and support through medication and weekly contact with a case manager and this made a research strategy based on identification with the group of clients ineffective. Third, the role as 'client' could have been bad for my health, since identification as 'mentally ill' in some instances can be inappropriately convincing (Estroff 1981; Scheff 1999). The final reason has a wider methodological implication for the ethnographic research strategy: I wished to gain an existential phenomenological (Csordas 2002; Merleau-Ponty 2002 [1945]) understanding of ways in which the intervention affected the clients in their particular life circumstances after having experienced serious mental illness for the first time. Not having had such extreme experiences myself, the mere assumption of the role as a 'client' would be lacking validity since the experiential depth of the experiences of the clients would be missing. For example, when a person engages in therapy and takes psychotropic drugs what is the personally felt reason for doing so? Ethnographic description of social interactional rules and cultural meaning needs to consider the existential position and biographical details of the individuals who take part. The life perspective of human beings is not restricted to the here-and-now but includes the persons' previous experiences and future hopes and expectations. For these reasons, my research did not allow a predominant reliance on an autoethnographic approach (Berger 2001; Ellis 2002) where the ethnographer primarily uses her or his personal experiences to gain insights into cultural meaning.

My solution to the methodological challenge was to take a person-centred approach which Hollan (2001) suggests and seek insight into the perspectives of the clients themselves. In the autumn and winter of 1998 I asked fifteen new clients if they would like to be interviewed. I approached them through their case managers and presented them with a letter of consent detailing the type and extent of their involvement and guaranteeing their right to withdrawal and anonymity in any subsequent publications. I had presented my research proposal to the Danish Medical Research Ethics Committee but was advised that the non-therapeutic and social science nature of my research did not require their approval (this would, however, be different if the research had been conducted in the UK where an extensive procedure of research ethics approval has to be completed prior to any research activity in a health-care setting). When selecting informants I followed a maximum variation strategy to consider gender, age and allocation to various case managers. Over a two-and-a-half-year period I arranged five series of interviews which were audio-recorded and transcribed. The last interview took place about six months after they had left the service and it allowed them to look back on the experience. The longitudinal design allowed me to ask questions as they were relevant to the phase they were going through in their engagement in the intervention and I could establish a biographical link between issues we had discussed previously (Larsen 2003). To engage less formally with my informants I invited them to take part in a book project where they could write about their experiences with mental-health problems and mental-health treatment. My role in this participatory project was that of a facilitator. Eight of my fifteen key informants came to at least one of the sixteen meetings we held in the book group during my last year of fieldwork and seven wrote about their personal experiences. An independent Danish publisher published six of the stories as a book (Larsen 2002b).

Multi-method approach

Throughout the period of fieldwork I used different methods of data generation. I obtained historical letter correspondence and early project drafts describing the intervention's institutional creation and I interviewed people from different organizations about their involvement and the political context. I sent out two series of surveys to question users and their relatives about their views on the treatment and support. I arranged for my colleagues to fill in time registration forms on their work as case managers, requested them to provide me with written narratives of their work and ran focus groups where staff exchanged views on various aspects of the intervention. I also carried out focus group interviews with clients and clients' relatives about their views on the intervention. I observed meetings between case managers and clients, and over a period of two months I took part in different types of therapeutic groups. These methods presented different perspectives on the intervention.

Data management

It helped me to manage the wealth of data by working towards the deadlines of the half-yearly evaluation reports I had to produce for the steering group. To clearly identify and separate the purposes of the evaluation and my research was also useful. The evaluation required factual data to describe activities and the views of different actors in the field and the analysis was purposively directed towards a clinical and political context. Information obtained through my key informants provided the core of my research, exploring their experiences with psychosis, hospitalization, relations to family and friends, psychotropic medication, various therapeutic interventions and their struggles to re-engage in their personal life projects (Larsen 2002a). In this way, the ethnography led to two different products – and a third was created through the participatory process in the book project.

Analysis and the role of theory

I used the computer software NVivo (Richards 1999) to manage the analysis of data by coding text sections from transcripts and comparing data over time as well as between individuals. This combination of case and cross-case analytic strategies (Patton 2001) allowed me analytically to construct general themes that became more apparent as I became increasingly familiar with literature on the history of mental-health treatment, and studies in the disciplines of Medical Anthropology and Medical Sociology. The theoretical perspectives and analytic concepts allowed me to identify structures and processes at work in the intervention. One example was the concept 'symbolic healing' which I first came across during my last year of fieldwork (Kleinman 1988; Csordas 1994, 2002; Helman 2000). The concept provides an analytic framework for understanding how non-medical therapies work in different cultural settings to influence individuals to experience recovery and hope for their future lives. Stages in the process of symbolic healing and the strategies of the healers clearly described what was going on in Danish mental-health intervention. The theoretical perspectives allowed me to demonstrate how the intervention influenced the clients on an individual level, not only by giving them treatment and support to control symptoms and avoid relapse, but also by changing their understandings of experiences of mental-health problems and treatment (Larsen 2004b). The new understanding worked through minimizing their ontological insecurity by developing their sense of biographical continuity and establishing a new sense of self and their future lives (Larsen 2004a).

Conclusion

Ethnography can be used in health-care research as a means of problem solving as well as comparison and evaluation, its role being to illuminate, understand and ultimately interpret and present a range of perspectives – patients', carers', practitioners' and commissioners'. It is powerful in demonstrating cultural and social dynamics in social settings and can thereby uncover implicit values and unspoken rules of social interaction, presenting challenges for issues of access, applicability, ethics and funding. Ethnographers do not claim to reveal 'the truth', but aim to represent and provide a window to experiences, cultural values and social interaction in an honest and accessible way.

It is perhaps appropriate to conclude with the view of the editors of one of the most comprehensive books written on ethnography, *Handbook of Ethnography* (Atkinson *et al.* 2001). Given the diversity of approaches, methods and applications in ethnography, the editors do not feel that it is useful to try and equate ethnography with one disciplinary tradition, indeed, flexibility is seen as one of its core strengths. They remind readers of the utility of ethnographic methods across many fields of research – health, education, social care. Not all researchers claim to be undertaking 'ethnographies' while using methods familiar to ethnographers – participant observation, interviews, diaries and focus groups and the editors of *Handbook of Ethnography* reaffirm the centrality of participant observation in the method, the rooting of ethnography in 'first hand exploration of research settings' (p. 5). This is what sets it apart from other qualitative methods.

References

Adler, P.A. and Adler, P. (1987) *Membership Roles in Field Research*. Newbury Park, CA: Sage.

Adler, P.A. and Adler, P. (1994) Observational techniques. In Denzin, N.K. and Lincoln, Y.S. (eds) *Handbook of Qualitative Research*. Thousand Oaks, CA: Sage, 377–392.

Ardener, E. (1987) Remote areas: Some theoretical considerations. In Jackson, A. (ed.) *Anthropology at Home*. London: Tavistock, 38–54.

Atkinson, P., Coffey, A., Delamont, S., Lofland, J. and Lofland, L. (eds) (2001) *Handbook of Ethnography*. Thousand Oaks, CA: Sage, 177–187.

Aunger, R. (1995) On ethnography: storytelling or science? *Current Anthropology*, 36 (1): 97–130.

Berger, L. (2001) Inside out: narrative autoethnography as a path towards rapport, *Qualitative Inquiry*, 7 (4): 504–518.

Berger, P. and Luckmann, T. (1967) *The Social Construction of Reality: a Treatise in the Sociology of Knowledge*. Hamondsworth: Penguin.

Bloor, M. (1997) Addressing social problems through qualitative research. In Silverman, D. (ed.) *Qualitative Research, Theory, Method and Practice*. Thousand Oaks, CA: Sage, 221–238.

Bloor, M. (2001) The Ethnography of Health and Medicine. In Atkinson, P., Coffey, A., Delamont, S., Lofland, J. and Lofland, L. (eds) *Handbook of Ethnography*. Thousand Oaks, CA: Sage, 177–187.

Blumer, H. (1954) What is Wrong With Social Theory? *American Sociological Review*, 19 (1): 3–10.

Blumer, H. (1969) *Symbolic Interactionism*. Englewood Cliffs, NJ: Prentice Hall.

Bourdieu, P. (1990) *The Logic of Practice*. Cambridge: Polity Press.

Campbell, M., Fitzpatrick, R., Haines, A., Kinmonth, A.L., Sandercock, P., Spiegelhalter, D. and Tyrer, P. (2000) Framework for design and evaluation of complex interventions to improve health, *BMJ*, 321: 694–696.

Csordas, T.J. (1994) *The Sacred Self: A Cultural Phenomenology of Charismatic Healing*. Berkeley, CA: University of California Press.

Csordas, T.J. (2002) *Body/Meaning/Healing*. Basingstoke and New York: Palgrave Macmillan, 100–137.

Denzin, N.K. (1997) *Interpretive Ethnography*. Thousand Oaks, CA: Sage.

Denzin, N.K. and Lincoln, Y.S. (1994) (eds) *Handbook of Qualitative Research*. Thousand Oaks, CA: Sage.

Ellis, C. (2002) Shattered lives: making sense of September 11th and its aftermath, *Journal of Contemporary Ethnography*, 31 (4): 375–410.

Ellis, C. and Bochner, A.P. (2003) Autoethnography, Personal Narrative, Reflexivity: Researcher as Subject. In Denzin, N.K. and Lincoln, Y.S. (eds) *Collecting and Interpreting Qualitative Materials*. Thousand Oaks, CA: Sage, 119–258.

Emerson, R.M., Fretz, R.I. and Shaw, L.L. (2001) Participant observation and fieldnotes. In Atkinson, P., Coffey, A., Delamont, S., Lofland, J. and Lofland, L. (eds) *Handbook of Ethnography*. Thousand Oaks, CA: Sage, 352–368.

Estroff, S.E. (1981) *Making it Crazy: An Ethnography of Psychiatric Clients in an American Community*. Berkeley: University of California Press.

Fielding, N. (2001) Computer applications in qualitative research. In Atkinson, P., Coffey, A., Delamont, S., Lofland, J. and Lofland, L. (eds) *Handbook of Ethnography*. Thousand Oaks, CA: Sage, 453–467.

Fine, M. (1994) Working the hyphens: Reinventing self and other in qualitative research. In Denzin, N.K. and Lincoln, Y.S. (eds) *Handbook of Qualitative Research*. Thousand Oaks, CA: Sage, 70–82.

Gadamer, H.-G. (1989 [1960]) *Truth and Method*. London: Sheed & Ward.

Geertz, C. (1973) *The Interpretation of Cultures*. London: Fontana Press.

Glaser, B. and Strauss, A. (1967) *The Discovery of Grounded Theory*. Chicago: Aldine.

Glaser, B. and Strauss, A. (1968) *Time for Dying*. Chicago: Aldine.

Goodwin, D., Pope, C., Mort, M. and Smith, A. (2003) Ethics and ethnography: An experiential account, *Qualitative Health Research*, 13 (4): 567–577.

Greene, J.C. (2003) Understanding Social Programs Through Evaluation. In Denzin, N.K. and Lincoln, Y.S. (eds) *Handbook of Qualitative Research*. Thousand Oaks, CA: Sage, 981–999.

Guba, E.G. (1990) (ed.) *The Paradigm Dialog*. Newbury Park, CA: Sage.

Hammersley, M. (1992) *What's Wrong with Ethnography?* London: Routledge.

Hammersley, M. (1995) *The Politics of Social Research*. London: Sage.

Hammersley, M. and Atkinson, P. (1995) *Ethnography. Principles in Practice*, 2nd edn. London: Routledge.

Harper, D. (2003) Reimagining visual methods: Galileo to Neuromancer. In Denzin, N.K. and Lincoln, Y.S. (eds) *Collecting and Interpreting Qualitative Materials*. Thousand Oaks, CA: Sage, 176–198.

Helman, C.G. (2000) *Culture, Health, and Illness*, 4th edn. Oxford: Butterworth Heinemann.

Heyl, B.S. (2001) Ethnographic interviewing. In Atkinson, P., Coffey, A., Delamont, S., Lofland, J. and Lofland, L. (eds) *Handbook of Ethnography*. Thousand Oaks, CA: Sage, 369–383.

Hodder, I. (2003) The interpretation of documents and material culture. In Denzin, N.K. and Lincoln, Y.S. (eds) *Collecting and Interpreting Qualitative Materials*. Thousand Oaks, CA: Sage, 155–175.

Hollan, D. (2001) Developments in person-centred ethnography. In Moore, C.C. and Mathews, H.F. (eds) *The Psychology of Cultural Experience*. Cambridge: Cambridge University Press, 48–67.

Hornberger, C.A. and Kuckelman, C.A. (1998) A rural vision of a healthy community, *Public Health Nursing*, 15 (5): 363–369.

Jenkins, R. (1996) *Social Identity*. London: Routledge.

Jenkins, R. (2002) *Foundations of Sociology: Towards a Better Understanding of the Human World*. Basingstoke and New York: Palgrave Macmillan.

Kelleher, H. and Verrinder, G. (2003) Health Diaries in a Rural Australian Study, *Qualitative Health Research*, 13, 435–443.

Kleinman, A. (1988) *Rethinking Psychiatry: From Cultural Category to Personal Experience*. New York: Free Press.

Larsen, J.A. (2002a) Experiences with Early Intervention in Schizophrenia: An ethnographic study of assertive community treatment in Denmark. PhD thesis, Department of Sociological Studies, University of Sheffield.

Larsen, J.A. (2002b) (ed.) *Sindets Labyrinter – Seks beretninger fra mødet med psykiatrien*. København: Hans Reitzels Forlag.

Larsen, J.A. (2003) 'Identiteten: Dialog om forandring'. In Hastrup, K. (ed.) *Ind i Verden: En grundbog i antropologisk metode*. Copenhagen: Hans Reitzels Forlag, 247–271.

Larsen, J.A. (2004a) Becoming mentally ill: existential crisis and the social negotiation of identity. In Jenkins, R., Jessen, H. and Steffen, V. (eds) *Managing Uncertainty: Ethnographic Studies of Illness, Risk and the Struggle for Control*. Copenhagen: Museum Tusculanum Press.

Larsen, J.A. (2004b) 'Finding meaning in first episode psychosis: experience, agency, and the cultural repertoire', forthcoming in *Medical Anthropology Quarterly*, 18 (4).

Leininger, M.M. (1985) *Qualitative Research Methods in Nursing*. Philadelphia, PA: W.B. Saunders.

Leyser, O. (2003) Doing masculinity in a mental hospital, *Journal of Contemporary Ethnography*, 3 (23): 336–359.

Lofland, J. and Lofland, L. (1995) *Analysing Social Settings: A Guide to Qualitative Observation and Analysis*, 3rd edn. Wadsworth.

Malinowski, B. (1922) *Argonauts of the Western Pacific*. London: Routledge & Kegan Paul.

Manias, E. and Street, A. (2000) Legitimation of nurses' knowledge through policies and protocols in clinical practice, *Journal of Advanced Nursing*, 32 (6): 1467–1475.

Merleau-Ponty, M. (2002 [1945]) *Phenomenology of Perception*. London and New York: Routledge Classics.

Meyerhoff, B. and Ruby, J. (1982) Introduction. In Ruby, J. (ed.) *A Crack in the Mirror: Reflexive Perspectives in Anthropology.* Philadelphia: University of Pennsylvania Press, 1–35.

Morse, J.M. (1994) (ed.) *Critical Issues in Qualitative Research Methods.* Newbury Park, CA: Sage.

Morse, J.M. and Johnson, J.L. (eds) (1991) *The Illness Experience: Dimensions of Suffering.* Newbury Park, CA: Sage.

Murphy, E. and Dingwall, R. (2001) The ethics of ethnography. In Atkinson, P., Coffey, A., Delamont, S., Lofland, J. and Lofland, L. (eds) *Handbook of Ethnography.* Thousand Oaks, CA: Sage, 339–352.

Oakley, A. (1990) Interviewing women: a contradiction in terms. In Roberts, H. (ed.) *Doing Feminist Research.* London: Routledge & Kegan Paul, 30–61.

Patton, M.Q. (2001) *Qualitative Evaluation and Research Methods,* 3rd edn. Newbury Park, CA: Sage.

Pols, J. (2003) Enforcing patient rights or improving care? The interface of two modes of doing good in mental health care, *Sociology of Health and Illness,* 25 (4): 320–347.

Richards, L. (1999) *Using NVivo in Qualitative Research,* 2nd edn. Melbourne: Qualitative Solutions and Research.

Richardson, L. (2003) Writing: A method of inquiry. In Denzin, N.K. and Lincoln, Y.S. (eds) *Collecting and Interpreting Qualitative Materials.* Thousand Oaks, CA: Sage, 499–541.

Robson, C. (1995) *Real World Research.* Oxford: Blackwell.

Robson, C. (2002) *Real World Research,* 2nd edn. Oxford: Blackwell.

Rock, P. (2001) Symbolic interactionism and ethnography. In Atkinson, P., Coffey, A., Delamont, S., Lofland, J. and Lofland, L. (eds) *Handbook of Ethnography.* Thousand Oaks, CA: Sage, 26–38.

Rose, D. (1990) *Living the Ethnographic Life.* Newbury Park: Sage.

Ryan, G.W. and Russell, H. (2003) Data management and analysis methods. In Denzin, N.K. and Lincoln, Y.S. (eds) *Collecting and Interpreting Qualitative Materials.* Thousand Oaks: Sage, 259–309.

Sanders, C.R. (1999) Prospects for a post-postmodern ethnography, *Journal of Contemporary Ethnography,* 28 (6): 669–675.

Savage, J. (2000) Ethnography and health care, *BMJ,* 32: 1400–1402.

Scheff, T. (1999 [1966]) *Being Mentally Ill: A Sociological Theory,* 3rd edn. New York: Aldine de Gruyter.

Schwandt, T.A. (1994) Contructivist, Interpretivist Approaches to Human Inquiry. In Denzin, N.K. and Lincoln, Y.S. (eds) *Handbook of Qualitative Research.* Thousand Oaks, CA: Sage, 118–137.

Sharkey, S. (2004) *An exploration of the experiences of family carers of people with serious mental health problems living in the Highlands of Scotland.* Final Report, University of Stirling.

Spradley, J.P. (1979) *The Ethnographic Interview.* New York: Holt, Rinehart & Winston.

Spradley, J.P. (1980) *Participant Observation.* New York. Holt, Rhinehart & Winston.

Spradley, J.P. and McCurdy, D.W. (1972) *The Cultural Experience: Ethnography in Complex Society.* Chicago: Science Research Associates.

Strauss, A. and Corbin, J. (1998) *Basics of Qualitative Research: Techniques and Procedures for Developing Grounded Theory.* Thousand Oaks, CA: Sage.

Thomas, J. (1993) *Doing Critical Ethnography.* Newbury Park, CA: Sage.

Trujillo, N. (1999) Teaching Ethnography in the Twenty-first Century Using Collaborative Learning, *Journal of Contemporary Ethnography*, 28 (6): 705–719.

World Health Organization (1993) *The ICD-10 Classification of Mental and Behavioural
Disorders: Diagnostic Criteria for Research.* Geneva: World Health Organization.

Zimmerman, D.H. and Wieder, D.L. (1977) The Diary: Diary–Interview Method, *Urban
Life*, 5 (4), 479–498.

11

ANDREW C. SPARKES
Narrative analysis: exploring the *whats* and *hows* of personal stories

Introduction

According to Lieblich *et al.* (1998: 1), 'During the last 15 years, the concepts of narrative and life story have become increasingly visible in the social sciences.' Likewise, Roberts (2002: 115) states that the narrative study of lives 'has become a substantial area for analyses of life experience and identity as connected to social groupings, situations and events'. All of this has led Denzin (2003: xi) to suggest the following:

> We live in narrative's moment. The narrative turn in the social sciences has been taken ... Everything we study is contained within a storied, or narrative representation. Indeed, as scholars we are storytellers, telling stories about other people's stories. We call our stories theories.

Not surprisingly, for Horrocks *et al.* (2003) these developments in the social sciences have led to a growing interest in narrative theorizing and a recognition of the value of this kind of research in a range of health arenas, such as nursing, primary care, psychotherapy, and bioethics. Indeed, for Riessman (2003), the last decade has seen a burgeoning literature on the illness narrative in the social sciences. For her, this development recognizes 'the importance of subjective reality in adaptation to chronic illness: how disease is perceived, enacted and responded to by the "self" and others' (p. 7). In support of this, Bury (2001: 263) points out that 'Illness narratives, particularly those of patients or lay people, are a particular focus in health related setting.'

As part of the 'narrative turn' scholars have begun to treat seriously the view that people structure experience through stories, and that a person is essentially a storytelling animal. This has led to a more sophisticated appreciation of people as active social beings and focused attention on the way personal and cultural realities are constructed through narrative and storytelling. Indeed, Somers (1994) notes that scholars have suggested that social life is itself storied and that narrative is an *ontological condition* of social life.

Their research is showing us that stories guide action; that people construct identities (however multiple and changing) by locating themselves or being located within a repertoire of emplotted stories: that 'experience' is constituted through narratives; that people make sense of what has happened and is happening to them by attempting to assemble or in some way to integrate these happenings within one or more narratives; and that people are guided to act in certain ways, and not others, on the basis of the projections, expectations, and memories derived from a multiplicity but ultimately limited repertoire of available social, public, and cultural narratives.

(Somers 1994: 614)

Narrative analysis and qualitative research

Qualitative researchers have become increasingly interested in narrative forms of inquiry because, according to Polkinghorne (1995: 5), narrative is the 'linguistic form uniquely suited for displaying human existence as situated action. Narrative descriptions exhibit human activity as purposeful engagement in the world.' For Cortazzi (1993), McAdams (1993), McLeod (1997), Murray (1999) and Crossley (2000) a story not only imparts information about the inner world of the storyteller or the person(s) about whom the story is being told but it also reveals a great deal about the identity, intentions, and feelings of the person telling the story.

Indeed, as Murray (2003: 116) points out, narratives also provide a structure for our very sense of selfhood and identity, 'we tell stories about our lives to ourselves and to others. As such we create a narrative identity.' Furthermore, Miller (1994) argues that personal stories, based on remembered experiences, are an important site for the social construction of self in which facets of self and various identities are projected and maintained over time. For her, selves, like cultures, 'are not so much preserved in stories as they are created, reworked, and revised through participation in everyday narrative practices that are embedded in and responsive to shifting interpersonal conditions' (pp. 175–176).

Of course, as Lieblich et al. (1998) acknowledge, the relationship between identity and narrative is extremely complex and multifaceted. They emphasize that no story is unidimensional in its voices, and identity can have many components and layers. Despite this complexity they argue that since identity is a narrative construction, then narrative forms of analyses are well suited to understanding this phenomenon. As such, Riessman (2002) suggests, narrative analysis allows for the systematic study of personal experience and meaning and is very useful for exploring the active, self-shaping qualities of human thought, and the power of stories to create and refashion identity. She goes on to point out that, 'Narratives are a particularly significant genre for representing and analyzing identities in its multiple guises and different contexts' (p. 707).

In a similar fashion, Cortazzi (1993: 2) argues that narrative analysis can be seen as 'opening a window on the mind, or, if we are analysing narratives of a specific group of tellers, as opening a window on their culture'. Therefore, a focus upon narrative can be used to explore individual *and* group subjectivities. As Riessman (1993) notes, for the sociologically orientated investigator, studying narratives is useful for what they reveal about social life in that culture 'speaks itself' through an individual's story: 'It is possible to examine gender inequalities, racial oppression, and other practices of power that may be taken for granted by the individual speakers. Narrators speak in terms that seem natural, but we can analyse how culturally and historically contingent these terms are' (p. 5). This is because, as Murray (1999: 53) points out, 'Narratives do not, as it were, spring from the minds of individuals but are social creations. We are born into a culture which has a ready stock of narratives which we appropriate and apply in our everyday social interaction.'

The potential for narrative studies to explore the links between identities and culture has been recognized in the field of health and illness. For example, Robinson (1990: 1173) notes, with regard to individual subjectivities, 'Narrative analysis of personal accounts provide valuable access to the personal world of illness.' Steffen (1997: 99), in discussing illness narratives, supports this view but also suggests that by contextualizing meaningful events 'personal narratives contribute to the understanding of individual experience as part of general social relations and cultural values, making them useful as cultural data in general'. In summarizing the analytic possibilities, Bury (2001: 264) states 'on the one hand the exploration of chronic illness narratives may throw light on the nature of disrupted experience, its meanings and actions taken to deal with it. On the other hand, the study of such narratives has the potential to reveal a wider set of important issues to do with the links between identity, experience and "late modern" cultures.'

In emphasizing the dialectic between the individual and the cultures they inhabit, Frank argues that while people tell their own unique illness stories, they compose these stories by adopting and combining narrative types that cultures make available to them. In commenting on this social aspect of narrative he states:

> The ill body's articulation in stories is a personal task, but the stories told by the ill are also *social*. The obvious social aspect of stories is that they are told *to* someone, whether that other person is immediately present or not ... From their families and friends, from the popular culture that surrounds them, and from the stories of other ill people, storytellers have learned formal structures of narrative, conventional metaphors and imagery, and standards of what is and is not appropriate to tell. Whenever a new story is told, these rhetorical expectations are reinforced in some ways, changed in others, and passed on to affect others' stories.
>
> (Frank 1995: 3)

Personal stories of health and illness, therefore, are both personal and social at the same time. As Coffey and Atkinson (1996: 61) pointed out, 'Although the reported biographical events may be unique to the individual, they are structured according to socially shared conventions of reportage.' They go on to argue that qualitative analysis is as much about *how* things are said as about *what* is said, and emphasized that 'storytelling is culturally situated and relies for its success on culturally shared conventions about language and the hearing of stories' (p. 77).

This view is supported by Gubrium and Holstein (1998, 2000), and Holstein and Gubrium (2000). In making their case for a better understanding of *narrative practice*, they advocate a reflexive analytic approach that enables us to focus alternately on the *what*s and the constitutive *how*s of social life, allowing us to shift our attention from the substantive or the contextual to the artful components of reality construction and back again. For them, a focus on narrative practice allows us to maintain a focus on the interactional accomplishment of local realities in terms of, for example, the ways in which stories about experience are presented, structured, and made to cohere, while also allowing us to maintain an awareness of the institutional and cultural conditions that shape this accomplishment. Thus, questions about why a story is told in certain ways (the *how*s) are asked in relation to questions about its plot and content (the *what*s), as these are equally important in understanding how meaningful interaction transpires.

With the above points in mind, attention can now be turned to the delights and dilemmas of narrative *analysis*. First, it needs to be recognized that there are a number of ways to analyze the stories we collect as researchers. As Coffey and Atkinson (1996: 80) remark, 'There are no formulae or recipes for the "best" way to analyse the stories we elicit and collect. Indeed, one of the strengths of thinking about our data as narrative is that this opens up the possibilities for a variety of analytic strategies. Such approaches also enable us to think beyond the data to the ways in which accounts and stories are socially and culturally managed and constructed.' Indeed, a number of excellent texts are now available that not only introduce the philosophical and literary background to the concept of narrative, but also illustrate a number of different ways to analyze narrative material (e.g. see Riessman 1993, 2002; Lieblich *et al.* 1998; Crossley 2000; Roberts 2002; Murray 2003).

Accordingly, in the sections that follow my aspirations will be modest. The focus will be on personal accounts or stories told about disruptive life events, such as illness. Painting with broad strokes, I will consider three ways in which these stories can be analyzed to incorporate the *what*s and the *how*s of their telling. These are an analysis of structure and form, an analysis of content, and an analysis of how the narrative operates and is performed. In each section, exemplars will be provided to give a flavour of how each kind of analysis works. The first two sections of what follows consider the analysis of structure and form along with the content analysis. Here, the focus is mainly on the *what*s of narrative. In contrast, the third section, considers approaches that focus on the *how*s of narrative. Having said this, the boundaries I have created, and the sections I have allocated specific studies to are rather artificial as many of the studies called upon use more than one lens for their analytical purposes.

Analysis of structure and form

According to Riessman (1993: 18), 'Like weight bearing walls, personal narratives depend on certain structures to hold them together.' Likewise, Coffey and Atkinson (1996: 57) point out that 'narratives have rather specific, distinct structures with formal and identifiable properties.' Thus, for Murray (2003), a particular concern in narrative analysis is how the narrative is structured or organized. Addressing issues of structure and form are important because, as Lieblich *et al.* (1998) remind us, the formal aspects of structure, as much as the content, express the identity, perceptions, and values of the storyteller, 'analysing the structure of a story will therefore reveal the individual's personal construction of his or her evolving life experience' (p. 88). Furthermore, the choice of narrative genre a person adopts can have a strong influence on the kind of story he, she or they are likely to tell.

One scheme for analyzing the structure of a narrative is provided by Gergen and Gergen (1983). For them, one essential aspect of narrative is the capacity to generate directionality among events; that is, 'to structure events in such a way that they move over time in an orderly way toward a given end' (p. 257). They take as their starting point four basic forms or genres of narrative: the *romance*, the *comedy* or *melodrama*, the *tragedy*, and the *satire*. According to Lieblich *et al.* (1998: 88) these can be described as follows:

> In the 'romance,' a hero faces a series of challenges en route to his goal and eventual victory, and the essence of the journey is the struggle itself. The goal of 'comedy' is the restoration of social order, and the hero must have the requisite social skills to overcome the hazards that threaten that order. In 'tragedy', the hero is defeated by the forces of evil and ostracised from society. Finally, the 'satire' provides a cynical perspective on social hegemony.

Exploring the sequential shifts found in each of these four basic forms, Gergen and Gergen (1983) note that what they have in common are shifts in the evaluative character of events over time. With this as their starting point, they proceed to identify three forms of narrative in relation to the development of the plot over time. These are the *stability, progressive* and *regressive* narratives as represented in Figure 11.1. In the *stability* narrative, the plot is steady and does not change over time. In the progressive narrative, the plot advances steadily over time. In contrast, the plot of the regressive narrative indicates deterioration and decline over time.

For Gergen and Gergen (1983: 259), 'Theoretically one may envision a potential infinity of variations on these rudimentary forms. However ... the culture may limit itself to a truncated repertoire of possibilities.' For example, the tragedy tends to be a progressive narrative followed by a rapid regressive narrative, while the comedy–melodrama is the reverse: A regressive narrative is followed by a progressive narrative. Accordingly, as Murray (2003: 121–122) emphasizes, this classification scheme is a useful analytic tool, 'but it is important not to apply it in a schematic way but in a flexible manner so as to encapsulate the various shifts in any narrative account'.

Structure and form analysis in action

An example of the flexible use of the scheme developed by Gergen and Gergen (1983) is provided by Robinson (1990) in his study of the personal narratives of fifty people with multiple sclerosis (MS). Importantly, having taken the three

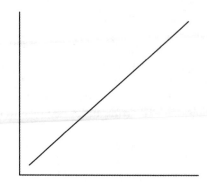

Progressive narrative

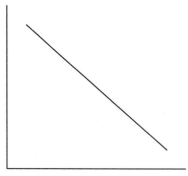

Stability narrative

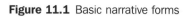

Regressive narrative

Figure 11.1 Basic narrative forms

LIBRARY
EDUCATION CENTRE
PRINCESS ROYAL HOSPITAL

broad forms of the stable, progressive and regressive narratives to provide an initial framework for his analysis, he proceeds to reveal that the patterning of the life stories of those with MS involves considerable sophistication and complexity both within and beyond these three broad narrative forms. His findings are also surprising. For example, the most frequently expected narrative in relation to life stories centred on a chronic condition like MS is the *tragedy*. Here, the progressive achievement of life goals, is interrupted and dramatically reversed following the onset of chronic illness. However, Robinson found that only 10 per cent of the accounts embodied such a narrative. Furthermore, within this narrative type, he found that three of the five told a variation called a *sad* narrative: 'Such narratives have a continuously negative slope away from life goals, perhaps accelerating as they progress' (p. 1183).

In contrast, Robinson (1990) found that the majority (52 per cent) of his sample, told positive or progressive narratives, and that these contained a *range* of narrative patterns that related to positive views of the self. He identifies the *heroic* narrative, the *implicitly heroic* narrative, the *detective* story, and four narratives frames that centred on the intervention of the supernatural. Against this, 20 per cent of his sample told stable narratives, while 18 per cent could not be classified as using any form. For Robinson, the value of the kind of analysis he applied lies in its ability to reveal how the meaning of illness is constructed over time and the ways in which this shapes how people live their lives. As he suggests, understanding the frameworks or structures of personal narratives 'is a way of both providing a complementary and insightful analysis of illness in relation to sickness and disease, and of clearly indicating the close association between illness and life' (p. 1185).

More recently, against the backdrop of heroic, tragic, ironic and comic, and regressive/progressive narratives, Bury (2001) offers a framework for studying chronic illness narratives that suggests three broad forms or types that need to be considered. The first of these is the *contingent* narrative. This involves explanations of illness onset that deal with its 'proximate' causes, and the practical and disabling effects of symptoms on the body, self and others. *Moral* narratives provide accounts of the changing relationships between the person, the illness and social identity, introducing an *evaluative* dimension into the links between the personal and the social. Here, Bury notes, 'valuations enter the picture, as sufferers seek to account for and perhaps justify themselves in the altered relations of body, self and society brought about by illness' (p. 274). Finally, *core* narratives reveal the connections between the layperson's experience and deeper cultural levels of meaning attached to illness and suffering. A focus on the core form brings to our attention what is explicit and what is hidden in narratives in ways that may not always be comprehended by those constructing them.

A focus on the *form* of illness narratives is also evident in the work of Frank (1995). For him, a narrative type is the most general storyline that can be recognized underlying the plot and tensions of particular stories. Three typical narratives types or genres are identified. The first, most prominent, and culturally preferred narrative in Western cultures is the *restitution* narrative. Here, the plot has the basic storyline: 'Yesterday I was healthy, today I'm sick, but tomorrow I'll be healthy again.' According to Frank, this storyline is filled with talk of tests and their interpretation, treatments and possible outcomes, the competence of doctors, and alternative treatments: 'Metaphoric phrases like "good as new" are the core of the restitution narrative. Such phrases are reflexive reminders of what the story is about: health' (p. 77). The teller of this kind of narrative wants the former predictability of the body back and with it the former sense of self that they had about themselves. Within the story, the body tends to be viewed as a machine in need of fixing. Thus, the temporarily broken-down body becomes an 'it' to be fixed and the self is dissociated from the body.

As Frank (1995: 90) points out: 'The purpose that restitution narratives aim toward is twofold. For the individual teller, the ending is to return to just before the beginning: "good as new" or status quo ante. For the culture that prefers restitution stories, this narrative affirms that breakdowns can be fixed.' Not surprisingly, therefore, as Kleinman and Seeman (2000) suggest, this narrative emphasizes positive responses and outcomes, 'it is a story of coping with illness, rebuilding the body self, and remoralisation. It may also be evoked in the construction of patients or, even more, of doctors as heroes of the illness experience. These are stories with happy real or projected endings' (p. 238).

The second narrative type identified by Frank (1995) is the *chaos* narrative. The plot of this narrative imagines life never getting better and so it is the opposite of the restitution narrative. Such stories are chaotic in their absence of narrative order and lack of plot. They are anxiety provoking and threatening both for the teller and the listener. Often, the ill person telling chaos stories defines him or herself as being swept along, without control, by life's fundamental *contingency*. For sure, efforts have been made to reassert the predictability of the former bodyself but these efforts have failed, and each failure has had its costs. Therefore, while contingency is not exactly accepted, it is taken as *inevitable*. Thus, the characteristics of chaos narratives are disorder, distortion, fragmentation, threat, anguish, and uncontrollability.

In contrast to the restitution narrative that attempts to outdistance mortality by rendering illness transitory, and the chaos narrative that is sucked into the undertow of illness and the disasters that attend it, is the *quest* narrative. According to Frank (1995: 115), 'Quest stories meet suffering head on; they accept illness and seek to *use* it. Illness is the occasion for a journey that becomes a quest. What is quested for may never be wholly clear, but the quest is defined by the ill person's belief that something is to be gained from the experience.' Here, the biographical disruption or disruptive life event is reframed as a challenge and an opening to other ways of being. Such stories often tell of the search for alternative ways of being ill.

As the ill person comes to realize a sense of purpose, Frank (1995: 117) argues, then the idea that illness has been a journey emerges: 'The meaning of the journey emerges recursively: the journey is taken in order to find out what sort of journey one has been taking.' Importantly, quest stories are about being transformed, and the teller being given something by the experience of illness, that is then passed on to others in the telling. As Kleinman and Seeman (2000: 238) note, these narratives emphasize either the 'search for cure (sometimes expressed through the turn towards experimental treatment of non-biomedical alternatives) or the search for meaning and transcendence within and through illness'.

Reflecting on his proposal that there are 'types' of illness narrative that individual stories somehow fit into, Frank (1995) is aware of the risk of creating yet another 'general unifying view' that subsumes the particularity of individual experience. Thus, he cautions that no actual telling of an illness experience conforms exclusively to any of the three narrative types, and that in any illness *all* three narrative types can be told, alternatively and repeatedly. He feels that the advantage of using his typology is that it encourages closer attention to the stories that ill persons tell. That is, they are to be used as *listening devices*, as an aid to listening to the ill: 'Listening is difficult because illness stories mix and weave different narrative threads. The rationale for proposing some general types of narratives is to sort out those threads' (p. 76).

Kleinman and Seeman (2000) also suggest that these narrative types are best understood as guideposts rather than rules to which every narrative must conform. As they point out, 'individuals' narratives may even participate in different genres at different points in their telling. In addition, it is important to understand that this shifting emplotment of different narrative genres may actually help to transform illness experience over time' (p. 238). This said, they emphasize that from a clinical perspective, it is important to understand what conventions of genre a patient may be presuming and how that may affect her or his outlook and actions.

The benefits for the care of others that can accrue from soliciting, listening to, and recognizing the *form* of illness narratives has been noted by others, such as Brock and Kleiber (1994), who focus on the narrative structure of the illness stories told by seventeen injured, elite collegiate athletes. Their analysis suggests that if health-care professionals are open to hearing the injured athlete's complete illness narrative, they could expect a story structure that approximates the following:

A prologue – includes some form of celebration of the athlete's gifts, the recognition of high school performance.

Chapter 1 – choosing the university at which best to express athletic gifts; usually preparing for a future self as athlete, sometimes pursuing education toward an additional possible future self.

Chapter 2 – collegiate participation in sport and the injury episode – either the injury is incremental and invisible or sudden and apparent (with consequences for the themes in later chapters).

Chapter 3 – rehabilitation and the decision about, and attempts to return to, active sport participation.

Chapter 4 – the recognition of the career-ending nature of the injury/disease and the decision to stop.

Chapter 5 – the experience of loss – with feelings of confusion, isolation, guilt, bitterness, disconnectedness (in various combinations and degrees), along with the feeling of relief for some ... The stories told by those currently in college end with chapter five, leaving it to the reader/listener to imagine a future resolution.

Chapter 6 (in stories told from a distance of nearly 20 years from the injury episode) – places the injury in a context and addresses how this disruption to their then-life-narrative has influenced its authorships since.

(Brock and Kleiber 1994: 417–419)

For Brock and Kleiber (1994), an awareness of this narrative structure and where the athlete is positioned in it, has the potential to enhance the clinician's ability to identify those whose illness experience will be most problematic. This, in turn, would allow them to anticipate the shape of that problematic experience so that prompt interventions to modify the course of distress could be made and thereby allow for more rapid rehabilitation. Brock and Kleiber's analysis of a particular illness narrative points to the more general benefits of a narrative perspective for medicine to complement the biomedical view. For them like the other scholars considered above, 'taken together as complimentary, an analysis of the patient's illness narrative and a biomedical assessment can bring the suffering person fully into clinical focus and anticipate roadblocks to and avenues for healing' (p. 427).

Content analysis

According to Lieblich et al. (1998), the narrative materials of life stories may be processed analytically by breaking the text into relatively small units of content and submitting them to either descriptive or statistical treatment. This is normally called *content analysis* in which 'the original story is dissected, and sections or single words belonging to a defining category are collected from an entire story or from several texts belonging to a number of narrators' (p. 12). This said, Lieblich et al. note that the method of content analysis has many variations, depending on the purpose of the study and the nature of the narrative materials. Preference for one variation or another is also related to the researcher's adherence to 'criteria of objectivity and quantitative processing, on the one hand, as opposed to hermeneutic and qualitative perspectives on the other' (Lieblich et al. 1998: 112).

Importantly, as Holloway (1997: 35) emphasizes, 'It is not easy to distinguish between different forms of content analysis.' Likewise, various kinds of content analysis can be used in conjunction with an analysis of the form and structure of narratives as described in the previous section of this chapter. These points need to be born in mind in reflecting on the following exemplars.

Content analysis in action: exemplars of narrative research

Davies (1997) provides the first exemplar in her study of one of the main existential problems faced by people living with an HIV positive diagnosis. This involves the disruption of their routine orientation towards time, and the ways in which this has the capacity to affect their lives more generally.

As part of a larger study, Davies (1997) draws on data generated by semi-structured interviews with thirty-eight participants who have been living with an HIV positive diagnosis for at least five years. The existential temporal dimension of these participants' situation was explicitly addressed in one question within the interview schedule but was also 'implicitly evident over the whole course of the interview due to the overwhelming influence of temporal assumptions' (p. 564). Accordingly, the first step in her analysis entailed a careful reading of the transcripts with a view to capturing the essence of this experience. The second step involved categorizing each individual in terms of one of three predominant forms of temporal orientation discernible from the interviews. Thus, 55 per cent of her participants were deemed as having experienced a renewed understanding of their concepts of time, meaning, and values so as to be *living with a philosophy of the present.*

In contrast, 18 per cent of the participants embodied a strategy of minimization that involved 'active denial' insofar as they were determined not to let their HIV positive diagnosis 'ruin' the plans that they had in the past, and held for the future. This temporal orientation was classified as *living in the future.* Finally, a substantial proportion of the participants, 26 per cent, had not been able to compensate for the loss of their routine understanding of themselves and their place in it by adopting either of the previously mentioned temporal orientations. Rather, these people were *living in the empty present.* As part of her interpretation, Davies (1997) points out that the 'empty present' perspective is less conducive to effective adaptation than either the 'philosophy of the present,' or the 'future orientated' perspectives. Furthermore, she argues, it is likely that those who operate with an 'empty present' temporal perspective will be in most need of help in adapting to life with an HIV positive diagnosis.

The way that time operates within life stories in relation to disruptive life events or biographical disruption has been explored using a content analysis *and* an analysis of form by Sparkes and Smith (2003). Drawing on data from a life history study of a small group of fourteen men who have experienced spinal cord injury and become disabled through playing sport, they focus on the lives of three of the men. Utilizing concepts and models of time from a range of scholars within biographical research and narrative studies, they examined the transcripts of the thematic interviews to see when and where they were evident in the data. They illustrate how the three men experienced time in a similar *cyclical* fashion prior to SCI when they inhabited disciplined, dominating, and able bodies, were physically active, and heavily involved in the contact sport of rugby football union. Likewise, each experienced the moment of their SCI as *immortalized* time, and their period in rehabilitation as *ruptured* time.

Beyond the context of rehabilitation, however, the three men experienced time in very different ways. Sparkes and Smith (2003) suggest that at this point, each of the men adopts a different narrative form that exerts a powerful influence on how they story and understand time in their lives post-SCI as disabled men. The narrative forms identified are those of restitution, chaos, and quest as defined by Frank (1995) and discussed earlier in this chapter. Thus, time is experienced variously within the restitution narrative as *waiting* time and *consumed* time. A *philosophy of the future* also operates that can incorporate the time tenses of the *past in the future*, the *present in the future*, and the *future in the past*. Time experienced in such ways connects the individual to notions of a restored and entrenched self that has its reference point firmly in the past.

In contrast, shaped by the chaos narrative, time is experienced as *static*, biographical time *stops*, and life is understood as occupying an *empty present*. Within this narrative, the time tense of the *future in the present* predominates. In these circumstances, characterized by narrative wreckage, constructing any sense of self or exploring any other identity becomes extremely problematic as the individual has lost the sense of temporality that is a key resource in restorying a life. Finally, the quest narrative provides an opportunity for time to be *reclaimed* in ways that link the individual to a *fragmentary* model of autobiographical time, and the time tenses of *past in the past*, the *present in the present*, and the *future in the future*. In combination, these enable a developing self and a more communicative mode of embodiment to emerge that is willing to explore different identities and possible selves as the need arises and circumstances allow (also see Sparkes and Smith 2002; Smith and Sparkes 2004).

Finally, a content analysis is evident in the work of Sparkes (1998) in his biographical study of one elite athlete whose career was prematurely terminated by illness. Having transcribed the eighteen hours of interview with this athlete, Sparkes first assumed the posture of indwelling and immersed himself in the data in order to understand the athlete's point of view from an empathetic position. Next, he read through the transcripts again and identified narrative segments and categories within it. Simultaneously, he wrote analytic memos that began to make tentative and preliminary connections to various theoretical concepts that he thought might be related to issues emerging from the athlete's story. These memos and codes helped frame the questions and themes that were explored in the interviews as part of a cyclic process. This same procedure was applied to pieces of reflective writing that the athlete undertook. As the interviews progressed and data were accumulated, Sparkes searched for connections across the narrative segments and themes in an attempt to identify patterns and meanings as they emerged in the athlete's story.

Based on this content analysis, Sparkes (1998) explores the emergence of a high-performance body and how this shapes a particular sense of self and a strong, exclusive, athletic identity that can operate as an 'Achilles' Heel' when biographical disruption is encountered. Following this, he reveals how, as the athlete descends from the heights of the extraordinary into the mundane world of ordinariness, the loss of certain selves enforces a heightened reflexivity and awareness of previously taken-for-granted aspects of the body–self relationship that are no longer attainable. The manner in which certain selves at the apex of an identity hierarchy exert pressure on the athlete to seek a restored self rather than opt for more attainable or realistic identities is highlighted. Finally, his analysis reveals the problems of restorying the self when an individual is constrained by limited narrative resources. He concludes that an awareness of such issues, and a greater understanding of the processes involved, would benefit the care of seriously injured athletes by enabling effective, multidimensional programmes to be developed that link the timing of the transitional experience, like career-ending injury or illness, to an appropriate intervention.

Analyzing the *hows*

As noted in the introduction to this chapter, qualitative analysis is as much about *how* things are said as about *what* is said. Asking *how* questions about the narrative initiates reflection on the performative dimensions of storytelling and draws attention to the manner in which they are artfully constructed for particular purposes, at particular times, in specific contexts. Thus, rather than ask 'what does the story tell us about X?' the question becomes, 'how is X constructed in the telling?'

Analyzing the *hows* in action

Adopting this kind of stance, Smith and Sparkes (2002) explore the manner in which coherence is constructed in the life stories told by two men who have acquired a spinal cord injury through playing sport. Rather than ask 'What do these stories tell us about coherence?', they direct their attention towards the *artful* practices through which these men as storytellers *do* coherence. Their question then becomes 'How is coherence achieved and constructed in the telling?' In answering the *how* question they demonstrate that various narrative practices inform this process and reveal how they are framed by the local and cultural conventions of telling. As such, coherence is not seen as an inherent feature of the stories told by the men, but as something that is both artfully crafted in the telling and drawn from the available meanings, structures and linkages that comprise stories.

The two life stories told by the men are identified by Smith and Sparkes (2002) as being framed respectively by the *restitution* narrative and the *quest* narrative as described by Frank (1995). Drawing a number of concepts from the phenomenology and sociology of the body, Smith and Sparkes proceed to link these to the framework for analyzing narrative practice provided by Gubrium and Holstein (1998, 2000) and Holstein and Gubrium (2000). Accordingly, they utilize the notions of narrative composition, linkage, slippage, shift, editing, footing, elasticity and control to explore how these are used in combination to construct coherence and maintain specific, but often contradictory, body–self relationships within the different storylines told by the men within the framework of the restitution and quest narratives.

For example, according to Gubrium and Holstein (1998), a narrative footing provides clues to listeners about the kinds of stories that could be told and possible points to make. Such a footing reveals the positions from which storytellers can offer their narratives. Smith and Sparkes (2002) illustrate this move by using extended interview extracts from each of the participants in which a narrative footing is constructed for the rest of their stories in relation to the restitution and quest narrative respectively. Extracts from interviews with the two men are also used to illustrate how each edits their story as part as an active process of composition in which they constantly monitor, manage, modify, and revise the emergent story they are telling, particularly when facets of this story are contradictory.

Narrative slippage is also revealed in each of the stories told. This refers to the discontinuities between received cultural scripts or maps like the restitution and quest narratives, and the ways these scripts are applied by the individual. Thus, while each of the stories told is clearly framed by a powerful narrative form, this does not determine how the story is composed and the teller is capable of fashioning diverse themes pertinent to their life story and biographical particulars. As part of this creative and artful construction the teller gains a degree of narrative ownership.

Acknowledging this creative element in the storytelling opens up the possibilities for bringing about change in the form and content of the narrative for both narrators and the health professionals involved with them.

The *hows* of narrative practice are also brought into focus when questions are asked regarding *therapeutic emplotment*. According to Brooks (1984) *emplotment* is an active process by which people creatively engage with and make sense of a story so as to determine what is really going on and what is likely to happen as the story progresses. This concept has been applied to making sense of illness by Del Vecchio *et al.* (1994) who focused on people learning to live with a cancer diagnosis. They defined therapeutic emplotment as 'the interpretive activity, present in clinical encounters, through which clinicians and patients create and negotiate a plot structure within clinical time, one which places therapeutic actions within a larger therapeutic story' (p. 855). They concluded that the emplotment of illness and the therapeutic course constitutes a major task in the treatment of cancer. They proceeded to illustrate how this operates from the perspective of oncologists, and revealed how they attempt to formulate experiences for patients by structuring time and horizons in ways that instilled hope, encouraged investment in arduous and toxic treatments, and avoided a sense of despair.

More recently, Crossley (2003) has drawn on the analysis provided by Del Vecchio *et al.* (1994) to focus on what it is like to have to live as a cancer *patient* following diagnosis. Specifically, she focuses on the autobiographical account, in the form of diary extracts from the time of his suspected diagnosis of oral cancer in September 1996 until the week before his death in March 2001, of John Diamond in his book entitled *Snake Oil and Other Preoccupations* (Diamond 2001).

Drawing on the diary extracts, Crossley (2003) divides the time between suspected diagnosis and death into six main stages in order to depict the dominant themes and underlying temporal structure characterizing Diamond's attempts to adapt to the reality of oral cancer. These stages include: (1) pre-cancer: touch wood; (2) learning to live in 'therapeutic emplotment'; (3) in limbo: holding one's breath; (4) recurrence: 'therapeutic emplotment' cont.; (5) through the mirror: the 'unspoken narrative' and (6) endings or the end? Her analysis of each stage illustrates the ways in which Diamond's narrative very quickly appropriates the characteristic form of therapeutic emplotment used by oncologists. For example, Del Vecchio *et al.* (1994) note one narrative strategy oncologists use that expresses time within specific or highly foreshortened horizons in order to create an experience of immediacy, of 'living for the moment' rather than trivial chronology. Likewise, Crossley notes how Diamond, from his early diagnosis to first recurrence, is largely focused on the 'immediacy' of specific treatments, expressing (in retrospect) a naïve faith in their efficacy. However, she goes on to show how, as time progressed, Diamond questioned the surgical story, and a largely 'unspoken narrative' of fear and uncertainty emerged that began to supersede the therapeutic plot.

Thus, Crossley's (2003) detailed case study of one individual illustrates *how* the process of therapeutic emplotment implicitly worked to structure the narrative produced by one man attempting to adjust to the reality of life with oral cancer. Importantly, in asking questions about the *hows* of therapeutic emplotment, Crossley emphasizes that personal accounts provided by people living with illness 'constitute a form of life in their own right, a constitution of reality in which the individual ongoingly makes sense of and struggles to adapt to what is happening in their life' (p. 3).

In her discussion of the analysis of personal narratives, Riessman (2002) also asks a number of 'how' questions in relation to the *performative* aspects of narration. She emphasizes that when people tell stories about their lives they perform their (preferred) identities. Therefore, given that personal narratives contain many performative features that enable the local achievement of identity, precisely *how* narrators accomplish their situated stories conveys a great deal about the presentation of self. This is not to say that the identities constructed are inauthentic, but rather to acknowledge that they are situated and accomplished in social action. Consequently, for Riessman, approaching identity as a performative struggle over the meanings of experience, 'opens up analytic possibilities that are missed with static conceptions of identity and by essentializing theories that assume the unity of the inner self' (p. 701).

The performative approach advocated by Riessman (2003) emphasizes narrative as action and an intentional project: 'Analysis shifts from the "told" – the events to which language refers – to include "the telling", specifically the narrators' strategic choices of illness narrative about positioning of characters, audience, and self' (p. 8). She suggests that, in a general sense, a performative approach asks the following questions: Why was the illness narrative developed that way, and told in that order? In what kinds of stories does the narrator place him/herself? How does he/she locate him/herself in relation to the audience, and vice versa? How does he/she locate characters in relation to one another and in relation to him or herself? How does he/she strategically make preferred identity claims? What other identities are performed or suggested? What was the response of the listener/audience, and how did it influence the development of the illness narrative, and interpretation of it?

To illustrate what her angle of analytic vision offers, Riesmann (2003) develops two case studies based on illness narratives. Each man involved carries a diagnosis of multiple sclerosis and each performs a version of masculinity that is agentic and positive. Importantly, the narratives of these two men were first collected and analyzed twenty years previously in the 1980s as part of a study of marital dissolution in the USA. As such, this contemporary analysis is a rare example in the social sciences of a researcher returning to previous data to reinterpret them in the light of new conceptions, theoretical developments, and methodological advances. Thus, Riessman's article involves *new* case studies constructed from research materials she worked with differently many years ago.

Importantly, by examining the performative aspects of the interviews with these men she highlights how their illness narratives differ in fundamental and critical ways. That is, the men *do* illness differently. In addition, her analysis reveals how these men *do* gender in vastly different ways with contrasting versions of masculinity being performed in the illness narratives.

Like the previous work mentioned in this section, the cases presented by Riessman (2003) highlight how the telling of personal stories, like other artistic performances, is a dynamic and fluid process composed in the spaces between performer and audience. They are *not* fixed texts composed by speakers and enacted similarly for different audiences. As such, the study of narrative as performance has much to offer, particularly with regard to interrogating how both the teller and the audience (researcher) are active agents in the production of, and reaction to, illness narratives.

Reflections

My intentions in this chapter have been to give a flavour, albeit limited, of various forms of narrative analysis and their potential to assist us in understanding the social world of health and illness in different ways. As Murray (2003) reminds us, the opportunities provided by narrative research are extensive and still being developed. With this in mind, Riessman (2002: 706) suggests that narrative analysis 'is a useful addition to the stockpot of social research methods, bringing critical flavours to the surface that would otherwise get lost in the brew'. This said, Riessman makes it clear that narrative analysis is one approach, suitable for some situations and not others, it is *not* a panacea.

> Its methods are not appropriate for studies of large numbers of nameless, faceless subjects. The approach is slow and painstaking, requiring attention to subtlety: nuances of speech, the organisation of a response, relations between researcher and subject, social and historical contexts. It is not suitable for investigators who seek a clear and unobstructed view of subjects' lives, and the analytical detail required may seem excessive to those who orient to language as a transparent medium.
>
> (Riessman 2002: 706)

For those who do feel drawn towards narrative forms of analysis the emphasis should be on the plural. That is, there is no one 'best way' to conduct a narrative analysis. The approach chosen will depend on the purposes of the research and the questions being asked. Accordingly, in this chapter, I have not privileged one form of analysis over any other. An awareness of both the *whats* and the *hows* of storytelling are equally important in understanding how meaningful interaction transpires and both need to be considered whenever possible. This is particularly so given their relative strengths and weaknesses.

For example, content analysis is very useful for examining the thematic similarities and differences between narratives provided by a number of people. This kind of analysis focuses on the *whats* rather than the *hows* of the telling. The strength of this form of analysis lies in its capacity to develop general knowledge about the core themes that make up the content of the stories collected in an interview context.

Despite the recognizable strengths of content analysis its use in isolation can lead to an over-determination of the themes identified in the data, seemingly 'ironing out the pleats'. This is particularly so given the diversity of the stories that researchers get told, and the contradictions and tensions contained within them. Such concerns appear warranted given Faircloth's (1999) belief that core themes can often be underscored at the expense of variation and difference which, in turn, leads the researcher to under-appreciate the heterogeneity of experience and the storied quality of data. For him, with content forms of analysis 'there is a narrative detachment from the artfulness of storytelling' (p. 210). Since this form of analysis remains abstract and formal, it often, therefore, misses the uniqueness of each story because it relies on the preconceived categorizations of the researcher. Consequently, as Sparkes notes (1999: 21), 'by seeking common themes in the stories there is the danger of missing other possible messages that individual stories might hold'.

Conclusion

Given the situation as described, there is a need to be wary of approaches that focus exclusively on the *whats* of narrative and ignore the *hows* of social interaction. Of course, we should be equally wary of approaches that focus exclusively on the *hows* of narrative at the expense of the *whats*. This is not to suggest that any one researcher can focus on both simultaneously. As Gubrium and Holstein (1998, 2000) emphasize, because interpretive practice is two-sided there is an inescapable analytic tension within it that needs to be accepted but cannot be completely resolved. This is because to designate an analytic point of entry and foreground one side of the practice, e.g. the *hows*, means that the other side, the *whats*, is placed in the background. The process Gubrium and Holstein advocate for moving back and forth between the components that compromise interpretive practice is that of *analytic bracketing*.

> Analytic bracketing amounts to an orientating procedure for alternately focusing on the *whats* and then the *hows* of interpretive practice (or vice versa) in order to assemble both a contextually scenic and a contextually constructive picture of everyday language-in-use. The objective is to move back and forth between discursive practice and discourses-in practice, documenting each in turn and making informative references to the other in the process. Either discursive machinery or available discourses becomes the provisional phenomenon, while interest in the other is temporarily deferred, but not forgotten.
> (Gubrium and Holstein 2000: 500)

Importantly, this alternating movement does not privilege one form of analysis over another. Indeed, it suggests the need for analytic diversity when considering narratives. This need for pluralism is supported by Lieblich *et al.* (1998) who repeatedly return to the same life history data from a variety of angles with 'different hearing aids, lenses, which produced a myriad of readings' (p. 167). These different readings reveal similarities as well as contradictions and conflicts, which for them are part and parcel of any narrative inquiry that seeks to understand the multi-layered and complex nature of human identity.

In this regard, Coffey and Atkinson (1996) suggest that qualitative researchers should consider using a variety of analyses in order to understand their data in different ways. Analytical diversity is useful, they argue, because researchers 'can use different analytic strategies in order to explore different facets of our data, explore different kinds of order in them, and construct different versions of the social world' (p. 14). For them, the juxtaposition or combination of different analytical techniques does not reduce the complexity of our understandings. Rather, they emphasize, the more we examine our data from different viewpoints, 'the more we may reveal – or indeed construct – their complexity' (p. 14). Revealing and constructing the complexity of personal stories told about illness and health are worthy goals and, as this chapter has attempted to illustrate, narrative forms of analysis have an important contribution to make in this area.

References

Brock, S. and Kleiber, D. (1994) Narrative in medicine: The stories of elite college athletes' career-ending injury, *Qualitative Health Research*, 4 (4): 411–430.

Brooks, P. (1984) *Reading for the Plot*. New York: Vintage.

Bury, M. (2001) Illness narratives: fact or fiction? *Sociology of Health and Illness*, 23 (3): 263–285.

Coffey, A. and Atkinson, P. (1996) *Making Sense of Qualitative Data*. London: Sage.

Cortazzi, M. (1993) *Narrative Analysis*. London: Falmer.

Crossley, M. (2000) *Introducing Narrative Psychology*. Buckingham: Open University Press.

Crossley, M. (2003) 'Let me explain': Narrative emplotment and one patient's experience of oral cancer, *Social Science and Medicine*, 56 (3): 439–448.

Davies, M. (1997) Shattered assumptions: Time and the experience of long-term HIV positivity, *Social Science and Medicine*, 44 (5): 561–571.

Del Vecchio Good, M., Munakata, T., Kobayashi, Y., Mattingly, C. and Good, B. (1994) Oncology and narrative time, *Social Science and Medicine*, 38: 855–862.

Denzin, N. (2003) Foreword: Narrative's moment. In Andrews, M., Sclater, S., Squire, C. and Treacher, A. (eds) *Lines of Narrative*. London: Routledge, xi–xiii.

Diamond, J. (2001) *Snake Oil and Other Preoccupations*. London: Vintage.

Faircloth, C. (1999) Revisiting thematisation in the narrative study of epilepsy, *Sociology of Health and Illness*, 21 (2): 209–227.

Frank, A. (1995) *The Wounded Storyteller*. Chicago: The University of Chicago Press.

Gergen, K. and Gergen, M. (1983) Narratives of the self. In Sarbin, T. and Scheibe, K. (eds) *Studies in Social Identity*. New York: Praeger, 254–273.

Gubrium, J. and Holstein, J. (1998) Narrative practice and the coherence of personal stories, *The Sociological Quarterly*, 39 (1): 163–187.

Gubrium, J. and Holstein, J. (2000) Analysing interpretive practice. In Denzin, N.K and Lincoln, Y.S. (eds) *Handbook of Qualitative Research*. London: Sage, 487–508.

Holloway, I. (1997) *Basic Concepts for Qualitative Research*. Oxford: Blackwell Science.

Holstein, J. and Gubrium, J. (2000) *The Self We Live By*. New York: Oxford University Press.

Horrocks, C., Kelly, N., Roberts, B. and Robinson, D. (2003) Introduction. In Horrocks, C., Kelly, N., Roberts, B. and Robinson, D. (eds) *Narrative Memory and Health*. Huddersfield: University of Huddersfield Press, xv–xx.

Kleinman, A. and Seeman, D. (2000) Personal experience of illness. In Albrecht, G., Fitzpatrick, R. and Scrimshaw, S. (eds) *Handbook of Social Studies in Health and Medicine*. London: Sage, 230–242.

Lieblich, A., Tuval-Mashiach, R. and Zilber, T. (1998) *Narrative Research: Reading, Analysis, and Interpretation*. London: Sage.

McAdams, D. (1993) *The Stories We Live By*. London: The Guilford Press.

McLeod, J. (1997) *Narrative and Psychotherapy*. London: Sage.

Miller, P. (1994) Narrative practices: Their role in socialisation and self-construction. In Neisser, U. and Fivush, R. (eds) *The Remembering Self*. Cambridge: Cambridge University Press, 158–179.

Murray, M. (1999) The stories nature of health and illness. In Murray, M. and Chamberlain, K. (eds) *Qualitative Health Psychology*. London: Sage, 47–63.

Murray, M. (2003) Narrative psychology. In Smith, J. (ed.) *Qualitative Psychology*. London: Sage, 111–131.

Polkinghorne, D. (1995) Narrative configuration in qualitative analysis. In Hatch, J. and Wisniewski, R. (eds) *Life History and Narrative*. London: Falmer Press, 5–23.

Riessman, C. (1993) *Narrative Analysis*. London: Sage.

Riessman, C. (2002) Analysing personal narratives. In Gubrium, J. and Holstein, J. (eds) *Handbook of Interview Research*. London: Sage, 695–710.

Riessman, C. (2003) Performing identities in illness narrative: Masculinity and multiple sclerosis, *Qualitative Research*, 3 (1): 5–33.

Roberts, B. (2002) *Biographical Research*. Buckingham: Open University Press.

Robinson, I. (1990) Personal narratives, social careers and medical courses: Analysing life trajectories in autobiographies of people with multiple sclerosis, *Social Science and Medicine*, 30 (11): 1173–1186.

Smith, B. and Sparkes, A. (2002) Men, sport, spinal cord injury, and the construction of coherence: Narrative practice in action, *Qualitative Research*, 2 (2): 143–171.

Smith, B. and Sparkes, A. (2004) Men, sport, and spinal cord injury: An analysis of metaphors and narrative types, *Disability and Society*, 19 (6): 613–626.

Somers, M. (1994) The narrative constitution of identity: A relational and network approach, *Theory and Society*, 23: 635–649.

Sparkes, A. (1998) Athletic identity: An Achilles' heel to the survival of self, *Qualitative Health Research*, 8 (5): 644–664.

Sparkes, A. (1999) Exploring body narratives, *Sport, Education and Society*, 4 (1): 17–30.

Sparkes, A. and Smith, B. (2002) Sport, spinal cord injury, embodied masculinities and the dilemmas of narrative identity, *Men and Masculinities*, 4 (3): 258–285.

Sparkes, A. and Smith, B. (2003) Men, sport, spinal cord injury and narrative time, *Qualitative Research*, 3 (3): 295–320.

Steffen, V. (1997) Life stories and shared experience, *Social Science and Medicine*, 45 (1): 99–111.

12

DAWN FRESHWATER
Action research for changing and improving practice

Introduction

This chapter, drawing upon the contemporary developments in health care, aims to illustrate the role of action research in changing and improving practice. Importantly, it identifies the potential of action research in supporting practitioners to manage seemingly competing agendas. I also attend to the concepts of power and oppression, specifically focusing on the generation of knowledge. I purposely draw upon the theory of action research as it has been defined in education; the discipline of education has much to offer in the understanding and application of this particular methodology, with many of its early exponents coming from an educational background. Having outlined the philosophical underpinnings and origins of action research, I then go on to clarify some of the aims and objectives, referring to the collaborative, reflective and cyclical nature of the process. Specific concerns relating to the estimations of rigour of these processes and action research as a whole are addressed within a concluding critique. This is followed with an extended exemplar of an ongoing action research project within the context of prison health care. The project involves the development of an educational intervention that has an impact on clinical practice, clinical leadership and clinical governance agendas in a vastly marginalized group of practitioners, marginalized that is, both in terms of research and development, and in respect of their isolation from professional colleagues.

Action research has been described as a tool to change society and generate knowledge, which, at its best, is emancipating and empowering. Traditionally, action research has been used within educational settings to help teachers cope with the challenges of change, enabling them to carry through innovation in a reflective way (Freshwater 2000; Kemmis and McTaggart 2000; Zeichner 2001). A decade ago, Altrichter *et al.* (1993) related this to the prevailing climate of rapid social change, which they argued, apart from challenging stability, provided exciting possibilities for building more dynamic educational systems. While there have been many changes in education over the past ten years, they have been even more dramatic in health care. It would seem that the only constant has been change itself. In fact, it would seem that the pace of change within the health service 'industry' is incongruent with one of the fundamental drivers of that change, that is the requirement for evidence-based practice, and this within a coherent and stringent governance structure (DoH 2001, 1998). In other words, the fundamental principles of evidence-based practice are almost impossible to achieve in a climate of such dramatic continuous change, unless the notion of evidence-based practice is viewed within a framework of change itself. One of the many challenges that health professionals face in such a climate is how to progress existing, and generate new knowledge, while simultaneously delivering, monitoring and evaluating the day-to-day work of high quality patient-centred care.

A further concern lies in the question of who is directing and influencing the development of knowledge for practice, and how this serves to either empower or disempower those involved in the process. The concept of power is significant in any discussion relating to the process of action research; Lewin (1946), the founding father of action research, viewed it as a democratic approach to researching and changing behaviour, not because it introduced democracy, but because it embodied democratic principles. That action research is carried out, in the main, by practitioners directly concerned with the clinical situation, points not only to the importance of ownership of change but also to the power of practice-generated theories. This emphasis on power within knowledge is a theme that will be revisited throughout the chapter and is central to the case study exemplar.

Many writers identify action research as an activity that is an integral part of professional work, thus avoiding the split between theoretical and practical understanding (Kemmis and McTaggart 2000; Rolfe *et al.* 2001; Winter and Munn-Giddings 2001; Zeichner 2001; Holloway and Wheeler 2002). This is reflected in perhaps the shortest and most straightforward definition of action research provided by Elliott (1991: 69) who states that action research 'is the study of a social situation with a view to improving the quality of action within it'. Action research has the potential therefore to act as a bridge between research, theory and practice (Somekh 1995). It is not surprising then that it has been widely, and sometimes uncritically, embraced particularly by those working in the health- and social-care disciplines. Such professions are not only faced with constant change, as already mentioned but are also familiar with the theory–practice and research–practice gaps that have dominated the health science literature for over three decades. Take, for example, Greenwood (1984), a particularly strong advocate of action research, who claims that it is the most appropriate method for the discipline of nursing. Critical of the poor uptake of research by nurses, she believes that action research is the way to address the theory–practice gap. These comments have been echoed by other nursing authors including Miller (1989), LeMay *et al.* (1998), Freshwater and Rolfe (2001) and Rolfe (2002). Other health-related disciplines concur with these sentiments, colleagues in psychology, physiotherapy and general practice have all expounded the value of action research in bridging the divide (see, for example, Higgs and Titchen 2001). Importantly, action research is useful in its ability to identify and work with numerous splits and divides.

Philosophy and origins of action research

Exploring and understanding the philosophical basis for any research method is a necessary and important part of the research process, not least because of the requirement for philosophical, theoretical and methodological congruence (McKenzie 2002). While this is not the place to examine the philosophical basis of action research in depth, what follows is a brief overview of both the philosophical underpinnings and theoretical origins of the method.

Truth and action research

Rorty (1979) argues that philosophical inquiry can never be more than a 'conversation' motivated by the 'hope' for mutual understanding. Further it is dependent on the recognition of the differences between individuals and groups. Rorty's argument contains elements of both the pragmatic and the postmodern, turning against the correspondence theories of truth, towards coherence theories. The emphasis on a philosophical truth that is based on coherence theory provides strong grounds for the context bound, action oriented work of action research (Stringer 1996). Postmodernist perspectives challenge the notion of a 'grand narrative', arguing for local and contingent knowledge, this being based in a pragmatic epistemology that focuses on practically effective knowledge. However, it should be remembered that the philosophical view of truth taken here is only an emphasis, for if truth is totally dependent upon context and multiple realities then it makes it very difficult to formulate inquiry at all. As Winter and Munn-Giddings (2001: 258) comment: 'for action research, at least (with its concern for the improvement of human well-being), the debate about the validity of the outcomes of social inquiry needs to be moved away from a simple opposition between "absolute, objective truth" and total relativism in which each local "reality" has its own "subjective" or culturally determined truth criteria'.

Drawing upon the work of Putnam (1987) they argue instead for statements about the world that are empirically established and are true under 'normal conditions'. Hence truth, rather than being polarized as *either* objective *or* culturally relative, is placed on a continuum where differing statements can be ordered according to the process that is needed to create a consensus regarding the conditions needed to verify them. This however has implications for the researchers involved in the process. Not least the fact that each person is required to be mindful not only of the conditions within which the process of change is taking place, but also the values, beliefs, norms and level of consciousness that they bring to bear on the process. That is to say that all change, when viewed from an action research perspective is *intentional*, *deliberative*, *conscious* and importantly *reflexive*. The issue of reflexivity will be addressed at a later point in the chapter, for now the focus remains with the philosophy and theory that underpins the action research method, taking the concept of consciousness further.

Consciousness and power

Paulo Freire (1972) introduced the world of education to the notion of con-scientization, presenting it as the ability to become critically conscious. This is not simply examining an event to see how it could have been done differently; critical consciousness is linked to critical awareness and implies political, social and ethical dimensions which enable assumptions inherent in ideologies to be challenged (Freshwater and Rolfe 2001). Critical consciousness is derived from the theory of critical social science, a science that aims to foster enlightenment, empowerment and emancipation from culturally induced consciousness, for example, dominant discourses such as positivistic science, or, in the case of health care, that of medical hegemony. Hegemony, in this context, refers to the extent to which there is uncritical acceptance of the dominant groups' meaning systems within the health-care culture (Grundy 1987).

Freire, a social activist as well as an educationalist, suggested that 'false con-sciousness' in the Marxist sense, that is consciousness that is culturally induced within individuals, could be transcended by education. Roberts (1983: 24) counters this, asserting that the education system is one of the mechanisms that reinforces the position of false consciousness, stating: 'if the education is controlled by the powerful and limited to the curricula that support their values, little conflict occurs'. The central tenet of Freire's pedagogy (1972) was the practice of trans-cending false consciousness in order to achieve conscientization; interpreted by Askew and Carnell (1998: 65) as: 'coming to a consciousness of oppression and a commitment to end that oppression'. Developing consciousness of one's influ-ences is relatively straightforward; however, taking action to challenge, change or destabilize those influences, requires a degree of risk taking and an openness to being destabilized oneself. Mezirow (1981) referred to this process of con-scientization as perspective transformation. Becoming conscious of one's oppression and making the commitment to end it require two different shifts. I would argue (as does Menzies-Lyth in 1988, using many health-related case examples as evidence) that there is an enormous resistance to coming to con-sciousness and ending uncritical acceptance within the health professions.

Socialized into a culture of uncritical acceptance or received wisdom as it is sometimes termed, practitioners might not necessarily be aware of any conflict or dissonance. Indeed practitioners may find it preferable to remain anaesthetized to conflict. Conflict does occur, although not necessarily overtly. For example, individuals may not be aware that some internalized self-criticism originates in uncritical acceptance and unexpressed conflict in relation to feeling oppressed. Thus, a false consciousness develops, sometimes without the individual knowing that there may be a different consciousness, although they may be aware of some degree of cognitive dissonance, however, it is not always linked to oppression. Dissonance is not comfortable, but often comes before action, and can be the motivating force to encourage the practitioner to move beyond routinized and habitutalized practices to a more conscious reflexive occupation of their position.

It could be argued then that dissonance precedes action, which in turn demands further action and a shift in consciousness (Festinger 1957; Joyce 1984).

Action does not always equate with taking responsibility for the self against the perceived oppressor (reclaiming power explicitly); it may in fact mean choosing to remain powerless or consciously playing the power game (playing with the implied power). The latter is particularly employed by doctors and nurses at all levels; Down illustrates a good example of this in her research into critical care (Down 2002).

Action research is also a process of conscientization at differing levels, for the researcher it brings to awareness the conflict between the inner and the outer dialogue, which is often suppressed within the work setting, making the private knowledge public. Just as in reflective practice, an experience or awareness of discrepancy is often found to be the motivating force behind an action research question. These might be discrepancies between espoused theories and theories in action, between the way in which a group of people view a situation (for example, shared values or philosophy of care), or discrepancies between what has happened and what was intended. Discrepancies and contradictions, once they are consciously recognized, provide food for thought, inviting differing starting points for the research process. Dadds (1985) suggests these might come from an interest (trying out a new idea or developing a strength); a difficulty (compensating for a deficiency or trying to solve a problem or an unclear situation (attempting to understand the unexpected or seeing how one intervention interfaces with another).

Aims, purpose and processes

The specific aims, purpose and process of action research are to some extent determined by the type of action research being utilized. There are several forms of action research. Three main types have been identified within the literature; these are technical and positivist; practical and interpretive; critical and emancipatory (Zuber-Skerritt 1991; McTaggart 1992), although, in describing participatory action research, Kemmis and McTaggart (2000) develop a further typology that moves beyond the traditional notions of action research to include a reflexive–dialectical perspective.

Zuber-Skerritt (1991) explicates three basic levels of action research, briefly summarized here:

- Technical action research aims at effectiveness and efficiency in performance, that is, changes in social practices. Participants are often co-opted and rely on an outside expert.

- Collaborative practical action research involves transformations of consciousness of participants as well as change in social practices. The expert acts as a process consultant, engaging in dialogue to encourage both the cooperation of the participants and self-reflection.

- Emancipatory action research includes the participant's emancipation from tradition, self-deception and coercion. The expert is a process moderator, collaborating and sharing equal responsibility with the participants. Having more involvement with the participants' emancipatory action research has the potential to generate and test action theories, thereby developing and empowering practitioners. (Interestingly, Carr and Kemmis (1986) suggest that emancipatory action research is the only true action research.)

These three types are not mutually exclusive, and as the Kemmis and McTaggart (2000) model of reflexive dialectical research demonstrates, there is a place for all three approaches in a broader framework of historical, social and discursive construction and deconstruction. Kemmis and McTaggart (2000) also clarify a number of variations of action research, each of which has a specific emphasis, but that broadly use similar processes, namely:

- Participatory action research.
- Critical action research.
- Classroom action research.
- Action learning.
- Action science.
- Soft systems approach.
- Industrial action research.

While the processes may be similar, what tends to be different across all the typologies is the role of the researcher, be that, for example, a more authoritarian and rigid director of research, or a more democratic and appreciative co-partici-pant who focuses on implicit wisdom, situational intelligence and emergent knowledge. It is interesting to note that in discussing the three types of action research Zuber-Skerritt (1991) does not make it clear what she means by the term 'expert', and this can lead to some confusion, not least because action research is more often deemed to be not only participative, but also collaborative. This is not a moot point, as the notion of 'expert' and 'expertise' links closely with the concepts of power, oppression and knowledge. Cohen and Manion (1989) contend that while all action research is situational, concerned with diagnosing a problem in a specific context and attempting to solve it in that context, it is not always colla-borative. This, of course, is more of a contentious issue when viewed in the current climate of multiprofessional collaboration and when professionals and researchers attempt to achieve definition, ownership and commitment to local improvements that are crucial to the effective implementation and evaluation of national policies. Winter and Munn-Giddings observe this collaborative process, linking it with improving practice thus: 'Action research inquiries are closely bound up with criteria for "good practice", and this obviously entails a strong link between the rationale for the inquiry process and a "reality" that is fully (officially and inten-sively) shared between practitioners, service-users and accountable managers at local and national level' (2001: 258).

Aims and purpose

As already mentioned action research is primarily concerned with the management of change. However, any research process can bring about change, what is important here is the issue of improvement. An action research project might have brought about change in a situation, but what is often forgotten in the evaluative process is whether that change has actually led to an improvement. Such improvement may not always be directly related to practice, for example, a specific patient intervention, an improvement in team-working, or ownership of shared values can ultimately lead to an impact on patient care.

However, it cannot be assumed that this will automatically be the case, and even if it is, the process does not end there. One might ask how an improvement might also lead to further change, thus engaging in a cycle of continuous reflection and dialogue with practice and the research question. The aims and purposes then of action research can be described as improving practice through dynamic focused inquiry. Here we already encounter a difficulty, for despite the ubiquity of practice, it holds different meanings for different people. Kemmis and McTaggart (2000) reason that this is perhaps due to the fact that those who examine practice do so from different intellectual traditions and naturally tend to focus on different aspects of practice when they investigate it.

In summarizing the aims and purpose of action research it is perhaps pertinent to return a question posed by Kemmis and McTaggart: Is the research only concerned with efficiency, leaving basic values unquestioned, or is it really committed to social improvement? Essentially emancipation is at the heart of action research and as such it further aims to liberate individuals from the constraints placed upon them both by themselves and the dominant discourses they perpetuate.

Processes

Action research has been described as a cycle or a spiral of steps (Lewin 1946). Lewin, renowned not just for his work on action research, but more significantly for his development of field theory, first (1946) identified these steps as planning, acting, observing and reflecting (see Figure 12.1).

Over the years Lewin's theories have been adopted (and adapted) into a variety of contexts, including management and consultancy, community development, responsive evaluation, aviation and the world of business and commerce and, of course, health care. The four stages in the action research approach comprise a careful and systematic approach to developing changes and innovations in the social world. The initial step in the cycle is to design a plan of action; after the action has been executed it is followed by a period of reflection. Changes and modifications are made to the plan, and the cycle is then repeated. It is important to note, however, that reflection also occurs continuously throughout the cycle. Generally it is claimed that in action research any phase of data gathering and interpretation can only be a tentative step forward and not a final answer; this is congruent with the postmodern viewpoint that all work is in process, is

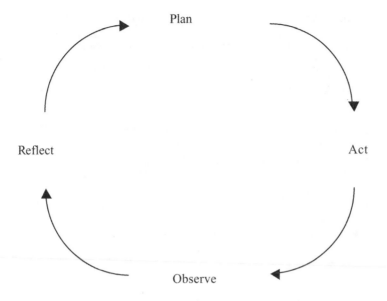

Figure 12.1 Action research cycle (Lewin 1946)

incomplete and requires a response from others positioned differently (Rolfe *et al.* 2001). It is worth noting here the links between action research and postmodern and poststructural thinking, feminist theory, realist evaluation (Kazi 2003) and real world research (Robson 2002). All of these point to the fact that any end point is arbitrary; it is, instead, a reflection of the point in time at which the knowledge was generated. This mirrors the dynamism of health-care practices themselves, and indeed many theories of health are closely aligned to this dynamic idea of *becoming*.

Unlike some approaches to research, action research does not use its own particular research techniques. It is not technique that distinguishes action research from other research approaches; what distinguishes action research from other methodologies is its process, that is, the process of critical reflection and a commitment to the improvement of practice. Once again we come back to the fundamental guiding principles previously described that define the uniqueness of action research. Hart and Bond (1995) devised a useful action research typology in order to make this point, asserting that action research is able to retain a distinct identity while simultaneously stretching across the spectrum of research approaches. This typology of action research spans from experimental to organizational to professionalizing and empowering.

Hence, action research uses a variety of methods from both the quantitative and qualitative paradigms and yet remains distinct (see Table 12.1). Action research can draw upon multiple methods of data collection, enriching the perspectives that the researcher has on the phenomenon. The methodological mix can occur either sequentially or simultaneously, combining either a quantitative and a qualitative method or two or more methods within the same methodology (Holloway and Wheeler 2002). The nature of action research means that it is largely self-evaluative with modifications continuously made within the ongoing situation.

Table 12.1 Approaches to research (adapted from Askew and Carnell (1998))

	Action research	Qualitative research	Quantitative research
Purpose	To bring about informed change	To illuminate meaning and understanding	To increase knowledge and find universal laws and generalizations
Framing	Concerned with the whole picture	Concerns understanding phenomena	Focus on behaviour not context
Rationale for planning	Research planned to investigate practice	Research planned to investigate phenomena	Research planned to test hypotheses
Techniques	Draws on qualitative and quantitative	Ethnography, case study, phenomenology	Uses measuring techniques
Rigour	Based on logical coherence, interpretations in the reflections	Through discussion of bias and constraints	Statistical analysis and meta techniques for establishing validity and reliability
Objective–subjective dichotomy	Enables practitioners to clarify values on which research is built	Recognition of the subjective nature of research	Sets out to be objective and value free
Evaluation	By reflective questions	Evaluated by questions related to meaning and understanding	Evaluated by questions referring to reliability and duplication

Thus action research is essentially developmental, longitudinal and multi-dimensional, necessitating reflection at different levels. The evaluation itself consists of two stages, firstly a diagnostic stage in which the problems are analyzed and hypotheses are developed and secondly a therapeutic stage when the hypotheses are tested by a consciously directed change experiment. A robust and substantial action research study demands a great deal of reflexivity and rigour, made explicit through the transparency of the audit trail.

Establishing the rigour of action research

Action research has been heavily criticized for its apparent lack of scientific rigour, and for confusing social activism and community development with research. Kemmis and McTaggart (2000: 569) capture these criticisms succinctly when they comment: 'Critical action research may be regarded as a "dangerous" vehicle for importing "radical" ideology into social settings.' Dangerous for whom, one might ask, perhaps for those who perpetuate and depend on the influence of the dominant discourse and culturally induced consciousness? One might be justified in challenging whether or not research carried out by the practitioner and involving self-evaluation can ever be reported in an unbiased or undistorted way. Indeed

Kemmis and McTaggart (2000) ask the question (of participatory action research): Is this defensible as research? The answer is always going to be dependent on the criteria by which the research is judged; one such criterion is the level of reflexivity.

Research that simultaneously describes and constitutes a social setting has been termed reflexive (Alvesson and Sköldberg 2000; Freshwater and Rolfe 2001; Rolfe 2002). Reflexivity is an important concept, not only in critical science to ensure that the object of critical intent is as far as possible critically appraised, but also in the carrying out of action research and reflective practice. The idea of reflexivity was central to the development of George Kelly's personal construct theory (1995). As Kelly says: 'We can turn our mind back on to itself and contemplate our own contemplations' (1995: 60). Reflexive research then does not only necessitate thinking about practice, it also requires practitioners to reflect on how they are thinking about practice.

Rather than attempting to eliminate the effects of the researcher, reflexive researchers try to understand them, the objective–subjective dichotomy is seen as unproductive (Kemmis and McTaggart 2000; Freshwater and Rolfe 2001; Rolfe 2002). Kemmis (1993: 257) points out that it is impossible to analyze 'praxis' from a value free, neutral stance. Lather (1991) agrees stating that: 'just as there is no neutral education, there is no neutral research'. Further, it could be argued that viewing action research as biased or distorted, misses the purpose of action research as facilitating self-reflection in the practitioner (and research team), who will therefore discover previously unrecognized distortions of action and in turn endeavour to make changes to practice (thus engaging in the process of conscientization). It could be argued that all interpretations of meaning from action would be relative, and as such always have to be estimated in relation to the original question. Further, reflexivity demands that these interpretations are located in the wider social, political and ethical context (Freshwater and Rolfe 2001), thereby enabling theoretical generalization (Sharp 1998).

It has been mentioned that the cycle of reflection is a core component of the action research process. The processes of reflection and action learning are also major proponents of the transformatory approach to learning (Askew and Carnell 1998). While in action research the focus is external and usually on professional practice within a particular context, action learning is primarily a personal activity with an internal focus but always context bound. Using the self as a research instrument does invoke some criticism, not least when the researchers declare that the research is also a tool for *personal* and *professional* development. The validity is liable to be questioned if they are not able to demonstrate reflexive awareness of the factors influencing the various stages of the research activity (Freshwater and Rolfe 2001), what some authors describe as location and positioning (Koch and Harrington 1998). Achieving the balance between the internal and the external, the personal and the professional is a delicate procedure, for as Somekh (1995) warns, too much emphasis on self in action research distracts from the substantive focus of the study. The rigour then of action research: 'derives from the logical, empirical, and political coherence of interpretations in the reconstructive moments of the self-reflective spiral (observing and reflecting) and the logical, empirical, and political coherence of justifications of proposed action in its construction or prospective moments (planning and acting)' (Kemmis 1993: 185).

Critical reflection on action research

One of the major weaknesses of action research is that the findings cannot always be generalized to other situations, because action research deals with local problems. The word 'generalizability' is one that is imposed from the language of traditional science and as such is contentious in what is essentially a qualitative endeavour (even where quantitative methods of data collection are employed). It is generally assumed that findings that are not generalizable do not affect practice. There are, however, many ways to affect practice (Rolfe 1996). The broader context of the theory–practice gap in health-care practice and education is a problem that is recognized on a national scale. The social and political context will have some resonance with other organizations, while the local factors may differ slightly; the principles underpinning the transformatory approach to practice and research are transferable to any clinical situation. The outcomes however will always be different as the learning is unique to each situation and therefore cannot be replicated exactly. It is also worth noting here that while action research aims to develop practice within existing frameworks, it is also labour intensive, demanding a great deal of commitment from all those involved in the process.

Reporting and disseminating action research

Despite the argument that action research is about local and contingent knowledge, dissemination of learning and findings is crucial, not only in order to deepen the understanding of the project material itself, but also to add to the continual development of action research as a methodology. Thus action research reports function on at least two levels. Firstly, that of reflecting on the learning process within a particular context in order to better understand how to affect change/improvement and, secondly, to develop an understanding of the action research process and its value as a tool for professional development.

Reporting action research through the explication of processes, audit trails and outcomes enables other researcher-practitioners to resonate with relevant concerns of their own. Hence 'action research reports describe the local process (of challenge and negotiation) whereby eventual agreement is reached concerning the generally shared truth criteria implicit in their various conclusions and outcomes' (Winter and Munn-Giddings 2001: 259).

Holloway and Wheeler note that 'The final report should reflect the variety of perspectives that were examined.' This is not an easy task given the multiple roles employed by researchers who might be 'research participants, change agents and evaluators of change' simultaneously (Holloway and Wheeler 2002: 197). Nevertheless this potential 'messiness' more closely reflects the everyday world of practice, in which health-care professionals are engaged in multiple roles and functioning at multiple levels concurrently (Schön 1987). What is required is the engagement of practitioners in a critical reflective dialogue both with themselves and their colleagues about the impact and influence of these different aspects on the research process and clinical situation.

Summary: action research as praxis

It is fundamental to the process of action research that it addresses the reality of practice, thereby bringing theory and practice more in relationship through the application of a pragmatic epistemology (Rorty 1979). Research that produces data as outcomes is not enough (Newman 1994), clinical research should also aim to help participants understand and act on their particular situations. This is often referred to as praxis research. Praxis is action informed by practical theory, which in turn may inform and transform theory.

Rolfe (1996) reminds us that the term 'praxis' had its origins in Greece where it was used by Aristotle to describe a 'doing' action and that Marx adopted the term to denote the unity of theory and practice. Newman (1994) and Rolfe (1996) seem to concur, saying that reflection and action are essential ingredients to the successful integration of research and theory with practice. Rolfe (1996) contends that research should not only be concerned with what he terms formal, generalizable theories, but also with changing and improving practice while at the same time generating micro, informal theory. Viewing research from this perspective is helpful in that it provides a shift away from the either/or debate of positivism or antipositivism, instead these are seen as valid and necessary steps on the way to operationalizing research findings.

Contemporary models of action research such as reflexive action research contribute to the reduction of the theory–practice gap by enabling practitioners to research their own practice; directly bringing about improvements in clinical practice by building positive change into the research process. Further, such approaches are premised on the value of action learning, that is the bringing together of people to learn from each other's experience, and as such they are closely linked to the implementation of reflective practice and clinical supervision and the drive towards work-based learning in health care.

Extended case study: clinical leadership in prison health care

This reflexive action research project aimed to establish a strategy for the effective implementation of a clinical supervision strategy across the prison health-care setting. The project is currently in its third action cycle, the first cycle consisting of a local pilot project, the second cycle focusing on the development of a national training programme and the third cycle shifting the emphasis back to regional leads for the prison service.

Background

Recent developments in health-care practice have included the implementation of clinical supervision and evidence-based practice (UKCC 1996). While clinical supervision is a relatively new concept in some health-related disciplines, it has long been an established part of practice in counselling, psychotherapy, social work and midwifery. Clinical supervision has been promoted as a method of ensuring safe and accountable practice, emphasizing standards and quality of care, patient safety and staff support.

Health care in secure environments requires a concentration of staff with specific expertise who have considerable continuing professional development needs and clinical supervision requirements. Nursing staff in the prison service comprises mainly health-care officers and civilian nurses. There are currently over 1000 registered nurses working in prisons in England and Wales. Nurses who work in these prisons undertake roles which incorporate both nursing and security thus demanding skills and competencies in both areas. Nurses, health-care officers and medical officers working in prison have to care for patients with a wide range of needs. The prison population can be viewed as a small community representative of the community outside the prison, hence the prison nursing staff has to manage chronic disease, mental illness, drug and alcohol abuse as well as acute medical problems and trauma. Additionally, nurses undertake health screening for new prisoners coming into prison. Many prisons also accommodate in-patient care in addition to primary care services. Primary care services are often provided by nursing staff working in treatment rooms in the residential area of the prison. GP surgeries are sited in most prisons within which nurses undertake a practice-nursing role.

The findings of a recently published UKCC report which examined nursing in secure environments (UKCC and University of Central Lancashire 1999) reached a number of conclusions and recommendations that were relevant to the development of clinical supervision within the prison service. It was reported that there was a low level of acceptance of clinical supervision, possibly because practical problems and lack of management support create difficulties in its implementation. In addition, clinical supervision was not readily available to practitioners working in conditions that test their professional resilience. The patient groups and professional isolation, in some instances, would suggest that this is an area where staff would benefit from the rigorous and systematic application of clinical supervision. In summary the report recommended that there should be a mandatory requirement for all health-care staff working in secure environments to receive clinical support and supervision on a regular basis (UKCC and University of Central Lancashire 1999).

In many (but not all) prisons and young offender institutions the health-care culture is influenced by traditional attitudes, with an emphasis on security and less on nursing practice and health. The care versus custody debate is one that continues, as does the clarification of the role of health-care professionals within secure environments. Many health-care staff experience cognitive dissonance as they find themselves pulled between acting as advocate and carer and custodian. Prison health care suffers from a difficulty in recruiting staff, and, once recruited, staff are quickly socialized into the dominant discourse. Working in under established health-care centres and with little support, and with only a relatively new structure for professional development, prison health-care professionals in the UK have been tasked with improving standards of care. Funding was sought and obtained to pump prime the development and implementation of a strategy to support prison health-care staff through clinical supervision.

The study

The focus of the initial phase of this project was on supporting practitioners to develop an awareness of the skills and competencies required to manage the complex environment within which they work through the process of clinical supervision and reflective practice. Thus the project aim was to implement and evaluate models of supervision appropriate to the needs of prison health-service staff. The first cycle took place over a period of twelve months. This phase was based within a small group of prisons and intended to make recommendations for good practice, identifying real and perceived barriers. Thirty-five health-care staff from five prisons were involved in a training programme that prepared staff to facilitate reflective practice through clinical supervision. The project was undertaken with practitioners and managers from five prisons (three inner city large local prisons; one high security prison and one young offenders' institution). Establishments were chosen and invited to participate in this study to enable the evaluation of models of clinical supervision across a variety of different contexts. They were then asked to identify staff interested in becoming clinical supervisors. The educational preparation of supervisors within four of these prisons was undertaken by the project team and comprised three days training over approximately one month.

Action research formed the broad methodological and philosophical framework; however, the project team also drew upon elements of ethnography and reflexivity (Rolfe 1998; Freshwater and Rolfe 2001) and the case study approach (Rolfe *et al.* 2001). Action learning was also used as the basis for the supervision training. This was chosen for its congruence with action research and its potential for enabling the group to develop an experiential responsive programme of training that could be locally owned.

Despite the formation of a working group (incorporating health-care staff and project team) and participants being asked to volunteer, initial acceptance of the project team into the prison system was problematic. We experienced a high degree of suspicion and paranoia about the 'real' reason for being invited into the project and also concern about the identity of those to whom we were reporting back. There was a distinct feeling of 'them' and 'us', with the health-care staff feeling oppressed by some unnamed authoritarian figure, embodied in the lead researcher, myself! It appeared at this early stage, that while we were hoping for a collaborative and practical action research model, there was some energy being invested in keeping me the expert, and the authority, pushing for the technical model.

While the participants were wanting to be involved, they were also resistant to any change that might challenge their current ways of working. The action learning model proved to be threatening to the participants, particularly because of its iterative and experiential nature. Being invited to reflect on themselves and their practice obviously necessitated some degree of revelation, and perhaps a confrontation with their own inner contradictions. The lack of imposed structure challenged the norms of the group and as such created a degree of instability and cognitive dissonance.

In order to minimize the feeling of clinical supervision being imposed, it was negotiated within the group that they were to have complete control over the development of a minimum standard for clinical supervision within their individual practice settings. This was to be based on their own experience of supervision and on their learning in the training programme. As a team we worked hard at acknowledging our differences and similarities and at identifying potential saboteurs among the team and within the prison system. The newly trained supervisors had access to an external supervisor who facilitated group supervision on a regular basis following the period of initial preparation. This support was provided in an attempt to augment the initial preparation with ongoing support to enhance the participants' confidence. Follow-up support sessions were provided by the project team subsequent to the training and interview processes.

Data collection

Initial demographic data of the sample of supervisors attending the training were collected through a brief survey questionnaire. Tape-recorded semi-structured interviews were the primary data collection method; in addition fieldnotes were taken in cases where tape recorders were prohibited and where interviews took place over the telephone. Interviews were tape recorded in all but two of the prisons (for security reasons). The Manchester Clinical Supervision Scale was used when interviewing all participants to ascertain attitudes and perceptions of clinical supervision following the project. Health-care managers, supervisors and supervisees were interviewed in each prison and the Manchester Scale questionnaire administered. All participants, including researchers, kept reflective diaries, and these were analyzed alongside fieldnotes and other relevant documents.

Data analysis

Demographic data obtained from the questionnaire and the Manchester Clinical Supervision Scale were analyzed using computer software packages (SPSS). Thematic analysis of all qualitative and quantitative data was undertaken using a phenomenological reduction adapted from Giorgi (1970). A comparative analysis of all data was carried out across the project team to illustrate and validate the main themes emerging from the data. Three main themes emerged from the data analysis these being *practice barriers, educational issues* and *resistance to change.* Barriers to change included individual concerns, cultural and institutional issues, operational and personnel difficulties, For example, although many participants felt the benefit of both the training and the supervision itself, many others expressed their concern that it felt like they were being watched by 'big brother' and that it was an 'excuse for time out and gossip'. (For an in-depth review of the project and outcomes see Freshwater *et al.* 2001, 2002.)

Despite a clear focus on the development of their own standards for supervision and a jointly generated definition of the same, the findings from the date still indicated the sense of clinical supervision being a surveillance technique (inter-estingly paralleling their role as practitioners). Practitioners spoke of feeling observed and of anxiety about the confidential nature of the supervisory process. Interestingly, the power was still located externally, although several staff members described supervision as potentially liberating and empowering because of its confidential nature and it being something specifically for them. What was noticeable is how infrequently this group of prison health-care staff congratulated or appreciated either themselves or each other, rather, they tended to focus on what was lacking or could be perceived to be a failure. This was one of the dominant themes to arise from the first phase of the project, as was the difficulty with effective and supportive clinical leadership in the management of localized change. Thus the focus of the second cycle work shifted slightly to incorporate these concerns.

When using a reflexive approach the investigator becomes part of the data rather than separate, hence the influence of the investigator on the data collection and analysis is acknowledged. As befitting the action research approach the researchers and participants worked together to critically review the current situation, identify and monitor the effect of any changes being made. As previously mentioned, action research has its own criteria for success, one of which concerns the absence of any unintended negative effects. With regard to this criterion it is important to consider the impact of the project on both the practitioners and the patients. One of the most prominent ethical issues to have arisen from this project was the effect on patients as a result of removing the staff from the establishments to provide training away from the prisons. While there was little doubting the benefit of providing the training outside of the workplace and with other practi-tioners, as a consequence patients may have spent longer in their cells due to the shortage of staff. Thus in the immediate short term it could be argued that patient care actually suffered as a result of the project.

After discussion with the health-care staff a number of recommendations were outlined from the first phase of the work. These included:

- Leadership programmes for nurses and health-care officers in prison health care should be based on a model that includes clinical supervision.

- The significance of clinical supervision as a tool for the development of leadership needs to be highlighted.

- On induction into prison, health-care nurses and officers should be given the opportunity to embark on clinical supervision either within the establishment or from an external source.

- Governors and non-nurse health-care managers need to be appraised of the need for and benefits of clinical supervision and of the recommendations from such documents as *The Future Organization of Prison Healthcare*, *Nursing in Prisons* and *Making a Difference*. Appropriate training should be provided for both supervisors and supervisees in line with other national developments; this includes reflecting on the process of being in supervision as a learning and teaching approach, for example, utilizing action learning sets.

As a result of the ongoing reflection and evaluation of the supervision programme and its impact on practice the subsequent training programme was modified and transformed. Hence the revised aims of the project became:

- To effectively develop participants' knowledge and skills in facilitating reflection with supervisees.
- To promote an understanding of the nature and purpose of clinical supervision within the context of prison health care and wider.
- To enable participants to develop appropriate strategies to establish constructive, ethical, appreciative relationships.
- To enable participants to critically assess their own ability to balance challenge with support.

This project is now in its third phase, during which the project team members have managed to relinquish their part in the process. Training and supervision is now being provided at regional level by health-care staff, with the project team supporting the evaluation at a local and national level through action learning sets.

Conclusion

Critique of health-care practices is obviously important and is highlighted in many health-care initiatives, specifically those related to governance. However, it is also crucial to enable a process of appreciation to take place through research. Action research has, as Gergen (1982) argues, the capacity to challenge the guiding fictions of the culture, to encourage a reconsideration of the ordinariness of daily practice and to ask fundamental questions regarding social life. Cooperrider and Srivastva (1987) and Luduma *et al.* (2001) also persuade us to think about the degree to which action research can be utilized to facilitate an appreciation of the life-giving essentials of social existence.

References

Altrichter, H., Posch, P. and Somekh, B. (1993) *Teachers Investigate their Work: An Introduction to the Methods of Action Research.* London: Routledge.

Alvesson, M. and Sköldberg, K. (2000) *Reflexive Methodology.* London: Sage.

Askew, S. and Carnell, E. (1998) *Transformatory Learning: Individual and Global Change.* London: Cassell.

Carr, W. and Kemmis, S. (1986) *Becoming Critical.* London: Falmer Press.

Cohen, L. and Manion, L. (1989) *Research Methods in Education.* London: Routledge.

Cooperrider, D.L. and Srivastva, S. (1987) Appreciative inquiry in organisational life. In Pasmore, W.A. and Woodman, R.W. (eds) *Research in Organisational Change and Development,* Vol. 1. Greenwich: JAI Press, 24–56.

Dadds, M. (1985) What is action research? Paper presented at: Schulentwicklung an der Basis. Klagenfurt University, Austria, Dec.: 16–20.

Department of Health (1998) *Clinical Governance: Quality in the new NHS.* London: The Stationery Office.

Department of Health (2001) *Research Governance Framework*. London: The Stationery Office.

Down, J. (2002) Therapeutic Nursing and Technology: Clinical Supervision and Reflective Practice in a Critical Care Setting. In Freshwater, D. (ed.) *Therapeutic Nursing*. London: Sage, 57–74.

Elliott, J. (1991) *Action Research for Educational Change*. Milton Keynes: Open University Press.

Festinger, L. (1957) *A Theory of Cognitive Dissonance*. New York: Harper and Row.

Freire, P. (1972) *Pedagogy of the Oppressed*. Harmondsworth: Penguin.

Freshwater, D. (2000) *Transformatory Learning in Nurse Education*. London: Nursing Praxis International.

Freshwater, D. (ed.) (2002) *Therapeutic Nursing: Improving patient care through self-awareness and reflection*. London: Sage.

Freshwater, D. and Rolfe, G. (2001) Critical Reflexivity: A politically and ethically engaged research method for nursing, *NT Research*, 6 (1): 526–537.

Freshwater, D., Walsh, L. and Storey, L. (2001) Developing leadership through clinical supervision in prison healthcare, *Nursing Management*, 8 (8): 10–13.

Freshwater, D., Walsh, L. and Storey, L. (2002) Developing leadership through clinical supervision in prison healthcare, *Nursing Management*, 9 (1): 16–20.

Gergen, K.J. (1982) *Toward Transformation in Social Knowledge*. New York: Springer Verlag.

Giorgi, A. (1970) *Psychology as Human Science: A Phenomenologically Based Approach*. New York: Harper and Row.

Greenwood, J. (1984) Nursing research: A position paper, *Journal of Advanced Nursing*, 9: 77–82.

Grundy, S. (1987) *Curriculum: Product or Praxis?* London: Falmer Press.

Hart, E. and Bond, M. (1995) *Action Research for Health and Social Care. A Guide to Practice*. Buckingham: Open University Press.

Higgs, J. and Titchen, A. (eds) (2001) *Professional Practice in Health, Education and the Creative Arts*. Oxford: Blackwell Science.

Holloway, I. and Wheeler, S. (2002) *Qualitative Research in Nursing*, 2nd edn. Oxford: Blackwell.

Joyce, B.R. (1984) Dynamic disequilibrium: The intelligence of growth, *Theory into Practice*, 23 (1): 26–34.

Kazi, M.A.F. (2003) *Realist Evaluation in Practice*. London: Sage.

Kelly, G.A. (1995) *The Psychology of Personal Constructs*. New York: Norton.

Kemmis, S. and McTaggart, R. (2000) Participatory action research. In Denzin, N.K. and Lincoln, Y.S. (eds) *Handbook of Qualitative Research*, 2nd edn. London: Sage, 567–603.

Kemmis, S. (1993) Action research. In Hammersley, M. (ed.) *Educational Research: Current Issues*. Milton Keynes: Open University Press.

Koch, T. and Harrington, A. (1998) Reconceptualizing rigour: The case for reflexivity, *Journal of Advanced Nursing*, 28 (4): 882–890.

Lather, P. (1991) *Getting Smart: Feminist Research and Pedagogy within the Postmodern*. New York: Routledge.

LeMay, A., Mulhall, A. and Alexander, C. (1998) Bridging the Research–Practice Gap: Exploring the research cultures of practitioners and managers, *Journal of Advanced Nursing*, 28 (2): 428–437.

Lewin, K. (1946) Action research and minority problems, *Journal of Social Issues*, 2 (4): 34–46.

Ludema, J.D., Cooperrider, D.L. and Barrett, F.J. (2001) Appreciative Inquiry: the power of the unconditional positive question. In Reason, P. and Bradbury, H. (eds) *Handbook of Action Research*. London: Sage.

McKenzie, R. (2002) The importance of philosophical congruence for therapeutic use of self in practice. In Freshwater, D. (ed.) *Therapeutic Nursing*. London: Sage, 22–38.

McTaggart, R. (1992) Action research: Issues in theory and practice. Paper presented to Methodological Issues in Qualitative Health Research Conference, Deakin University.

Menzies-Lyth, I.E.P. (1988) *Containing Anxiety in Institutions*. Selected essays. London: Free Association Books.

Mezirow, J. (1981) A critical theory of adult learning and education, *Adult Education*, 1: 3–24.

Miller, A. (1989) Theory to practice: Implementation in the clinical setting. In Jolley, M. and Allan, P. (eds) *Current Issues in Nursing*. London: Chapman Hall.

Newman, M. (1994) *Health as Expanding Consciousness*, 2nd edn. New York: National League for Nursing Press.

Putnam, H. (1987) *The Many Faces of Realism*. Lasalle: Open Court.

Roberts, S.J. (1983) Oppressed group behaviour: implications for nursing, *Advances in Nursing Science*, July: 21–30.

Robson, C. (2002) *Real World Research*, 2nd edn. Oxford: Blackwell.

Rolfe, G. (1996) *Closing the Theory Practice Gap. A New Paradigm for Nursing*. Oxford: Butterworth Heinemann.

Rolfe, G. (1998) *Expanding Nursing Knowledge*. Oxford: Butterworth Heinemann.

Rolfe, G. (2002) Reflexive Research and the Therapeutic Use of Self. In Freshwater, D. (ed.) *Therapeutic Nursing*. London: Sage, 197–194.

Rolfe, G. Freshwater, D. and Jasper, M. (2001) *Critical Reflection for Nursing and the Helping Professions: A User's Guide*. Basingstoke: Palgrave.

Rorty, R. (1979) *Philosophy and the Mirror of Nature*. Princeton: Princeton University Press.

Schön, D.A. (1987) *Educating the Reflective Practitioner*. San Francisco: Jossey-Bass.

Sharp, K. (1998) The case for case studies in nursing research: The problem of generalisation, *Journal of Advanced Nursing*, 27: 785–789.

Somekh, B. (1995) The contribution of action research to development in social endeavours: A position paper on action research methodology, *British Educational Research Journal*, 21: 339–355.

Stringer, E. (1996) *Action Research: A Handbook for Practitioners*. London: Sage.

United Kingdom Central Council for Nurses, Midwives and Health Visitors (1999) *Nursing in Secure Environments*. London: UKCC.

United Kingdom Central Council for Nurses, Midwives and Health Visitors (1996) Position Statement on Clinical Supervision for Nursing and Health Visiting. London: UKCC.

Winter, R. and Munn-Giddings, C. (2001) *A Handbook for Action Research in Health and Social Care*. London: Routledge.

Zeichner, K. (2001) Educational action research. In Reason, P. and Bradbury, H. (eds) *Handbook of Action Research*. London: Sage.

Zuber-Skerritt, O. (1991) *Action Research for Change and Development*. Aldershot: Avebury.

13

KATHLEEN GALVIN
Navigating a qualitative course in programme evaluation

Theoretically, evaluation methodology presents a confusing, if not contradictory, mosaic of possibilities, rather than a unified and coherent set of
principles.

Prout 1992: 76

Introduction

Evaluation is ubiquitous in nature, referring to *the purpose* of the research which
subsequently draws upon a diverse range of research strategies, since there is no
unique research approach for evaluation research (Robson 2002). In its widest
context evaluation is concerned with systematic collection of information to
explore effectiveness and characteristics of programmes, to improve outcomes and
to examine worth and value (Suchman 1967; Rossi and Freeman 1993; Patton
1997; Weiss 1998). Long-standing debates within the evaluation literature concern
its emergence as a separate discipline. Some argue (House 1993; Scriven 1995)
that evaluation represents a distinct research school with its own identity, others
consider it a specialism within social science, placing emphasis upon meeting the
information needs of decision-makers and therefore policy (for example Patton
1997, 2002). There is no shortage of literature critiquing evaluation typologies
(Scriven 1967, 1991; Patton 1982, 1996; Chen 1996; Ovretveit 1998; Lazenbatt
2002). Additionally, numerous authors have drawn attention to debates about
various approaches within evaluation (Shadish *et al.* 1991; Chen 1996; Ong 1996;
Pawson and Tilley 1997; Shaw 1999; Tones and Tilford 2001; Robson 2002) and
others have analyzed the contribution of influential evaluation theorists and the
congruence of their theoretical positions (Shadish *et al.* 1991; Clarke with Dawson
1999; Shaw 1999).

Evaluation is often laden with high and sometimes contradictory aims and
expectations, sometimes ethical and political tensions are played out in the evaluation activity itself, sometimes they are embedded below the surface of research
project management activity. Inevitably the politics of evaluation and the role of
the researcher are further strands that are revisited later in this chapter.

There are several qualitative approaches viable in evaluation, related to a number of influential theoretical frameworks that form the focus of this chapter. I aim, firstly, to describe the major qualitative evaluation frameworks signposting further readings, and, secondly, to explore issues about qualitative evidence in the context of policy making. Patton (1997) offers an evaluative process, strategy and framework for deciding the focus and methods of an evaluation project in his 'utilization-focused' evaluation model. A key tenet concerns the intended use of the evaluation by intended users and outlines methodological strategies available which 'should include but not be limited to qualitative methods' (Patton 2002: 174). He suggests that the evaluator's task is to explore with evaluation users the design and data biases in an attempt to ensure that the evaluation generates knowledge that is credible and of value to all concerned. The credibility of qualitative evaluations in the context of policy-making is a theme I return to later in this chapter. It is important to note that the underpinning paradigm debate within evaluation literature has been heavily contested, and not all theorists agree that differing philosophical stances within research can be synthesized within one evaluation. That historical debate is ongoing; what follows here is a signposting of evaluation approaches that hold interpretive or humanistic values (some of which are dialectically opposed), while others are more pragmatic in their stance. These include several influential participatory frameworks such as cooperative inquiry (Heron 1996); empowering evaluation (Guba and Lincoln 1989); action research (Titchen and Binnie 1993; Stringer 1996; Greenwood and Levin 1998); case study/responsive evaluation (Stake 1975; 1995); rapid participatory appraisal (Lazenbatt 2002); rapid appraisal (Ong 1996). They either share some historical roots, overlap philosophically and/or draw upon qualitative method within their evaluative process.

Several related strands within the literature are drawn upon: key tenets of influential theoretical positions; participatory evaluation frameworks which have developed within and across a wide range of disciplines; qualitative methodology and its utility in policy-making; practical and political concerns.

Qualitative evaluation is naturalistic in that it is undertaken in 'real' and practice settings, the evaluator does not attempt to control or manipulate the setting being evaluated, and the findings unfold or emerge as there is generally no predetermined course or structured data collection controlled by the evaluator.[1] The naturalistic stance proposes that the social world cannot be reduced to that which is observable: rather, the social world is constructed and reinterpreted by people themselves. Knowledge of our world must facilitate key actors' accounts; people exist in a social context which is both material and bounded, and which influences their interpretations. Evaluation within a naturalistic stance requires analysis and description of people's meanings and interpretations of the social world examined within the natural 'real' world settings they occupy (Brewer 2003). The imperative for such an evaluation is to ask people their views; to ask in ways which facilitate a descriptive account of their meanings in their own words; to examine in-depth because meaning is embedded, complex and problematic; to emphasize social context which provides meaning and substance to the ideas which emerge.

In summary, qualitative evaluation strategies include methods that allow access to both meaning and context and which facilitate in-depth rich accounts. Patton (2002) provides an overview of the range of qualitative inquiry traditions that can be employed within evaluation frameworks (including ethnography; autoethnography; phenomenology; ethnomethodology; symbolic interactionism; hermeneutics; narrative analysis; grounded theory and critical theory) which can be drawn upon in evaluations that require in-depth and contextual accounts. Williams (1986), later summarized by Shaw (1999), provides a useful synthesis of criteria which characterize such approaches in evaluation.

Qualitative evaluation may be appropriate when:

- issues under scrutiny are not defined in advance;
- insider ('emic') perspectives are required to understand the subject of the evaluation;
- outcome relates to complex happenings in their natural setting;
- intensive scrutiny of the programme or intervention in its natural state and cycle is possible;
- multiple sources of data are available;
- a desire and consent to explore negative aspects and contrary evidence is apparent;
- some agreement with recipients of the intervention or programme about the methodological approach is desirable.

Patton (2002: 177) summarizes common principles underpinning this 'real' world philosophy which include the uniqueness of individuals; that people and communities should be understood holistically and in context; the need for equity, fairness, transparency and mutual respect; the requirement to negotiate change processes and the importance of person-centredness. In simplistic terms, qualitative evaluative research means transforming human processes into advantage by using them in research approaches that are sensitive to both context and vulnerability[2] of people, which are likely to produce shared insights into the evaluand from the perspectives of all those involved, rather than removing or controlling human actions and context.

Influential evaluation genres

An important but contested philosophical backdrop concerns 'the hierarchy of evidence' with claims that the strongest evaluations are experimental in nature. Early critiques of historically prevailing experimental and quasi-experimental evaluation approaches have been provided (House 1980; Hammersley and Atkinson 1983; Greenwood 1984; Cook 1985; Wilson-Barnett 1991; Greenwood and Levin 1998) and 'comparative' methods within evaluation in particular have been critiqued at philosophical and methodological levels by Pawson and Tilley

(1997), in the context of realism. Other examples rooted in educational and health promotion literature include Tones and Tilford's (2001) outline of characteristics of evaluation, which emphasizes the role of evaluation in informing health promotion policy, simultaneously drawing attention to the increasing need to adopt methods to study *process* as well as outcomes. Also, the seminal work of Parlett and Hamilton (1977) and Parlett (1981), offer a contrast to 'narrower' impact and outcome evaluation (prevailing at that time) by focusing upon the *illumination* of process and to the wider social context within which the evaluation takes place. Illuminative evaluation has its origins within educational evaluation and places emphasis upon interpretation and context, heavily relying upon participants' perceptions and experiences. 'Illuminative evaluation takes account of the wider contexts in which educational programs function. Its primary concern is with description and interpretation rather than measurement and prediction' (Parlett and Hamilton 1976: 144).

Stake (1975, 1980, 1995) drew attention to the potential use of qualitative methods within *responsive* evaluation, and in the context of case study methods, places emphasis upon the interests of the stakeholders. He pioneered humanization of the evaluation process, by seeking out stakeholders perspectives and concerns, through 'a plan of observations and negotiations' (Stake 1975: 14). The emphasis here is upon facilitating the evaluation to emerge from observation and engagement with participants. Both illuminative evaluation and responsive evaluation have been labelled 'transaction models of evaluation' in that they draw upon informal methods of inquiry, and focus upon the transactions between the evaluator and the participants (House 1978). Stake was one of the first theorists to place qualitative methods and participation at the centre of an evaluation framework, as such responsive evaluation was influential in the work of naturalistic evaluators, Guba and Lincoln (1988) who later referred to their stance as within the *constructivist* tradition.

The constructivist stance is built upon the premise that the study of the social world requires an approach which allows access to people's interpretations of their world, because human beings can interpret and construct 'realities', which are shaped and perceived by cultural and linguistic meanings. A key assumption underpinning *constructivist* evaluation is that people construct their own reality and therefore evaluators' interactions with their participants and subject of evaluation is itself part of the evaluation exercise. Therefore the 'issues', 'concerns' and 'claims' of stakeholders determine what evaluation information is needed and how it is collected (Guba and Lincoln 1989).

Patton (2002: 98) asserts that the constructivist evaluator 'would examine the implications of different perceptions (or multiple realities) but would not pronounce which set of perceptions was "right" or more "true" or more "real" however the "constructivist evaluator could compare clients" perceptions and social constructions with those of funders or program staff and could interpret the effects of differences on attainment of stated program goals, but they would not value staff perceptions as more real or meaningful.'

Guba and Lincoln (1989) critique evaluative techniques that have characterized the literature for the last 60 years ('First' – the 'measurement' generation;

'Second' – the 'goal achievement' generation and the 'Third' generation – 'management technique' evaluations). They draw attention to a tendency towards managerialism, where commissioners of research determine what is to be evaluated and what will happen to the findings and consequently disempower other stakeholders. They suggest that evaluation should acknowledge and address pluralistic values, they highlight problems of 'context stripping' by overuse of the positivist approach and 'objective' measurement. There are strong parallels between Guba and Lincoln's arguments and those within health- and social-care policy, specifically, for example, within health promotion, health and community development literature. For instance, the ideological basis of health promotion as embodied in the Ottawa Charter (WHO 1996) reflects an ecological approach to health promotion whereby health education and healthy public policy contribute to the promotion of health. The principles underpinning this model are voluntary participation (Tones 1987) and empowerment in the achievement of equity in power and resources (Tones and Tilford 2001), so it follows that community participation is therefore a prerequisite of healthy public policy. These ideas are revisited in participatory evaluation frameworks that have emerged within community development work.

Guba and Lincoln (1989) reflect these principles in their *Fourth Generation Evaluation* framework. Pluralistic evaluation in this sense involves responding to stakeholders and allowing the focus of the research to emerge rather than being predetermined by the researcher. The methodological framework is interpretive. The role of the evaluator is to provide a methodology (dialectic/hermeneutic) through which different claims, concerns and constructions of stakeholders can be understood and critiqued. Unresolved claims and concerns are further investigated and suggest what action is to be taken. This approach therefore allows a range of stakeholders, for example, policy-makers, health service managers, those involved in the delivery of an intervention or service, beneficiaries of the evaluation (users of services) and subjects of the evaluation (who are normally excluded) to confront and deal with issues together. Negotiation among the stake holding groups using the information collected to reach consensus has benefits for the development of local services and policy. Another genre in this generation includes the muliplist model (Cook 1985).

There are also some relevant parallels to be drawn with action research and participatory frameworks which have their roots in community development, initiatives for equalizing access to health (for example, the Primary Health Care (PHC) approach forged by the World Health Organization and UNICEF in the 1970s) and historically in the work of Paulo Freire. These include 'Rapid Appraisal' and 'Rapid Participatory Appraisal'. The purpose of rapid appraisal is to involve communities in setting priorities and to influence policy-making. It brings with it a need for resource managers to respond to change as generated by community concerns (Ong 1996). In a similar vein, the purpose of rapid participatory appraisal is to study factors that contribute to community and individual health (Lazenbatt 2002). Lazenbatt argues that 'Rapid Participatory Appraisal' has the potential to demonstrate the power of significant user involvement in equalizing access to services and therefore to health as it can:

- facilitate an exploration of the locality and its community;
- illustrate the nature and extent of working relationships between agencies working in the same locale or sector;
- help to identify local health issues and issues of access;
- provide focus to link health needs with socio-economic inequality;
- facilitate the involvement of local service users and individuals from communities;
- facilitate a coordinated interagency responses.

The key tenets of both frameworks are that the activity has to be rapid to ensure findings are relevant and timely. The concerns of the community are at the heart and therefore the approach needs to be highly flexible and pragmatic to facilitate ideas and creative endeavour with all stakeholders. A key desire is that the outcomes should be sustainable (Ong 1996). The process includes formulating a list of community needs, developing priority-setting mechanisms with ongoing feedback to participants and development of a programme of change.

By their nature a range of methods may be used within the overall rapid appraisal design, 'methods will be selected according to local circumstances . . . and will be based upon dialogue with local communities' (Ong 1996: 75). However, as in all participatory approaches, observation and interviewing methods, in particular focus groups, will be a cornerstone of facilitating such dialogue within a participatory evaluation. The notion of dialogue has been further developed as the centrepiece of participatory evaluation by among others Guba and Lincoln (1989); House and Howe (1999); Abma (2001); Greene (2001); Widdershoven (2001).

> It is through the defining lens of value commitments, rather than methodology or purpose, that dialogue in evaluation is most meaningfully understood and discussed. For dialogue in evaluation most fundamentally means a value commitment to *engagement*, engagement with problems of practice, with challenges of difference and diversity of practices and their understandings, and thus with the relational, moral and political dimensions of our contexts and our craft.
>
> (Greene 2001: 181)

In a further example of inquiry, with dialogue at its core, *cooperative* inquiry (Reason 1994; Heron 1996), allows individuals in the inquiry group to explore their perceptions and shared meanings about a project or change under evaluation. The experience of engaging with a new way of working or living could be explored by reflective methods ('experiential knowing') and ways of dealing with barriers, difficulties and negative feelings could be recorded ('practical knowing') as outlined by Heron (1996). The findings generated could provide propositions about the various stages in the process of change and add valuable insights from the perspective of those either trying to deliver the new service or those at the receiving end. This approach offers a window for exploring the shared meanings embedded in practice. Another advantage is that power and control are shifted between *all* those involved in the research, rather than resting solely with the researcher.

Drawing upon collaborative evaluation literature, Robson (2000) compares three approaches to collaborative evaluation: stakeholder evaluation; participatory evaluation and practitioner centred action research. These three frameworks can be considered as a spectrum of 'involvement' (see Table 13.1).

Table 13.1

	Stakeholder evaluation	Participatory evaluation	Practitioner-centred action research
Study driven by	Evaluator	Evaluator guided and assisted by practitioners	Practitioners with assistance of evaluator
Involvement of practitioners/ users	Consultative role, provide information on context and key data	Active role engaged in key components of the evaluation	Fully involved and actively in control of the research process
Who is involved?	Large number of varied stakeholders and any groups with a stake in the programme/service	Small number of programme users/ practitioners	All practitioners and users involved as action researchers/'co-researchers'

$\longrightarrow$

Increased involvement and control of collaborators

$\longleftarrow$

Decreased 'control' of the evaluator

Adapted from Robson (2000) Table 2.1, p. 21

Shaw (1999) also distinguishes four areas of practitioner evaluation reflecting similar cross-cutting themes, these include: research and evaluation carried out *by practitioners*; participatory research; evaluation as a dimension of practice, e.g. reflective inquiry and evaluation for practitioners carried out *by researchers*. There are clear overlaps and parallels with the philosophy underpinning action research and reflective inquiry (see Chapter 12 on action research).

Within all these genres of evaluation, methods from qualitative inquiry schools are drawn upon to uncover and provide accounts of participants' perceptions and interpretations. This characteristic is overlaid by the context and nature of participation and how it is to be facilitated within the evaluation. Inevitably the context of the evaluation 'project' such as political issues, ownership of the evaluation, nature and extent of funding and the evaluation's ultimate purpose are considerations which may shape the evaluation approach but are also aspects that the evaluator may have little control over. An important feature is the intended use of the findings in informing policy.

Utility in policy and role of mixed methods

Diversity at method level is commonly discussed in the evaluation literature. Ovretveit (1998) describes many diverse evaluation types, two of which in particular necessitate a qualitative research perspective; these include process evaluation and pluralistic evaluation. *Process* evaluation uses qualitative strategies, although not exclusively, to assess progress, gain insight how the programme or intervention works and includes how the programme or intervention is organized, perceived and received. Pluralistic evaluation is a term with ranging definitions in the literature. One definition (Lazenbatt 2002) suggests that pluralistic evaluation examines the perspectives of stakeholders about success and the achievement or not of that success, by providing an ethnography of the intervention and explanation of processes involved in the light of interests and definitions of participating groups. However, most literature focuses on the potential of wide ranging methodology (a plurality of method) and its role in evaluation (for instance, Cook 1997; Ovretveit 1998; Greene *et al.* 2001).

Within evaluation traditions there exist differences of opinion about the role of qualitative and participatory evaluations play in wider policy-making and whether or not it is appropriate to mix methods. That said, it can be argued that robust evaluation, whatever the philosophical framework, provides policy-makers with an account, or accounts of what is going on, from the perspectives of those involved in the evaluation, within complex interventions, programmes or services at the very least, at local level.

However, if we accept that the challenge for researchers engaged in evaluation is to (a) develop appropriate methods that are trustworthy but at the same time produce findings which either transfer to real life contexts, and/or (b) have some utility in establishing the value of something, simultaneously informing future development or wider policy-making; then qualitative evaluation has to be examined within the context of paradigm issues.

The evaluation methods literature reflects the paradigm debate with increased 'legitimacy for qualitative methods' (Patton 2002: 584) evidenced through emphasis on methodological appropriateness, increased methodological sophistication, broader conceptual understanding of evaluation, and support for plurality of method from key institutions with vested interest in evaluation. However, there remain variances in credibility of qualitative evaluation between disciplines and countries (Patton 2002).

In the UK specifically there has been examination as to whether qualitative evaluations have any place within Health Technology Assessment and subsequently the wider evidence base of health care at all (Murphy and Dingwall 1992; Sassi 2000; Dingwall 2001; Murphy 2001). Murphy (2001) and Murphy and Dingwall (2001) conclude that qualitative methods do have an important role in terms of exploring areas inaccessible to other methods; shedding light upon the links between inputs and outputs through process illumination; generating hypotheses, understanding context of quantitative findings or as a precursor to quantitative research. Additionally, qualitative sampling strategies (in contrast to often misunderstood and ill-founded accusations of 'sampling error'; weak 'internal and external validity') are powerful aspects of qualitative method that can be positively harnessed to allow future application or transferability of findings and therefore increase utility in policy-making. Murphy and Dingwall (2001) make reference to Silverman (1989, 1993) suggesting that samples within a qualitative evaluation should be constructed in a systematic way, taking account of 'typicality' to facilitate future generalization. They also make the case that theoretical sampling lends itself aptly to technology assessment since it allows some *theoretical* generalization from one setting to another in addition to allowing evaluators to explore critical and contrary cases to modify or extend existing theory. Also Brewer (2003: 127) controversially claims that while qualitative methods are better at theoretical inference some

> . . . empirical generalisations to a wider population are feasible despite the limited number of cases if the cases permit comparisons and have been selected by a sampling procedure. There are two ways this can be done. First, it is possible to design the individual project in the mould of similar ones in different fields so that comparisons can be made across them and a body of cumulative knowledge can be built upon that is longitudinal, historical and comparative. The second way is to design the project as a series of parallel qualitative studies with different cases or with the same case in different fields, perhaps even using multiple researchers.

This is a debate which is contested as not all qualitative researchers agree that generalizability is possible or indeed a requirement (for example, Stake 1975). Unfortunately, however, the full potential of qualitative evaluation (embedded in its strengths of in-depth thick description, understanding of meaning, richness and ability to link complex chains of events, examination of multiple realities and so on) remains an 'Achilles heel' in the context of useful evidence as it is currently contended in such fields. Qualitative evaluation still carries with it a stigma of being 'soft' 'especially with the media and among policy-makers, creating what has been called the tyranny of numbers (Eberstadt *et al.* 1995; Patton 2002: 573). To add to evaluators' troubles any critique of qualitative evaluation in the health technology sense is set against a backdrop that 'is committed to pursuing **truth** as a secure basis for action' (Murphy and Dingwall 2001: 167, my emphasis).

Bate and Robert (2002) similarly conclude that within the UK Health Service a traditional mainstream approach to evaluation is favoured (summative, non-interventionist evaluation), therefore evaluation which has a 'technical–rational' research approach at its foundation. It seems then that the long-standing philosophical debate between Idealism and Constructivism is alive and well. At the methods level claims have been made that any qualitative evaluation is of limited value to policy-making due to lack of generalizability, reliance upon purposive sampling, the tendency to be small scale and in single setting, lack of statistical inference; that it is anecdotal and lacks precision (Murphy and Dingwall 2001). These assertions are not new, with philosophical and methodological counter arguments well rehearsed in this book and elsewhere. However, the mixed methods debate is more sophisticated than methodological 'trading' between approaches within evaluation theory, as Greene *et al.* (2001: 41) caution:

> Designing and implementing a mixed method evaluation is not merely choosing from a smorgasbord of methods available. Whether an evaluator is mixing methods practically, dialectically, within the boundaries of program theory or within alternative paradigms, this approach demands a heightened reflexivity and responsiveness.

At the technical level there is widespread support for mixed methods evaluation (Cook and Reichardt 1979; Patton 1982, 2002; Ong 1996; Lazenbatt 2002), driven historically by the problems of experimental methods in applied settings such as programme evaluation and the insufficiency of traditional social science methods when applied during the 1960s and 1970s to poverty alleviation programmes (Cook 1985). This call for mixed methods is about increasing the emphasis upon participatory and humanistic evaluation.

At the philosophical level, evaluation proponents hold several world views. The 'purist' stance holds that mixed methods are inappropriate, the interpretive paradigm reflects a *distinctive* set of assumptions about knowledge. Lincoln and Guba (1985) and Guba and Lincoln (1998) argue that decisions at paradigm level have precedence over methodological decisions and as there is no reconciliation possible between paradigms, they cannot be combined or merged. Similarly, Stake (1975, 1995) argues that generalization is not an appropriate goal in qualitative evaluation and that any attempts for representation distort case studies, an argument that contests a position I have alluded to earlier concerning the desire and possibility of generalization.

Advocates of mixed method designs have been discussed by Greene *et al.* (2001) as the 'pragmatic' and 'dialectical' schools (the most prominent) and the 'substantive' and 'alternative' schools. Pragmatists, such as Patton (1988), purport that responsiveness to stakeholders and issues within the evaluation guides the methodological design. Patton (1990: 38) proposes a 'paradigm of choices', which represents opposing and competing traditions with different approaches used for different situations.

The dialectical stance holds that opposing paradigm views cannot be reconciled but that they can guide mixed methods within an evaluation, to enhance understanding of social settings (Greene and Caracelli 1997). The substantive theorists hold that the evaluation should be driven by the intended links and impacts of activities and outcomes in programmes, that is the evaluation should focus upon the meaningfulness and programme effectiveness within a given social context (Chen and Rossi 1983; Chen 1990; Weiss 1998). The 'alternative' (critical theory) paradigm proponents encompass action research (Stringer 1996; Greenwood and Levin 1998) and cooperative inquiry (Reason 1994; Heron 1996).

In conclusion, qualitative evaluation is not atheoretical, evaluators are called to reflect upon their methodological stance at a number of levels: the evaluation framework – collaborative or non-interventionist; whether they are working from a purist, dialectical, pragmatic, substantive or alternative stance; the evaluation problem itself – the evaluation agenda and who set it; the purpose of the evaluation, its key inquiry questions, the extent of stakeholder participation and desired outcomes, the role and independence or collaboration of the evaluator, the appropriateness of method and resources. It is more than technical strategy, but rather a state of mind or value-based attitude (Dingwall 1992) that may involve resolving political and philosophical tensions. Evaluators' choices may be driven as much by political imperatives as by philosophical ones and their subsequent actions may be determined or even undermined by the political context of the evaluation itself.

Political misgivings

Weiss (1999) describes evaluation activity as a value laden and deeply political process. Research in the 'real world' implies that most investigators will find themselves undertaking evaluation (particularly in discipline areas such as health, social care, practice and education) (Robson 2002) and in so doing, unavoidably entangled in deeply sensitive political and ethical issues. Ethical issues of consent, privacy, confidentiality and anonymity need addressing as in any research but are often compounded in an evaluation with greater potential for conflict and the nature of practical impacts since evaluations are carried out for a specific purpose, often by 'outsiders', sometimes commissioned by funders of the programme and undertaken for a wide variety of audiences, some advocates, others sceptical. Naturally not all stakeholders will have the same agenda or interests. While researchers may be able to demonstrate the value of qualitative findings to other evaluators in their reporting, the findings may be rejected or criticized on methodological grounds. Negative and unintended consequences are a risk in any evaluation, and service users and providers may find the process anxiety provoking. Some of these concerns may be mitigated by active involvement of stakeholders but it would be naïve to assume that stakeholder participation eliminates risks and political tensions. Indeed, Mark and Shotland (1987) assert that stakeholder participation may not give participants an influential voice, stakeholding groups may not have equal representation and may be socially controlled, evaluators may see some groups as more legitimate participants than others, the evaluator has an influential role in determining who are the stakeholders. Evaluators have to reflect upon tensions and power struggles so that they can be sensitive to how tensions affect the direction and use of the evaluation. Rather than creating a partisan approach, Patton (1982) argues that being aware and sensitive to personality conflicts, power struggles and mistrust 'is not the same as taking sides' (p. 93). Tensions can be reported as part of the evaluation process or after the event. For example, Lax and Galvin (2002) attempt to articulate the tensions and lessons learnt in a community-based evaluation. Some anticipated problems may include unknown or unacknowledged agendas, issues of cooperation, skills required in building relationships, trust, credibility and reaching agreed plans for dissemination and responsibility for acting upon findings. Bate and Robert (2002) provide an example of a reflexive account of one evaluation team's efforts to move away from a traditional objective evaluation to an action research framework within a health-service context. They illustrate dilemmas presented to qualitative researchers as data emerged to suggest that the programme was failing, and map out their experience in pressing for an interventionist evaluation with qualitative data being feedback to programme delivery teams, in the face of opposition from commissioners. They conclude that the process demanded a much more political role for evaluators in shaping the direction of a project. 'Our story highlights the potential power and significance of qualitative evaluation in organisation development and Action Research settings and how, if it had been placed at the center of the change and developmental process, it could have facilitated a more intelligent, critical and self-questioning approach by those involved' (p. 978).

Interestingly, beyond the political role of evaluators, the political issue has also been a key impetus within wider philosophical evaluation debate. Both Shadish *et al.* (1991) and Shaw (1999) have placed research by Weiss (1987) concerning the political context of evaluation as a watershed which made way for the shift which ultimately placed qualitative evaluation at the heart of the evaluation theory debate between idealism and pragmatism.

Example: a pragmatic evaluation of an arrest referral scheme (ARS) in drug related crime

Background

The project 'Second Chance' arrest referral scheme first became operational in 1996. The aim of the ARS was to target arrestees (in police custody) to counsel and refer them to drug treatment services and ultimately break the cycle of drug-related crime. The scheme was delivered by three trained project workers. This type of initiative first emerged in the UK in the late 1980s as a direct response to the evidence of a link between increasing crime and drug using. ARSs have been introduced throughout Britain taking a number of varied forms. Three models of arrest referral have been identified by Edmunds *et al.* (1998); this scheme was a proactive model characterized by its setting in a police custody suite where trained drugs workers liaise closely with police to target, counsel and make referrals for arrestees who have a drug problem.

Galvin *et al.* (1998) undertook an evaluation of a local arrest referral scheme (ARS). A drugs action team (DAT) who wanted to review the development of the service commissioned the evaluation. Specific aims were set by the commissioners and included:

- Description of the uptake of the scheme and referral patterns from it to local health- and social-care providers.
- Assessment of the impact of the intervention from the perspective of its users.
- Description of police perceptions about the scheme.

The agenda was made explicit by their chair who met the evaluation team frequently before the evaluation began: the scheme was already valued but in order to support it in the long term its impact needed description and documented evidence. Funding decisions had to be made about distributing resources to increase its capacity and to support complementary drug treatment services. The drug action team wanted information to help determine how resources should be distributed across types of drug treatment and support service and whether the scheme should be extended to other custody suites. Since the DAT expressed potential for the scheme to be expanded, the research team also added three aims:

1. To explore obstacles and opportunities for development of the scheme.
2. To explore the characteristics of the project and how the project workers delivered their service.
3. Identify areas and issues that may be insightful to other similar projects.

Design considerations

Three major considerations guided the evaluation design:

1. The commissioners wanted findings quickly, one year with interim feedback at six months (this was driven by their funding for evaluation). It was considered appropriate to involve as many stakeholders in the project as possible within the evaluation, to give depth to the evaluation and to explore the initiative from varied multiple institutional perspectives, this was particularly appropriate since it was a multisectoral initiative; including police, judicial system, health and social care and the voluntary sector.
2. Drug users are hard to access and their stories would be set within the context of crime, therefore the evaluation team were anxious that the evaluation should not 'deter' drug users from making full use of the ARS initiative.
3. The aims of the evaluation required methods which facilitated an examination of the project overall, in addition to providing accounts from multiple stakeholder perspectives as to how the scheme was delivered and received in practice. The evaluation framework was pragmatic in the sense that methods decisions were guided by the appropriateness of method (Patton 1997) to ensure generation of useful data. Figure 13.1 summarizes the data collection methods used and for the purposes of this chapter qualitative aspects of the evaluation are described (although both qualitative and quantitative procedures were used).

Fieldwork encompassed a short period 'shadowing' the project workers and undertaking 'tours' of the project setting. Individual conversational interviews were conducted with the three project workers; individual interviews with Second Chance clients at the project office; focus groups with court cell staff and probation officers; focus groups with custody staff and police operational officers; individual semi-structured interviews with supporting agency representatives including residential and day-care drug treatment providers; drug use advisory service; bail support service and social services. Interview and focus group guides are described in detail in the full report.

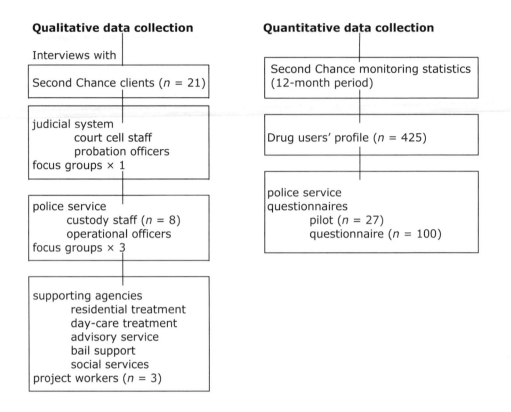

Figure 13.1 Summary of data collection methods used for case study evaluation

Practical and access issues tended to drive the sampling strategies used. For instance, a sequential sample of twenty-one Second Chance users was identified through brokerage by the project workers. The project workers approached clients at their meeting in the custody suite and asked for voluntary participation in an interview with a researcher 'from the university' in the local Second Chance office at a date and time convenient to them. Most often this was as soon as they were released from the custody suite on the same day and required the evaluation team to be 'on call' for interviews. Interviews with drug users were semi-structured and comprised participants with a history of drug use, history of offending, history of treatment, the interviewees' experience of the intervention by ARS, hopes for the future. Thematic content analysis was used to analyze the interview data.

Three focus groups were arranged with the assistance of a senior police officer which took place at the police station. Each focus group involved staff from different areas such as court cell staff, custody suite officers and operational drug officers. Staff at supporting agencies was contacted individually by phone to arrange an interview at their place of work. This purposive sample included seven agencies, representing residential and day-care services, advisory, support, probation services and social services. In three incidences, due to professional commitments, interviews were undertaken and recorded via telephone.

Our qualitative data analysis illuminated perceptions and views about the scheme, the style of the project workers, what clients valued, and how the scheme 'stood out' from other drug treatment related services. Agencies with whom the ARS worked viewed the project as positive, also alluding to its distinctive style and agency staff believed it was a very effective service. Interviews with project workers revealed a strong and shared commitment to the project, a common operational style and ability to be responsive and innovative which characterized their relationship with other agencies and clients. Generally the views of the representatives of the judicial system were supportive of the scheme and underlined the clear role for project workers. There was some negativity among custody staff which was often related to views about drug users as a group. Feedback to custody staff of the outcome of the ARS intervention was one area which emerged as needing attention. Two other difficulties were identified, the potential for clients to abuse the scheme with the intention of avoiding legal proceedings, and that the projects strength, its informal and flexible approach, sometimes led to problems when dealing with agencies which had a disciplinary and authoritarian approach.

The findings overall reflected other national data and studies that had been undertaken with similar schemes and links with existing literature and published evidence could be made. The scheme had impact and was highly valued by clients and respected by other agencies.

Overall outcomes of the evaluation were twofold: firstly, a set of recommendations to ease problems identified, to strengthen the scheme's monitoring and ongoing examination of its effectiveness and, secondly, a set of key points of best practice to inform future schemes. The aims of the evaluation were addressed within the report in the context of the sources of data. Overall the report was well received by its commissioners, but there were debates about the language used in the report. The commissioners agreed with the recommendations but wanted a role in how they should be expressed which was agreed with the evaluation team.

Throughout the evaluation the evaluators worked proactively in developing a relationship with the commissioners, met with them frequently, reviewed progress, discussed pragmatic solutions to methodological problems, time scales and funding. Within a pragmatic evaluation the team were keen that commissioners should be part of the decision-making as the evaluation unfolded. Additionally the DAT was made up of fifteen individuals representing ten organizations and a range of professional disciplines. Our stance aimed to be collaborative with commissioners and the wider project stakeholders. We were anxious not to get in the way of the work of the project during data collection; we aimed to be as flexible as possible in practical arrangements. As it turned out, at the final reporting stage there were still debates within the drug action team and with the evaluators about the ultimate value of the study, whether it was 'soft' and if it really demonstrated that the scheme was effective in encouraging drug-using offenders to access treatment. Later questions about the value of the ARS in helping clients *stay in* treatment and its impact on crime also emerged. The commissioners had from the outset been interested in an in-depth view from many perspectives, and we believed this paved the way for qualitative data collection (which we saw as essential to meet several of the aims), but such data alone would not have fully satisfied our commissioners, even when linked to aims about people's perspectives. Because an overall profile of the ARS was generated by quantitative data, and because we included a (limited quick and dirty) survey of police officers, the evaluation had something of interest for every organization. This necessity, we believe existed in the 'subtext' of working with a multisectoral commissioning body in this case. Around the same time other schemes had reported qualitative evaluations in the literature. Both these factors helped us in our defence of our overall evaluation design. It was agreed by all that the evaluation could only ever be a 'snap shot', but that it gave a rounded picture, illuminated ARS strengths and problems. As a result the drug action team funded a follow-up study which provided some evidence that the scheme was indeed 'working' in the long term (the findings suggested that over half of the original sample of clients had remained 'clean' following drug treatment which had been accessed via the ARS two years later (Crossen-White and Galvin 2002).

In conclusion, as we negotiated a contract and communicated the findings in an ongoing way, we embraced many roles to serve needs of our stakeholders. They included: scientific, consultative, diplomat, activist, communicator, and problem-solver roles. We needed to review our decisions often, to reflect upon our progress and likely nature of our written report throughout the evaluation project. This emerged as an essential activity, since as Ovretveit (1998) outlines there are commonplace difficulties such as fuzzy boundaries; for example, interventions have fuzzy boundaries, they can be wobbly, constantly changing and goals of the intervention may be unclear. Reflecting upon progress and negotiations with commissioners can facilitate an account of the flexibility required and its rationale in implementing a pragmatic evaluation, as choices cannot always be theoretically driven. Ovretveit (1998) suggests that the evaluators' response to problems will affect the value and use of the evaluation. In this case study our responsiveness to commissioners facilitated the findings to be taken seriously, because the value of the scheme was evidenced from a number of perspectives, ultimately the report influenced the DATS decision to continue to expand the ARS and award extra funding since it provided some documented evidence. If we had not engaged in a debate and responded to opinions about the nature of the evidence, the evaluation report may have been rejected.

Taut and Brauns (2003) discuss the complexity of psychological perspectives within evaluation such as power; reactance, control, competition and conflict and suggest that user-orientated, participatory approaches are supported by the theoretical analysis of these concepts and are less likely to increase resistance to evaluation. Within the 'confusing and contradictory' world of evaluation, a team approach with a commitment to a collaborative and pragmatic stance is a feature of the case study which we believe aided its success.

Conclusion

In this chapter I have described the varied but related theoretical frameworks which can inform qualitative evaluation and outlined the underpinning humanistic principles. Two prominent themes emerge within this discussion: participation and pragmatism. Additionally, both the role of qualitative evaluation within broader political processes and the political role of the evaluator are not only unavoidable, they are an aspect of explicit recognition of both conflicting values and plurality of values in any participatory or constructivist approach. To recap the purpose of evaluation, if it is to explore *effectiveness*, to examine worth and value, and to contribute to 'social betterment' (Marks *et al.* 2000), then 'The effectiveness requirement has been supplemented by other important requirements: justice, legitimacy, mutual understanding, integration of professional and experiential knowledge and democratic pluralism. The perception that evaluation is carried out with the explicit aim of finding an instrumental means–ends relationship is superseded by evaluation becoming part of the policy process' (Khakee 2003: 347). Qualitative evaluation is underpinned by appropriate values and has a clear and pertinent role in this process.

References

Abma, T.A. (2001) (ed.) Special Issue: Dialogue in Evaluation. *Evaluation*, 7 (2): 155–280.

Bate, P. and Robert, G. (2002) Studying health care 'quality' qualitatively: the dilemmas and tensions between different forms of evaluation research within the UK National Health Service, *Qualitative Health Research*, 12 (7): 966–981.

Brewer, J. (2003) Naturalism. In Miller, R.L. and Brewer, J.D. (2003) (eds) *The A–Z of Social Research*. London: Sage, 210–212.

Chen, H.T. (1990) *Theory Driven Evaluation*. Thousand Oaks, CA: Sage.

Chen, H.T. (1996) A comprehensive typology for program evaluation, *Evaluation Practice*, 17 (2): 121–130.

Chen, H.T. and Rossi, P.H. (1983) Evaluating with sense: the theory driven approach, *Evaluation Review*, 7: 283–302.

Clarke, A. with Dawson, R. (1999) *Evaluation Research: An Introduction to Principles, Methods and Practice*. London: Sage.

Cook, T.D. (1985) Post positivist Critical Multiplism. In Shotland, R.L. and Mark, M.M. (eds) *Social Science and Social Policy*. Thousand Oaks, CA: Sage, 21–62.

Cook, T.D. (1997) Lessons learned in evaluation over the past 25 years. In Chelimsky, E. and Shadish, W.R. (eds) *Evaluation for the 21st Century: A Handbook*. Thousand Oaks, CA: Sage, 30–52.

Cook, T.D. and Reichardt, C.S. (1979) *Qualitative and Quantitative Methods in Evaluation Research*. Beverly Hills, CA: Sage.

Crossen-White, H. and Galvin, K. (2002) A follow-up study of drug misusers who received an intervention from a locals arrest referral scheme, *Health Policy*, 61: 153–171.

Dingwall, R. (1992) 'Don't Mind Him, He's from Barcelona'. In Daly, J., McDonald, I. and Willis, E. (eds) *Researching Health Care: Designs, Dilemma, Disciplines*. London: Routledge, 161–165.

Eberstadt, N., Eberstadt, N. and Moynihan, D.P. (1995) *The Tyranny of Numbers: Mismeasurement and Misrule*. Washington DC: American Enterprise Institute Press, cited in Patton, M.Q. (2002).

Edmunds, M., May, T., Hearden, I. and Hough, M. (1998) *Arrest referral: emerging lessons from research*, paper 23. London: Home Office.

Galvin, K., Crossen-White, H. and Jackson, D. (1998) *An Evaluation of the Second Chance Arrest Referral Scheme: A Report Commissioned by the Dorset Drug Action Team*. Institute of Health and Community Studies, Bournemouth University, ISBN: 1-85899-061-0.

Greene, J. (2001) Dialogue in Evaluation: A Relational Perspective, *Evaluation*, 7(2): 181–187.

Greene, J.C. and Caracelli, V.J. (1997) Defining and Describing the Paradigm Issue in Mixed Method Evaluation. In Greene, J.C. and Caracelli, V.J. (eds) *Advances in Mixed Methods Evaluation: The Challenges and Benefits of Integrating Diverse Paradigms, New Directions for Evaluation*, Issue 74: 5–17. San Francisco: Jossey-Bass.

Greene, J.C., Lehn, B. and Goodyear, L. (2001) The Merits of Mixing Methods in Evaluation, *Evaluation*, 7 (1): 25–44.

Greenwood, J. (1984) Nursing Research: a position paper, *Journal of Advanced Nursing*, 9 (1): 77–82.

Greenwood, D. and Levin, M. (1998) *Introduction to Action Research: Social Research for Social Change*. Thousand Oaks, CA: Sage.

Guba, E.G. and Lincoln, Y.S. (1988) Do inquiry paradigms imply inquiry methodologies? In Fetterman, D.M. (ed.) *Qualitative Approaches to Evaluation in Education: The Silent Scientific Revolution*. New York: Praeger, 89–115.

Guba, E.G. and Lincoln, Y.S. (1989) *Fourth Generation Evaluation*. Newbury Park, CA: Sage.

Guba, E. and Lincoln, Y. (1998) (eds) *The Landscape of Qualitative Research Theories and Issues*. London: Sage, 195–220.

Hammersley, M. and Atkinson, P. (1983) *Ethnography: Principles in Practice*. London: Tavistock.

Heron, J. (1996) *Co-operative Inquiry: Research into the Human Condition*. Thousand Oaks, CA: Sage.

House, E. (1978) Assumptions Underlying Evaluation Models, *Educational Researcher*, 7: 4–12.

House, E.R. (1980) *Evaluating with Validity*, Beverly Hills, CA: Sage.

House, E.R. (1993) *Professional Evaluation: Social Impact and Political Consequences*. Newbury Park, CA: Sage.

House, E.R. and Howe, K. (1999) *Values in Evaluation and Social Research*. Thousand Oaks, CA: Sage.

Khakee, A. (2003) The emerging gap between evaluation research and practice, *Evaluation*, 9 (3): 340–352.

Lax, W. and Galvin, K. (2002) Reflections on a community action research project: interprofessional issues and methodological problems, *Journal of Clinical Nursing*, 11 (3): 376–386.

Lazenbatt, A. (2002) *The Evaluation Handbook for Health Professionals*. London: Routledge.

Lincoln, Y.S. and Guba, E.G. (1985) *Naturalistic Inquiry*. Beverly Hills, CA: Sage.

Mark, M.M., Henry, G.T. and Julnes, G. (2000) *Evaluation: An Integrated Framework for Understanding, Guiding, and Improving Policies and Programs*. San Francisco: Jossey-Bass.

Mark, M.M. and Shotland, L. (eds) (1987) *New Directions for Program Evaluation*. No. 35. San Francisco: Jossey-Bass.

Murphy, E. (2001) Micro-level qualitative research. In Fulop, N., Allen, P., Clarke, A. and Black, N. *Studying the Organisation and Delivery of Health Services*. London: Routledge, 40–55.

Murphy, E. and Dingwall, R. (2001) Qualitative Methods in Health Technology Assessment. In Stevens, A., Abrams, K., Brazier, J., Fitzpatrick, R. and Lilford, R. (eds) *The Advanced Handbook of Methods in Evidence Based Healthcare*. London: Sage, 166–178.

Ong, B.N. (1996) *Rapid Appraisal and Health Policy*. Cheltenham: Nelson Thornes.

Ovretveit, J. (1998) *Evaluating Health Interventions*. Buckingham: Open University Press.

Parlett, M. (1981) Illuminative evaluation. In Reason, P. and Rowan, J. (eds) *Human Inquiry: A Sourcebook of New Paradigm Research*. London: Wiley, 219–226.

Parlett, M. and Hamilton, D. (1976) Evaluation as Illumination. A new approach to the study of Innovatory Programs. In Glass, G.V. (ed.) *Evaluation Studies Review Annual*, Vol. 1. 140–157. Beverly Hills, CA: Sage.

Parlett, M. and Hamilton, D. (1977) Evaluation as illumination. In Hamilton, D. (ed.) *Beyond the Numbers Game*. London: Macmillan, 6–22.

Patton, M.Q. (1982) *Practical Evaluation*. Beverly Hills, CA: Sage.

Patton, M.Q. (1988) Paradigms and pragmatism. In Fetterman, D.M. (ed.) *Qualitative Approaches to Evaluation in Education: The Silent Scientific Revolution*. New York: Praeger, 116–137.

Patton, M.Q. (1990) *Qualitative Evaluation and Research Methods*, 2nd edn. Newbury Park, CA: Sage.

Patton, M.Q. (1996) A world larger than formative and summative, *Evaluation Practice*, 17 (2): 131–144.

Patton, M.Q. (1997) *Utilization Focused Evaluation*, 3rd edn. Thousand Oaks, CA: Sage.

Patton, M.Q. (2002) *Qualitative Research and Evaluation Methods*, 3rd edn. Thousand Oaks, CA: Sage.

Pawson, R. and Tilley, N. (1997) *Realistic Evaluation*. London: Sage.

Prout, A. (1992) Illumination, collaboration, facilitation, negotiation: evaluation the MESMAC project. In Aggleton, P., Young, A., Moody, D., Kapila, M. and Pye, M. (1992) *Does it Work? Perspectives on Evaluation of HIV/AIDS Health Promotion*, 77–92.

Reason, P. (ed.) (1994) *Participation in Human Inquiry*. London: Sage.

Robson, C. (2000) *Small-Scale Evaluation, Principles and Practice*. Thousand Oaks, CA: Sage.

Robson, C. (2002) *Real World Research: A Resource For Social Scientists and Practitioner Researchers*, 2nd edn. Blackwell: Oxford.

Rossi, P.H. and Freeman, H.E. (1993) *Evaluation: A Systematic Approach*, 5th edn (1st edn 1979). Newbury Park, CA: Sage.

Sassi, F. (2000) Methods for the Evaluation of Healthcare Interventions. In Cookson, R., Maynard, A., McDaid, D., Sassi, F. and Sheldon, T. (eds) *Analysis of the Scientific and Technical Evaluation of Health Interventions*. Report to the European Commission. July. http://www.lse.ac.uk/Depts/Isehsc/astec-report.htm.

Scriven, M. (1967) The methodology of evaluation. In Tyler, R., Gagne, R. and Scriven, M. (eds) *Perspectives on Curriculum Evaluation*. AERA Monograph Series on Curriculum Evaluation No. 1. Chicago: Rand McNally, 39–83.

Scriven, M. (1991) *Evaluation Thesaurus*, 4th edn. Newbury Park, CA: Sage.

Scriven, M. (1995) *Evaluation Thesaurus*, 5th edn. Newbury Park, CA: Sage.

Shadish, W., Cook, T. and Leviton, L. (1991) *Foundations of Program Evaluation: Theories of Practice*. Newbury Park, CA: Sage.

Shaw, I. (1999) *Qualitative Evaluation*. Thousand Oaks, CA: Sage.

Silverman, D. (1989) Telling Convincing Stories: a plea for cautious positivism in case studies. In Glassner, B. and Moreno, J.D. (eds) *The Qualitative–Quantitative Distinction in the Social Sciences*. Dordrecht: Kluwer Academic Publishers, 57–77.

Silverman, D. (1993) *Interpreting Qualitative Data: Methods for Analysing Talk, Text and Interaction*. London: Sage.

Stake, R.E. (1975) *The Art of Case Study Research*. Newbury Park, CA: Sage.

Stake, R.E. (1980) Program Evaluation, particularly responsive evaluation. In Dockrell, W.B. and Hamiliton, D. (eds) *Rethinking Educational Research*. London: Hodder and Stoughton, 72–87.

Stake, R.E. (1995) *The Art of Case Study Research*, 2nd edn. Thousand Oaks, CA: Sage.

Stringer, E.T. (1996) *Action Research: A Handbook for Practitioners*. Thousand Oaks, CA: Sage.

Suchman, E.A. (1967) *Evaluative Research*. New York, Russell Sage.

Taut, S. and Brauns, D. (2003) Resistance to evaluation: a psychological perspective, *Evaluation*, 9 (3): 247–264.

Titchen, A. and Binnie, A. (1993) Research partnerships: collaborative action research in nursing, *Journal of Advanced Nursing*, 18: 858–865.

Tones, B.K. (1987) Health promotion, affective education and personal–social development of young people. In David, K. and Williams, P. (eds) *Education in Schools*, 2nd edn. London: Harper & Row, 3–44.

Tones, K. and Tilford, S. (2001) *Health Education: Effectiveness, Efficiency and Equity*, 2nd edn. London: Nelson Thornes.

Weiss, C.H. (1987) Where politics and evaluation meet. In Palumbo, D. (ed.) *The Politics of Program Evaluation*. Newbury Park: Sage.

Weiss, C.H. (1998) *Evaluation*, 2nd edn. Upper Saddle River, NJ: Prentice Hall.

Weiss, C.H. (1999) The interface between evaluation and public policy. *Evaluation*, 5 (4): 468–486.

Widdershoven, G.A.M. (2001) Dialogue in Evaluation: A hermeneutic perspective, *Evaluation*, 7 (2): 253–263.

Williams, D.D. (1986) When is naturalistic evaluation appropriate? In Williams, D.D. (ed.) *Naturalistic Evaluation: New Directions in Program Evaluation*, No. 30, San Francisco: Jossey-Bass, 85–92.

Wilson-Barnett, J. (1991) The experiment: is it worthwhile? *International Journal of Nursing Studies*, 28 (1): 77–87.

World Health Organization (1996) Ottawa Charter for Health Promotion, An International Conference on Health Promotion, 17–21 November, Regional Office for Europe, Copenhagen WHO.

Notes

[1] However, sometimes a predetermined research process is a requirement of stakeholders.
[2] As the 'researched upon'.

14

DEBBIE KRALIK
Engaging feminist thought in research: a participatory approach

Introduction

I recall my introduction to feminism during my 1970s teenage years as repressive. As a young adult, my burgeoning social consciousness had led me to work voluntarily in a rape crisis centre. I found that the women with whom I worked held what I perceived to be inflexible views about women's social position and experiences. This experience made me conscious of the complexity of power relations. There seemed to be an alienating 'dress code' composed of combat gear that accompanied those women who identified themselves as 'feminists'. I do not recall the details of the feminist perspectives held by my co-workers as clearly as I recall the contradictions. Little discussion took place (with me) about what constituted feminist views. They espoused philosophy about inclusiveness but their practices were about exclusiveness. My own understanding about feminism has evolved since that time. I have come to understand feminism to be more than a set of rules, methods and ideas (Lumby 1997) but as a way of living that poses challenges to our everyday lives. One of the fundamental challenges that feminism puts to us is to be accountable for congruency between our feminist thinking and our daily behaviours (Maguire 1996).

In those early years I did not feel challenged by the feminist thought I had encountered as much as I felt ostracized by the rigidity of it. I wondered if others experienced feminism in the same way. I became acutely aware at that time that individualism within feminist thinking is something to be respected and acknowledged, because our thinking and reflections are not static. As our lives present us with challenges, changes and experiences, our perspectives also shift. Feminism is a dynamic and individual experience, as well as a social and political movement.

My interest in feminism developed further after I had studied at university. New learning opportunities led me to question my early experiences within a large, bureaucratic organization where the predominantly female profession of nursing was viewed as subservient to other male-dominated health professions. Even now, it is difficult to trace precisely how feminist thinking has influenced me. There was not one particular experience that led me to feminism, but rather through exploring feminist writings and working with women who identified with feminist thought, the influences have been like an unfolding or a dawning. Although my feminist position continues to evolve, I view my commitment to feminism as a commitment to humanity and the equality of all people. My feminism is about caring, a personal and professional commitment to care for and about others in a humanitarian way. It is about valuing women, their ideas, ideals and experiences and facilitating women towards taking meaningful action in their lives.

It is important for women to be inclusive of each other, and to be aware that there are many different forms of feminism and many ways of being feminist. Women living in diverse situations, with different religious and ethnic traditions have undertaken feminist theorizing, and therefore there is no one feminist perspective or theory. Given this, perhaps it is time to stop searching for a politically or theoretically pure position for feminism and instead embrace diversity as strength (Lumby 1997).

Adding to the diversity of feminist positions is the fact that the contours of feminist thought have shifted over time (Olesen 1994). I am conscious of participating in and learning from many dialogues. The historical context and development of the arguments that constitute feminist theory is important for gaining a sense of where we have been and how we have arrived at this point. Yesterday's understandings are replaced but not deleted. Theoretical history has meaning and purpose in connecting the old to the new as it allows us to record advances and lay the foundation for advancing inquiry. It is beyond the scope of this chapter, however, to represent the breadth of that historical feminist theorizing.

Feminist knowledge is not a 'given' but emerges from an exploration and unpacking of our own terms of reference. Rather than be preoccupied with discussion about what feminism 'is' (or is not), I aim to promote an unpacking of the assumptions and experiences that lead researchers to consider a feminist approach to research.

Each individual begins the process of engagement in feminist thinking at a unique level of awareness, with differences in experiences, perspectives and knowledge, which makes developing strategies for participation and transformation a necessary agenda (hooks 2000). Locating our own feminism is a dynamic process fired by reflection and a critical consciousness. Feminist inquiry is not an isolated scholarly exercise guided by theory, but is passionate, political, participatory and intensely personal. Feminist principles are intimately connected to our lives and the questions and events that confront us in our lives. Seeing and knowing through a feminist lens has implications for how we live and work, with whom and how we choose to be in our daily relationships, and whether we engage in feminist research (Maguire 1996).

Learning from my early experiences, I contend that feminism needs to be conscious of its own power and as such, in this chapter, I refrain from prescribing the 'rules' of feminist theorizing choosing instead to consider ways that feminist thinking may be engaged in qualitative research.

With the acknowledgement of diverse ways of feminist thinking, I begin by looking at some common feminist principles and tenets of feminist research. I then

LIBRARY
EDUCATION CENTRE
PRINCESS ROYAL HOSPITAL

consider how feminist principles can merge with a participatory research framework to engage women towards transformational action.

Feminist principles

What is feminism? Feminist theory is still emerging and does not have agreed upon answers for this question. There have been as many definitions of feminism suggested throughout the history of the feminist movement, as there are ways of being in the world. Feminism is a term that is grounded in knowledge, experience, awareness, action, culture, ideology and history. It is a term where the scope and boundaries depend upon who defines it, and why it needed to be defined in the first place. A 'grand' definition about 'what is feminism' becomes very difficult, if not impossible; however, two commonly used definitions of feminism are:

> ... a method of analysis as well as a discovery of new material. It asks new questions as well as coming up with new answers. Its central concern is with the social distinction between men and women, with the fact of the distinction, with its meanings and with its causes and consequences.
>
> (Mitchell and Oakley 1976: 14)
>
> ... theoretical constructions about the nature of women's oppression and the part that this oppression plays within social reality more generally.
>
> (Stanley and Wise 1983: 55)

The many diverse feminist theories demonstrate different views about the causes of women's oppression, what sustains it and consequently advocate different approaches to the social construction of inequality and the means by which justice (through action or change) may be achieved (Speedy 1991; Kolmar and Bartkowski 2000). There is some argument that diversity in theorizing is one of the weaknesses of feminism, however, I consider it also to be a strength because the many different voices and epistemologies enable feminism to be potentially relevant to all women across cultures, races and socio-economic situations.

There has also been a claim that the diversity of feminist orientations universalizes, over-generalizes or generates over-ambitious models of feminism (Clarke and Olesen 1999). Common in each of these feminist orientations, however, is the acceptance that women are oppressed by patriarchal power relations (Stanley and Wise 1983; Speedy 1991). Patriarchal power can be seen in relations where women's interests are subordinate to men and the role of women is defined in relation to the male norm. There is common understanding that at the basis of women's oppression is power inequity because the personal circumstances of women are consequences of the larger political realities in the world. Patriarchal relations exist in social and cultural practices and broad feminist theory can offer a framework to explain the oppressive structures and forces. However, when bringing patriarchal relations into view, it is important to acknowledge that a feminist perspective refrains from perpetuating the view of women as 'victims' of their circumstances, but instead celebrates women's diversity and strengths (Maguire 1996).

The aim of feminist theory is to transform the social world towards affirmation of women's lived experiences and participation in the construction of new realities (Smith 1991). Feminist theory examines and reshapes gender arrangements and the distortions created in women's lives by attempting to 'make the experiences and lives of women intelligible' (Frye 1983: xi). A woman-centred approach is fundamental to feminist scholarship, illuminating the life context and experiences of women, grounded by their frame of reference, experiences and language (DuBois 1985; Speedy 1991).

Feminist thinking develops through a critical awareness of experiences, values, ideologies and goals. It is through this awareness that consciousness raising and action becomes possible as women learn to view the world through a critical lens, and contradictions in their lives become illuminated. The generation of experiential knowledge and the creation of awareness provide possibilities for action and alternatives to oppression.

Some 'common threads in the tapestry of feminism' (Maguire 1996: 107) have been identified which include that:

- Feminism acknowledges that women face some form of oppression and exploitation.

- Women experience their oppressions, struggles and strengths in diverse ways because of the diverse realities and identities of women.

- Feminism is a commitment to uncover the forces that cause and sustain the oppressions.

- A commitment to feminism is a commitment to working *with* women (individually and collectively) towards challenging and transforming the oppressive structures and forces.

- Feminism encourages women to develop ways to create new structures or reshape existing forces so that women can 'live out new ways of being in relationship with the world' (Maguire 1996: 108).

My challenge to you as a researcher is to define your own feminist thought, to identify the assumptions that underpin your thinking and, just as importantly, your actions.

Some common principles that guide a feminist approach to research

There is no one kind of feminist research (or method) since feminist scholars are active in a variety of disciplines, social and cultural situations and influenced by different perspectives (Reinharz 1992; Webb 1993; Chinn 2003). Some authors have cautioned against strictly adhering to the rigidity of feminist research checklists (Harding 1987; Seibold *et al.* 1994), and others have called for creative and thoughtful interpretation of feminist research principles (Webb 1993; Carryer 1995).

When researching issues of concern for women, it is worthwhile to also focus attention towards our own research practices so that we can further develop an awareness of the way we approach research. We interpret the world though our personal perspectives, which have emerged from a collection of beliefs that are grounded in our own experiences and understandings. Feminist approaches to research bring personal perspectives to the surface (Chinn 2003). Our epistemology is influenced and shaped by our own life experiences, which we bring to research as well as the influences of the many voices and conversations within feminism. Our assumptions and personal belief system is likely to underpin the research process so identifying them prior to embarking on research and during the research process is fundamentally important. The challenge for us as researchers is 'to develop a kind of self reflexivity that will enable us to look closely at our own practice in terms of how we contribute to dominance in spite of our liberatory intentions' (Lather 1991: 150). Locating voice is a metaphor common in feminist research (Maguire 2001), and I suggest it applies to the researchers too, who through reflection create space for identifying their own voice in the research process as well as facilitating the voice of participants.

I have introduced the notion that feminism is more than a set of theories and ideas, because it bleeds into our everyday lives. This leads to the question that if feminist theory is so diverse, are there some common principles that offer guidance for feminist research?

Feminist inquiry has often been conceptualized as research *for* women and *with* women rather than research *on* women (Bunting and Campbell 1990; Anderson 1991; Campbell and Bunting 1991; Hall and Stevens 1991; Speedy 1991; Webb 1993; Olesen 1994; Scharbo-DeHaan 1994). Feminism has an intense interest in the way women are represented, and so the *way* in which knowledge is constructed is central to feminist debates (Rose 1983; Stanley and Wise 1983; Unger 1989; Duran 1990; Anderson 1991; Fonow and Cook 1991; Maynard and Purvis 1994; Griffiths 1995). Feminist inquiries have revealed that while most knowledge has been androcentric (generated and defined by males), the perspective they espouse is not the only one and not always appropriate (Speedy 1991). The experiences of men are not the experiences of women, nor are the experiences of women homogeneous. Feminists have challenged not only the view of the way in which knowledge is produced but also whose view of the world it represents.

> Very simply, to do feminist research is to put the social construction of gender at the centre of one's enquiries. Feminist researchers see gender as a basic organising principle which profoundly shapes/mediates the concrete conditions of our lives. The overt ideological goal of feminist research is to correct both the invisibility and distortion of female experiences in ways relevant to ending women's unequal position in society.
>
> (Lather 1988: 571)

There has also been a call for feminist research to extend further than the creation of knowledge, but to also have a commitment to social justice (Drevdahl 1999) and social change that will serve to enhance the lives of women.

Feminist research not only studies women and women's experience within the social context, but it also seeks to help women deal with the issues that are revealed as part of the process. Both the knowledge gained and the research process itself may serve as vehicles for creating social change that enhances lives of women.

(Ford-Gilboe and Campbell 1996: 173)

Feminism provides a framework by which socially constructed differences, such as gender and culture, may be incorporated into the design of research.

Feminist studies are designed, implemented and disseminated with the goal of providing for women explanations that they want and need about phenomena that affect their lives.

(Hall and Stevens 1991: 17)

Feminism is an openly political and transformative process and therefore feminist concepts are suitable for use where the aim of the research is to catalyze change (Jackson 1997). People grow and change within the realm of relationships. Feminist researchers are concerned with valuing and validating women's experiences and ideas, their position in the social structure and the desire to bring about social change of oppressive constraints (Hall and Stevens 1991).

After reviewing the characteristics of feminist research and feminist researchers, Speedy (1991: 201) identified three main principles inherent in feminist belief systems that inform feminist research. They were:

- A recognition that women are oppressed, which makes necessary an examination of the reasons for oppression in order that changes be made.
- That the personal is political which acknowledges the value of women's experiences.
- Consciousness-raising, which results in alternative views of the world from a woman's perspective.

Consciousness-raising has been advocated as involving the recognition of social, political, economic, and personal constraints on freedom, and it provides the forum in which to take action to challenge those constraints (Henderson 1995). By engaging in critical dialogue, individuals may discover the hidden contradictions within themselves that assist in sustaining an oppressive society (Freire and Ramos 1990). Furthermore, consciousness-raising challenges objectivity as the personal becomes privileged:

... women experience a shared sense of reality and a shared sense of oppression; they become conscious of their problems as group problems rather than as their own individual problems.

(Henderson 1995: 63)

Through consciousness-raising the opportunity may be created for women to learn how they have internalized the dominant view of their subordination (Henderson 1995). Identifying the contributors of their own oppression may lead women to a greater sense of empowerment as they understand that they both shape and are shaped by their reality. When researching 'with' people, it is in their actual experience that knowledge is created from their everyday lives. Taking a pragmatic stance, it surfaces the problem of connecting such knowledge with those for whom it might be useful and who might use it. This means seeking from a particular experience situated in the matrix of everyday life, to explore and display the relations, powers and forces that organize and shape it. Consciousness-raising enables women the opportunity to view the world in a different way and is based on knowledge gained. Feminist researchers use consciousness-raising within the context of women's experience as a tool for narrowing the distance between researchers and participants by generating reciprocity and collaboration (Lather 1986, 1988).

In feminist research, the questions that are asked are just as important as the data generated. Maguire (1996: 113) provided one example of researchers working in the field of domestic violence framing research by the question: 'why do women stay in violent relationships?' The research question stated in this way implied that something was intrinsically wrong with these women. The question was reframed to be: 'why do men brutalise women in so-called love relationships?' Clearly, values become evident in the generation of knowledge and the personal becomes highly political. This example adds credence to the argument that the personal values of the researcher, and how those values affect the research process, ought to be made explicit. The notion of researcher impact has been debated in qualitative research literature (Alvesson and Sköldberg 2000; Chesney 2000). The researcher's philosophy, beliefs, motivation and choice of orientation form the framework on which the choice of method and approach is based (Alvesson and Sköldberg 2000). In the creation of knowledge feminism prompts questioning of 'whose perspective? Whose voice? Whose knowledge?' (Maguire 2001: 63).

Although we have identified the diversity in feminist thinking, there are several important tenets of feminist research. There is a focus on exploring women's perceptions, feelings and experiences are valued and made visible (Delmar 1986; Harding 1987, 1989, 1991; Rosser 1987; Lather 1988, 1991; Ricketts 1989; Unger 1989; Fonow and Cook 1991; Crowley and Himmelweit 1992; Reinharz 1992; Maynard and Purvis 1994; Bowes 1996; Puwar 1997). The research focus is on topics that are of importance to women (Chinn 2003). The words 'feminism' or 'feminist' are used and feminist literature is cited (Duffy 1985). There is an emphasis on equality and mutuality that balances the relationship between researcher and researched, and uses consciousness-raising as a methodological tool to empower women (Lather 1988, 1991; Fonow and Cook 1991; Webb 1993; Bowes 1996; Millen 1997; Puwar 1997). Feminist principles are illuminated in the writing process. The research is reported in a way that the reader becomes engaged with the discourse as an active participant (Chinn 2003). Patterns and alternative explanations are the focus rather than prescriptive interpretation (Chinn 2003). This is particularly important because the written account of feminist research provides the vehicle for shaping social and political relations (Chinn 2003). Furthermore, researchers have an obligation to make the research findings available to those who participated in the generation of data, and disseminate them widely to women, otherwise there is little possibility of the findings being incorporated into their lives (Webb 1993). Given that feminist research promotes engagement between participants and researcher, facilitates participants to shape the research process and has liberation as an aim, it is important that researchers carefully consider ways of ending the research so that participants are unharmed and the benefits of the research sustained.

While the idea that feminist approaches to research may be framed by the tenets discussed so far, it is fundamentally important that feminist research also attempt to bring about progressive change in the interests of women. Feminist scholars and activists are inspired by a vision of the world where women can realize their potential (Chinn 2003). Action is the political side to feminist research; the side that says let us not simply observe and analyze these systems, but facilitate the action necessary for change to occur. This leads us to the question: 'how can action be facilitated in feminist research?'

Participation in action: an example of feminist qualitative research

Participatory research is conducive to the emancipatory goals of feminist theory because consciousness-raising provides the way in which a greater awareness is achieved and actioned as the researcher and researched engage in mutually educative and liberating encounters. In the study described below, I show the way that the principles of participatory action and feminism provided guidance in an inquiry that aimed to understand the impact of chronic illness on the lives of midlife women and share the ways that women incorporate chronic illness in their lives.

Illustration of the way feminist and participatory principles can guide research is provided by an inquiry (1996–2000) in which data were generated using correspondence between myself (as the researcher) and midlife women (participants) who had adult onset chronic illness (Kralik 2000, 2002; Kralik et al. 2000, 2001).

For the purpose of this inquiry the construction of the core middle years was defined as being between 30 and 50 years of age. The developmental tasks for women in this age group are considered to be assisting both younger and older generations, as well as being responsible for the growth and development of organizational enterprises. The core middle years have been identified as being the most productive stage of life for individuals in western society (Stevenson 1977). Understanding how women managed chronic illness during the core middle years was the focus of this inquiry. For twelve months, eighty-one midlife women explored with me aspects of their lives with chronic illness.

In my role as researcher, I acted as a conduit for the experiences of women, guided by carefully selected feminist principles. These principles: intersubjectivity, the centrality of women and action as a research outcome, underpinned the entire research process. Further to these principles, we embraced the actions of participating, sharing ongoing dialogue, sharing the ownership of the inquiry, reciprocating, self-reflecting, diminishing inequalities (through writing an accessible text), shaping the inquiry together, contributing to human growth and development, listening to each other's voices, privileging the experiences of women and lastly, taking action to improve their lives.

We initiated, developed and evaluated correspondence (email and letter writing) as an effective approach for data generation for qualitative inquiry (Kralik *et al.* 2000). Using correspondence we generated storied accounts of women's experiences, some of which were shared on a purpose-created website. The women's stories were evocative, full of passion, compassion and words of wisdom. Women related their experiences in a newly found voice that seemed to rise, sometimes gently, sometimes awkwardly and sometimes fiercely. Each woman had spoken independently of the other, yet similar themes emerged, creating a rich and complex pattern. Thirteen women volunteered to join me in the interpretation of the stories and together we shaped the inquiry.

The findings broadly revealed that women with illness were involved in an ongoing process of transition (Kralik 2002). The illness transition was a process that was non-linear, sometimes cyclical and potentially recurring throughout a woman's lifetime as changes in her life force new challenges. Our focus here, however, is on understanding the way the research was approached rather than the findings.

The inquiry was grounded in the actual experiences of the women and through reflection and interpretation, and the opportunity to have access to the research constructions, a consciousness-raising developed among many women. The goal was to understand the realities of experience constructed by this particular group of women, with the emphasis being on the context in which their lives were lived. With each woman's permission, excerpts of their letters were shared anonymously between women. At times it seemed like a chorus of voices brought life to a topic, as many women contributed to the conversation. Kerry reflected:

> Working with you has been so beneficial for me personally. I was thinking back to a time prior to my involvement in our project ... and all that has happened since then in terms of my understandings and perceptions...and I know I will be eternally grateful to you and to the other women for my growth.

Women revealed experiences with illness that were dynamic, emergent, changing and tension-filled, but which were central to lives that continue to be lived.

Three principles of feminist research

Three fundamental feminist tenets were incorporated into this research: intersubjectivity, the centrality of women and action as a research outcome (Speedy 1991). I will discuss and illustrate the way these characteristics were woven throughout the research process.

Intersubjectivity

Intersubjectivity means the dialectical relationship that the participants and the researcher share while engaged in research. The dialectical relationship refers to the way we (researcher and participants) were involved in the ethical, social and political implications of the inquiry. Intersubjectivity was central to the way that we communicated with each other, the language we used and the way in which together we created meaning out of the women's experiences of living with chronic illness. In this study, the dialectical relationship continued throughout the entire research process, as women were involved in the generation and interpretation of storied accounts of their experiences, and the confirmation and validation of the constructions. Several researchers (Buker 1987; Hammersley 1991; Reinharz 1992; Seibold *et al.* 1994) have expressed concern at the balance of power when the voices of women who have participated in research are analyzed and interpreted without their contribution. This issue was addressed by ensuring that women had the opportunity to be involved in the building of knowledge, by participating in interpretation of the storied accounts, and to read and make changes to the constructions as they emerged.

The dialectical relationship was enhanced when language common to the women was used to communicate their ideas, experiences and feelings. This enabled women to contribute to and understand the outcome of the research in which they had participated, and therefore claim ownership of their words. In these ways, the research process was collaborative and reciprocal, and the constructions were meaningful to the women. Rhondda, who participated in this inquiry, read the stories as they unfolded and reflected on being involved in a participatory feminist research process:

> You can do all the research in the world but without empathy, communication and excellent listening skills it just becomes another paper. You have captured insight into our lives and that came from listening, taking time to hear what we said, allowing us to talk, not belittling us, being non judgmental, gaining trust and treating us firstly as a person and not case number or diagnosis.

Intersubjectivity involves a complete rejection of the notion of distance between the researcher and the participants (Speedy 1991). In this inquiry, close bonds developed as, over time, we unveiled ourselves to each other. When discussing the researcher's involvement in an inquiry, Olesen (1994: 165) states:

> We cannot rid ourselves of the cultural self we bring with us into the field anymore than we can disown the eyes, ears and skin through which we take in our intuitive perceptions about the new and strange world we have entered.

The relationship between myself as the researcher and the women who participated was reciprocal rather than hierarchical. This sometimes surprised the women who participated. Rhondda wrote:

What I have found so nice about your study is that along the way you have revealed yourself, and that you are not just an academic asking questions.

I viewed my role as researcher to be inseparable from the personal values and assumptions, drawn from my life experiences that I brought to the study. Feminist principles in terms of sharing, collaborating and disclosure underpinned the intersubjectivity of the approach. In participatory feminist research the consciousness-raising is mutual, and it involves all engaged in the research process (Henderson 1995). Throughout this research I aimed to establish and foster a collaborative and non-exploitative relationship with women, to place myself within the inquiry to avoid objectification (Olesen 1994) and to enable the research to be transformative both to the lives of the women involved as well as for women who will follow in their paths of living through chronic illness.

The centrality of women

Centrality means that women's experiences are viewed as valid and privileged for study. This process involves three elements (Speedy 1991). The first is reflexive thinking by both the researcher and the participants. The second is that there is clearly an interpretation of events and experiences through immersion in the data. Third, the interpretation of the participants' realities must be evident (Speedy 1991). The process of centrality demonstrates the importance of the feminist concern that personal is political. The questions that feminist researchers pose relate to the centrality of gender in the shaping of our consciousness. The women's experiences of living with chronic illness were privileged in this inquiry. One important perspective in a feminist framework is to view gender as a basic organizing principle that shapes the condition of our lives (Wilkinson 1986; Lather 1991; Chinn 2003).

In this inquiry, the experiences of women living with chronic illness were clearly heard. The women's language was retained to avoid naming their experiences for them. Through written responses that actively embraced their issues and ideas, I made every effort to provide an atmosphere of engagement and trust which allowed women to develop their ideas and construct meaning, to share attitudes and experiences. Rhondda reflected:

> ... this has made me reflect on the last months of how I and all of us have bared our souls, how you as the researcher has brought that ease of sharing and talking and disclosing out in us. I, along with the others I am certain, have gained such an insight to who we really are and where we are heading ... anyone reading this paper could not help but be absorbed by the bonds formed, its clarity in how it has all happened, I truly love it. Nothing I have read in such a long time has touched me so much to make me cry. It has been a reflection of all our conversations, the every day things like pruning [the garden], to sharing our deepest thoughts ... So many of the lines written made me feel they were written just for me. The final line is what did it to me, 'many have become her friends', D ... you had to be a friend to gain us as friends, to get us to open up so freely.

Action as a research outcome

Action in this instance implies growth and development as new insights are gained through the consciousness-raising associated with our dialogue. The goal of feminist participatory research is to 'create individual and social change by altering the role relations of people involved in the project' (Reinharz 1992: 181), including recognizing the changes that occur in the researcher as well as those being researched. The process of writing held meaning for Rhondda, as it helped place events in her life into perspective, and create vision for the future:

It has meant a great deal to me in being able to truthfully write about all that I have been through and the aftermath. In a way it has given me a better understanding of who I am and where I am heading. I have got rid of some heavy baggage I was carrying around. Areas that had been put to rest but never resolved have had an airing. I can see by reading back that I am a worthy person, I have a fairly clear insight into where I get my strength from, how I have overcome tragedy and how I coped with a life threatening illness . . . It has been a long learning journey, one I wouldn't have missed for anything.

An important outcome of this inquiry has been that many of the women who participated were empowered through the process of telling their stories. Throughout this inquiry women shared their storied accounts with other women who participated, and in this way collective issues emerged. Women were active in the dissemination of the study findings. Some women who participated in our inquiry co-authored articles (Kralik *et al.* 2000, 2001). Throughout the research process, women had control over the way their words were used. Kerry shared:

Every step of the way in this [inquiry] you have had our interests at heart. It truly has been a feminist study and it has been a fantastic experience for me.
(Personal communication, 26 November 1999)

In line with feminist researchers who emphasize that women's lives and experience be valued, it was important that this research contribute to the improvement in the lives of women. This improvement has not always happened on a large scale, but some women acknowledged important changes at a personal level. Rhondda wrote:

It has been a learning and discovery time, time to reflect, time to make changes and like others in the study it has allowed plenty of debriefing and growth.

Rachel wrote after reading the research constructions:

I believe congratulations are in order. With a heated wheat bag on my neck I sat down and read it through last night. . . . Maybe it's time I should also thank you for providing a lifeline for me whilst I was living in Samoa. You might have thought I helped you in some small way, but the reality was you helped me deal with living in pain in an isolated country. I thank you so much!

This inquiry not only endeavoured to explore and share the health and illness experiences of midlife women, but also to raise consciousness and bring about changes to the health care of women by sensitizing health-care professionals to women's needs.

Throughout the entire research process I was conscious of the balance of power relations and its importance in ensuring women felt safe in the disclosure of their storied accounts of their experiences.

The centrality of power in feminist research

'We live in a world governed by the politics of domination' (hooks 2000: 432), one in which the belief is that the superior should rule over the inferior. There has been considerable debate among feminist researchers about the notion of empowerment and the balance of power relations within the research process. While immersed in this inquiry, I identified issues about the relations of power that require further discussion.

Participatory feminist research acknowledges the centrality of power in the construction of knowledge (Maguire 1996; Chinn 2003). Hence, almost every research text that discusses feminist research principles suggests that a leading goal of feminist research is empowerment of those participating in the research.

Empowerment occurs between the person who holds the power and those becoming empowered (Biley and Whale 1996) in a process of movement and change (Hutchinson *et al.* 1994). For empowerment to occur, both parties need to be equally participative in the process and share a common purpose. In this inquiry we had a common purpose to share and respond to each other. Let us turn our attention to some of the issues of power relations that confronted us during the course of the inquiry.

The position of the researcher

There has been considerable debate about the researcher's position in feminist research that appeared to begin with Oakley's (1981) and Finch's (1984) observations about interviewing women. They emphasized the use of qualitative research tools as a means of researching women's views. It has been proposed that in feminist research, the relationship between the researcher and the participants be non-hierarchical, reflexive and interactive, and cognisant of participants' feelings and values (Duffy 1985). A feminist research relationship ought to target collaboration and equality between the researcher and women participants. Of particular value in feminist qualitative research is the encouragement of interactive dialogue between the researcher and participants and the mutual creation of data (Webb 1993; Olesen 1994; FitzGerald 1997).

The personal experience and values of the researcher become an important component in feminist research. The feminist researcher is encouraged to describe and integrate their personal feelings and responses during the process of recounting and analyzing the research participants' experiences, pain and passions. One way of recording responses to research situations is to maintain a journal. During this research, I kept a reflexive journal in which I documented issues related to the research and which led me into a process of personal knowing.

> Written stories are in one sense limited in their capacity to convey the essence of the person, they are rich in conveying inner processes and meanings that are not easily perceived in the interpersonal experience. Written stories provide opportunities for response and reflection that are different from those provided by the self alone.
>
> (Chinn and Kramer 1999: 178)

During this inquiry, I often found myself pondering my carefully written replies to the women and deliberating over the exact words that conveyed the intended meaning out of concern that I might be misunderstood. The following is an example of one entry in my journal:

> It is difficult times. Jill has told me that she has now developed acute leukaemia in addition to osteosarcoma. As if she hasn't been through enough. I feel unprepared for this news and very inadequate. What do I say to her? How do I respond to her e-mail where I can feel that she is reeling from the shock of being told of a second cancer? This woman whom I have never met and yet feel so close to? I know that she is coming to the end of her life, and all I can offer her is written words. What should those words be?

The adoption of a feminist viewpoint involves challenging stereotypical assumptions and maintaining a critical awareness throughout an inquiry of ways in which the researcher may influence the work (Lawrence 1982; Opie 1992). I represented a privileged, white middle-class and often felt challenged, disrupted (Opie 1992) and sometimes silenced (Bhavnani 1988) by my involvement with women in this inquiry. I was challenged as my ways of seeing the world were expanded. I was disrupted as I came to understand the worlds of women, which were sometimes at odds with my own. I was silenced by their insight and wisdom developed from living a life with illness.

Participation and action in feminist research

Participation was central to the progress of our inquiry as together we created the storied accounts of women's lives with chronic illness. The central notion of participation encouraged a close relationship between action and research (Lather 1986; Cancian 1992; Maguire 1996). The development of our website and the collaborative development of papers for publication were displays of both passionate participation and action.

Change in the situations of women as an outcome of feminist research is also viewed as important. For many women, change began with reflection and experiencing doubt when interpreting their own experiences. The women learnt to doubt what seemed obvious or taken-for-granted in their lives. Experiencing doubt about one's world can be highly threatening. Certainly for some women in our inquiry, reflecting on past experiences was an uncomfortable process. The challenge for me as the researcher was to create the opportunity for reflective conversations, which induced some uncertainty through questioning the women's experiences without creating undue anxiety. Sensitive to create a context that was conducive to rich interaction, I had come to know each woman before reflective conversations took place. Too much threat and the women may have become overwhelmed and withdrawn from the process. Too little probing and the women may not be challenged sufficiently to take the leap into reflecting on their experiences.

Women engaged in reflective, written conversations about issues in which they made their reasoning explicit, critically inquired into their ways of framing issues and experimented with new ways of viewing and acting on those frames.

Throughout our inquiry, women participated in different ways and with different degrees of intensity and commitment. For some women, involvement was erratic because the time available to devote to writing was influenced by other events happening in their lives. For other women, a strong personal commitment to the inquiry was apparent. This commitment increased as women identified therapeutic benefits gained through reflective writing and their participation in this inquiry. The consequences of their involvement fit comfortably with the feminist requirement for participants to gain benefit from their research involvement.

The disclosure of experiences
In this inquiry, women revealed that the telling of one's story and the feeling that someone is listening could be an empowering and therapeutic experience. Many women expressed that they had lived with corrosive silence because they perceived that people had not wanted to hear their stories of illness. Other people were indifferent to the women's experiences of illness that had been so intense and personal for them. This silence had resulted in some women postponing any personal analysis of their experiences with illness. Through the course of this inquiry, their stories were finally told, the women found new meaning in their experiences. By giving voice to the voiceless, some women felt empowered and the increased self-awareness was often the impetus for change.

It is central to a participatory approach that the researcher finds ways to communicate with participants that both empowers and encourages them to speak in their own voice:

> When the balance of power is shifted, respondents are likely to tell 'stories' . . . interviewing practices that empower respondents also produce narrative accounts . . . Through their narratives people may be moved beyond the text to see the possibilities of action. That is, to be empowered is not only to speak in one's own voice and to tell one's own story, but to apply the understanding arrived at to action in accord with one's own interests.
>
> (Mishler 1986: 119)

It seems clear that the credibility of this research was enhanced by the reciprocal disclosure between all women who participated in the inquiry (researcher and participants). Some women responded with intensity about their experiences with illness and made known their strong desire to have their voices heard. This strong desire contributed to their disclosure of rich descriptions of their experiences. Women wrote that they were pleased they had the opportunity to share their experiences for the purpose of research so that other women who live with illness and health professionals may gain a greater understanding of their experiences. For some, it was evident that their experiences with illness had left them with a decreased self-esteem and a sense of inadequacy, and the opportunity to tell their story provided them with a sense of purpose which was experienced as empowering. They were elated that their story would be 'useful' and therefore their experiences were validated and had a purpose.

There were several instances throughout our inquiry when women disclosed highly personal information. Denise wrote after reading the constructions, 'I was thinking how amazing it is that people pour out their innermost, private and personal details to a stranger. I told you things I've told no-one!' This situation may be a dilemma in feminist research when women revealed intimate details to the researcher, and then have no control over analysis or how the researcher used their stories (Seibold et al. 1994). It was important for many women who participated in this inquiry that they had the opportunity to read the way that they were portrayed in the final report and in future publications and that they were aware that they would always have the opportunity to make changes to that text.

Consciousness-raising

Feminist research aims to raise the consciousness of people in general and of the women participants specifically (Stanley and Wise 1983). Consciousness-raising facilitates women to view the world in a different way and is based on knowledge gained.

In this inquiry, reciprocity abated the hierarchical nature of my position within the research. I used several strategies such as sharing my own experiences, assuring the women of their right to refuse to answer any questions, and sharing the writings of other women rather than imposing my own personal meanings on the women's experiences. Reciprocity affects all participants and gives individuals, including researchers a sense of their identity (Banister 1999). It is educative to consider the lives we have lived and the moments of particular significance within our lives, which play a part in shaping our ways of being in the world. Some women became aware of their social position through the research process and they then aimed to change their situation. The changes in the health situations of women, particularly in relationships with health professionals, became evident as women positioned themselves as central and in control of their health and illness care.

Women explained their social reality in personal accounts of their lives, and the themes emerged from their shared experiences (Holloway 1997). As the researcher, I read these accounts and while offering interpretation, gave a faithful picture of the personal histories and biographies of women who live with chronic illness, being conscious of their reality and guided women to see options for creating change in their lives.

Doing feminist research with non-feminist women

I became aware that my notion of power might not always be helpful to the women participating in the inquiry (Puwar 1997). Without the voice and direction from the women themselves, my ideas of power may be misconstrued as empowerment to do as I want, not empowerment to the women to express their own views, or take their own actions (Bowes 1996).

I became concerned that some women may actually be dis-empowered and further dis-organized in the short term by the reflective process. This situation may occur by undermining the woman's immediate coping strategies, which do not involve any long-term structural change. I contend that the women themselves have to be free to draw their own conclusions about their position in their lives. To impose feminist ideology on a woman may impose on their reality and forge changes for which she is not prepared.

I have come to understand through my own reality, that power is multi-layered and dynamic, and therefore empowerment is also situational and fractured. At the other end of the spectrum, it was essential that as a researcher, I understood that women experience patriarchy in different ways. These complexities in women's lives must be taken into account when considering the issue of the balance of power within feminist research.

Conclusion

Feminism acknowledges that women face some form of oppression and exploitation. Women experience their oppression, struggles and strengths in various ways because of the diverse realities and identities of women. Within this context of diversity, feminist research approaches inclusive of the principles of participation celebrate the practical and lived alongside the theoretical and dreamed about. Understandings and knowledge gained from this research approach are more than theory or description but based on people making sense of their own lives which facilitates collective action. Feminism and participation, when framed by authenticity, becomes a way of thinking, feeling and being in and of the world.

References

Alvesson, M. and Sköldberg, K. (2000) *Reflexive Methodology*. London: Sage.

Anderson, J. (1991) Reflexivity in fieldwork: toward a feminist epistemology. *Image*, 23 (2): 115–118.

Banister, E. (1999) Evolving reflexivity: Negotiating meaning of women's midlife experience, *Qualitative Inquiry*, 5 (1): 3–23.

Bhavnani, K. (1988) What's power got to do with it? Empowerment and social research, *Text*, 8: 41–50.

Biley, A. and Whale, Z. (1996) Feminist approaches to change and nursing development, *Journal of Clinical Nursing*, 5 (3): 159–163.

Bowes, A. (1996) Evaluating an Empowering Research Strategy: Reflections on Action-Research with South Asian Women, *Sociological Research Online*, 1 (1), http://www.socresonline.org.uk/socresonline/1/1/1.html.

Buker, E. (1987) Storytelling power: Personal narratives and political analysis, *Women and Politics*, 7 (Fall): 29–46.

Bunting, S. and Campbell, J. (1990) Feminism and nursing: historical perspectives, *Advances in Nursing Science*, 12 (4): 11–12.

Campbell, J. and Bunting, S. (1991) Voices and paradigms: Perspectives on critical and feminist theory in nursing, *Advances in Nursing Science*, 13 (3): 1–15.

Cancian, F. (1992) Participatory research. In Borgatta, E.F. and Borgatta, M. (eds) *Encyclopedia of Sociology* (1427–1432). New York: Macmillan.

Carryer, J. (1995) Feminist research: strengths and challenges, *Contemporary Nurse*, 4: 180–186.

Chesney, M. (2000) Interaction and understanding: 'me' in the research, *Nurse Researcher*, 7 (3): 58–69.

Chinn, P. (2003) Feminist approaches. In Clare, J. and Hamilton, H. (eds) *Writing Research*. London: Churchill Livingstone, 61–85.

Chinn, P. and Kramer, M. (1999) *Theory and Nursing, integrated knowledge development*, 5th edn. Missouri: Mosby.

Clarke, A. and Olesen, V. (1999) *Revisioning Women, Health and Healing*. New York: Routledge.

Crowley, H. and Himmelweit, S. (1992) *Knowing Women: Feminism and Knowledge*. Cambridge: Polity Press in association with The Open University.

Delmar, R. (1986) What is Feminism? In Mitchell, J. and Oakley, A. (eds) *What is Feminism?* New York: Pantheon.

Drevdahl, D. (1999) Sailing beyond: nursing theory and the person, *Advances in Nursing Science*, 21 (4): 1–13.

DuBois, E. (1985) *Feminist Scholarship: Kindling the Groves of Academe*. Urbana: University of Illinois Press.

Duffy, M. (1985) A critique of research: a feminist perspective, *Health Care for Women International*, 6: 341–352.

Duran, J. (1990) *Toward a Feminist Epistemology*. New York: Rowman and Littlefield.

Finch, J. (1984) It's great to have someone to talk to: the ethics and politics of interviewing women. In Bell, C. and Roberts, H. (eds) *Social Researching: Politics, Problems, Practice*. London: Routledge and Kegan Paul, 70–87.

FitzGerald, M. (1997) Nursing and researching, *International Journal of Nursing Practice*, 3, (1): 53–6.

Fonow, M. and Cook, J. (1991) *Beyond Methodology: Feminist Scholarship as Lived Research*. Bloomington, IN: Indiana University Press.

Ford-Gilboe, M. and Campbell, J. (1996) The mother-headed single-parent family: a feminist critique of the nursing literature, *Nursing Outlook*, 44 (4): 173–183.

Freire, P. and Ramos, M. (1990) *Pedagogy of the Oppressed*. New York: Continuum.

Frye, M. (1983) *The politics of reality*. Freedom, CA: Crossing Press.

Griffiths, M. (1995) *Feminisms and the Self: The Web of Identity*. London: Routledge.

Hall, J. and Stevens, P. (1991) Rigor in feminist research, *Advances in Nursing Science*, 13 (3): 16–29.

Hammersley, M. (1991) On Feminist Methodology, *Sociology*, 26 (2): 187–206.

Harding, S. (ed.) (1987) *Feminism and Methodology: Social Science Issues*. Bloomington, IN: Indiana University Press.

Harding, S. (1989) How the women's movement benefits science: Two views, *Women's Studies International Forum*, 12 (3): 271–284.

Harding, S. (1991) *Whose Science? Whose Knowledge? Thinking from Women's Lives*. Milton Keynes: Open University Press.

Henderson, D. (1995) Consciousness raising in participatory research: Method and methodology for emancipatory nursing inquiry, *Advances in Nursing Science*, 17 (3): 58–69.

Holloway, I. (1997) *Basic concepts for qualitative research*. Oxford: Blackwell Science.

hooks, b. (2000) Feminism: a transformational politic. In Kolmar, W. and Bartkowsli, F. (eds) *Feminist Theory*. London: Mayfield.

Hutchinson, S., Wilson, M. and Skodol Wilson, H. (1994) Benefits of participating in research interviews, *Image: Journal of Nursing Scholarship*, 26 (2): 161–164.

Jackson, D. (1997) Feminism: a path to clinical knowledge development, *Contemporary Nurse*, 6 (2): 85–91.

Kolmar, W. and Bartkowski, F. (2000) *Feminist Theory*. London: Mayfield.

Kralik, D. (2000) *The Quest for Ordinariness: midlife women living through chronic illness*. Unpublished PhD thesis, Flinders University of South Australia.

Kralik, D. (2002) The quest for Ordinariness: transition experienced by midlife women living with chronic illness, *Journal of Advanced Nursing*, 39 (2): 146–154.

Kralik, D., Koch, T. and Brady, B. (2000) Pen pals: Correspondence as a method for data generation in qualitative research, *Journal of Advanced Nursing*, 31 (4): 909–917.

Kralik, D., Koch, T. and Telford, K. (2001) Constructions of sexuality for midlife women living with chronic illness, *Journal of Advanced Nursing*, 35 (2): 180–187.

Lather, P. (1986) Research as praxis, *Harvard Educational Review*, 56 (3): 257–277.

Lather, P. (1988) Feminist perspectives on empowering research methodologies, *Women's Studies International Forum*, 56 (3): 257–277.

Lather, P. (1991) *Getting Smart: Feminist Research and Pedagogy Within/in the Postmodern*. New York: Routledge.

Lawrence, E. (1982) In the abundance of water, the fool is thirsty: sociology and black pathology. In Centre for Contemporary Cultural Studies (eds) *The Empire Strikes Back: Race and Racism in 70s Britain*. London: Hutchinson.

Lumby, C. (1997) *Bad Girls*. Sidney: Allen and Unwin.

Maguire, P. (1996) Considering more feminist participatory research: What's congruency got to do with it? *Qualitative Inquiry*, 2 (1): 106–118.

Maguire, P. (2001) Uneven ground: Feminisms and action research. In Reason, P. and Bradbury, H. (eds) *Handbook of Action Research*. London: Sage, 59–69.

Maynard, M. and Purvis, J. (eds) (1994) *Researching Women's Lives from a Feminist Perspective*. London: Taylor and Francis.

Millen, D. (1997) Some Methodological and Epistemological Issues Raised by Doing Feminist Research on Non-Feminist Women, *Sociological Research Online*, 2 (3), http://www.socresonline.org.uk/socresonline/2/3/3.html.

Mishler, E. (1986) *Research Interviewing: Context and Narrative*. Cambridge, MA: Harvard University Press.

Mitchell, J. and Oakley, A. (eds) (1976) *The Rights and Wrongs of Women*. Harmondsworth, Middlesex: Penguin.

Oakley, A. (1981) Interviewing women: A contradiction in terms. In Roberts, H. (ed.) *Doing Feminist Research*. London: Routledge, 30–61.

Olesen, V. (1994) Feminisms and models of qualitative research. In Denzin, N.K. and Lincoln, Y.S. (eds) *Handbook of qualitative research*. Thousand Oaks, CA: Sage, 158–174.

Opie, A. (1992) Qualitative research, appropriation of the 'other' and empowerment, *Feminist Review*, 40: 52–69.

Puwar, N. (1997) Reflections on Interviewing Women MPs, *Sociological Research Online*, 12 (1), http://www.socresonline.org.uk/socresonlin/2/1/4.html.

Reinharz, S. (1992) *Feminist Methods in Social Research*. Oxford: Oxford University Press.

Ricketts, M. (1989) Epistemological values of feminists in psychology, *Psychology of Women Quarterly*, 13 (December): 401–416.

Rose, H. (1983) Hand, Brain and Heart: A Feminist Epistemology for the Natural Sciences, *Signs*, 9 (1): 73–90.

Rosser, S. (1987) Feminist scholarship in the sciences: Where are we now and when can we expect a theoretical breakthrough? *Hypatia: A Journal of Feminist Philosophy*, 2 (Fall): 5–18.

Scharbo-DeHann, M. (1994) Connected knowing: Feminist group research. In Chinn, P.L. (ed.) *Advances in Methods of Inquiry for Nursing*. Maryland: Aspen Pub., 88–101.

Seibold, C., Richards, L. and Simon, D. (1994) Feminist method and qualitative research about midlife. *Journal of Advanced Nursing*, 19 (2): 394–402.

Smith, S. (1991) A feminist analysis of constructs of health. In Neil, R. and Watts, R (eds) *Caring and Nursing: Explorations in Feminist Perspectives*. New York: National League for Nursing, 209–225.

Speedy, S. (1991) The contribution of feminist research. In Gray, G. and Pratt, R. (eds) *Towards a Discipline of Nursing*. Melbourne: Churchill Livingstone, 191–210.

Stanley, L. and Wise, S. (1983) *Breaking Out: Feminist Consciousness and Feminist Research*. London: Routledge and Kegan Paul.

Stevenson, J. (1977) *Issues and Crises during Middlescence*. New York: Appleton-Century Crofts.

Unger, R. (1989) Psychological, feminist, and personal epistemology: Transcending contradiction. In Gergen, M. (ed.) *Feminist Thought and the Structure of Knowledge*. New York: New York University Press, 124–141.

Webb, C. (1993) Feminist research: definitions, methodology, methods and evaluation, *Journal of Advanced Nursing*, 18: 416–423.

Wilkinson, S. (1986) (ed.) *Feminist Social Psychology: Developing Theory and Practice*. Milton Keynes: Open University Press.

15

IMMY HOLLOWAY
Qualitative writing

> ... *To do research is to write, and the insights achieved depend on the right words and phrases, on styles and traditions, on metaphor and figures of speech, on argument and poetic image.*
>
> van Manen 2002: 237

Introduction

Whenever I read a qualitative study, I look for something different from other types of research report, something more than just a straightforward description of the things researchers have observed in the setting or heard from the participants in the study. The reader of a piece of qualitative research should be able to reconstruct a vivid picture of the world of the participants, therefore the research report must grip the reader's attention and imagination, and tell a compelling story. When I read the beginning of the chapter by Mattingley (2000) for instance, I could understand what qualitative writing is about (I also had instant information about narrative research).

> Suppose that some stories are not told so much as acted, embodied, played, even danced. On such occasions time itself takes on narrative shape. Actions acquire some of the formal and aesthetic qualities of the well-told tale: drama, suspense, risk, adventure, surprise, plot, a sense of the whole, and especially that sense that something significant is afoot.
>
> (Mattingley 2000: 181)

'Writing people' makes the emotions and thoughts of the participants come alive and readable. It has a feel of authenticity by which the reader can instantly recognize their social reality. Many qualitative texts include a chapter on writing-up; experts even devote whole books to it (for instance, Woods 1999; Wolcott 2001; Holliday 2002). The main principles of a report – be it a PhD thesis, an academic article or a report to a professional group, fund holder or policy-makers – are usually similar, regardless of the methodology used. Yet authors can be more flexible when reporting on a qualitative study and choose not to present a write-up on entirely traditional or conventional lines. An essential element in the qualitative text is, however, the ability of the writer to uncover the essence of the participants' emotions and perceptions as well as trying to find the meaning of their actions. The write-up of a qualitative study may also be seen as 'literary work' as Alasuutari (1995) calls it, and not just a way of reporting. One of my colleagues talks about what happened to her while learning about qualitative research: she had training in research methods, but she only ever found out about constructing reports on quantitative research rather than writing qualitative accounts (Lewis 2004), and these are, of course, very different. The write-up of qualitative research is crucial. Indeed, '. . . writing is the most important part of the research: when all is said and done, the world is left with nothing else but the text' (Alasuutari 1995: 177). Writing up a study is the culmination of a demanding research process and crucial to its success. In this chapter I am not concerned with the mechanics and procedures of writing a qualitative research report or thesis, for this is well described in most books on research; rather I wish to address what it means to write qualitatively. However, I shall first provide an overview of key aspects of the qualitative research account ('report' is not a wholly appropriate term for this type of writing).

In qualitative research in particular, writing does not start on completion of the inquiry but is a continuous process. It often requires several attempts at writing and rewriting before the writer is satisfied, not just with the content of the report but also with its coherence and eloquence. This means that the end product may be quite different from earlier drafts, and qualitative writing may be viewed as a narrative art form. Results are not just found, 'they are narrated into being' (Wetherall 2001: 396). Writers seek to describe, interpret or explain their findings and transform the data in writing up. Schostak (2002) points out that writing research has both political and ethical implications; it has the potential to affect the lives of those who participate and also those who read the story and are interested in the findings, their application and implications. Ethical issues (discussed in Chapter 2) are paramount, particularly in health research, and they permeate the whole of a well-written research study. Political issues are involved throughout the research by the choice of topic and participants as well as by the selection of particular items from the data and the interpretation of the findings. The author of the research story assists the reader in realizing these ethical and political implications.

The qualitative writer normally starts with an introduction that identifies a question, issue or problem, set in a particular context. Once the research has been completed, the researchers must construct and present a rationale that explicitly supports their selection of the topic and make a strong case for the use of the chosen methodology. This should be justified within the context in which the research takes place. The introduction is followed by a method section that provides a clear account of, and justification for, the methodology used, the participants included, ethical issues and details of the research procedures and processes. Ways of writing up method sections vary widely from the factual to the discursive – much depends on the discipline for which the research is intended. Throughout their journey, researchers have to be mindful of rigour and quality so that they produce a report of high standard that is valid and has credibility.

The main purpose of most research in health care is to contribute to knowledge and understanding of issues in the health arena and suggest solutions to problems. Therefore the author needs to present a conclusion that addresses the answers to the original research question, or indeed raises new questions. This conclusion is followed by recommendations or implications for practice. Some see qualitative findings as unscientific, yet qualitative research 'evidence' can have a great impact on practice. Guba and Lincoln (1989) went so far as to suggest that the research could assist the participants in decision-making and empower them by lending 'catalytic authenticity' to the study.

Researchers are often mindful of this as they reflect on the meaning of the data and construct and improve their line of argument. Through this process the data are transformed and a meaningful story generated. The researchers must, of course, convince the reader that their arguments are grounded in the data and communicate the thoughts and experiences of the participants rather than merely being a flight of their own fertile imaginations. Since the researcher is seen as the main research tool, he or she has to demonstrate through writing how the knowledge gained from participants is received, perceived and constructed.

Overall, qualitative researchers need to take account of a number of important factors when presenting their written report or thesis, including:

1. The development of coherent and persuasive arguments.
2. The readership to whom they address the report or thesis.
3. The context of the research: context sensitivity.
4. Their own stance and location as researchers: reflexivity.
5. The validity and credibility of the research: quality.
6. The form in which they present the study: language and style.

Perhaps the most important purpose of qualitative writing is to communicate the 'voices' – the feelings and thoughts – of the participants so that their experiences are heard and understood, and their actions made visible. It needs to be recognized, however, that the term 'voice' is not unproblematic. There is never a single voice or a single social reality; rather there is a multiplicity of perspectives including those of the reader, the researcher and the researched. I shall explore this in more detail in the following sections.

Developing the argument and transforming the data

As the research progresses, the research questions may change, and the researcher reaches the point at which previous arguments must be developed or changed. These changes are incorporated into the text to build a case for the conclusions based on the findings. Smith and Osborn (2003) explain that the process is interactive and iterative; the themes are formed into a narrative which itself contains expansions, illustrations, interpretations of the analysis; Charmaz (2003), too, suggests that the analytic process continues through the course of report

LIBRARY
EDUCATION CENTRE
PRINCESS ROYAL HOSPITAL

writing. Indeed, most qualitative researchers are unanimous about this: for instance, Morse and Richards (2002) suggest that qualitative research is rarely complete, as there is an ongoing engagement of the researcher with the topic; researchers ask questions throughout the research depending on what they have already discovered.

The qualitative writer starts by setting the scene, describing the setting and the arena and through this defines the scope of the research. A rationale is provided for the research, a line of argument or thesis developed and the approach taken to the research justified. This is what most researchers do in the course of their writing. But important differences between qualitative and quantitative research become clearer in the treatment of the literature. An initial literature review is essential to identify a gap in knowledge that needs to be filled, but the review is not exhaustive, nor should it force the researcher into a particular direction. In fact, most of the literature relevant to the study will eventually be integrated into the findings and discussion during the course of writing and rewriting or crafting the report. Indeed, Todres (in Chapter 7) suggests that the findings of the research be considered in dialogue with the literature and current research.

Many qualitative writers, including myself, prefer that the results and discussion be presented as an integrated whole, although some authors choose to separate them or use them in poetic presentation or alternative ways. This can be powerful and dramatic. Poetic presentation can truly 'transform' the meaning of the text for the reader. Indeed, the way the data are presented on the page affects the way they are read. Integration allows the writer to place the findings in the context of early and current literature that either confirms or challenges the findings of the research. It may also assist in providing the researcher with a language to label themes or categories generated by the inquiry.

In the final version of the research account, authors need to present their message or key argument in a coherent and persuasive way. They give evidence from the data to support this through quotes from the words of the participants and excerpts from observation notes. The writers will also show that there may be other, alternative interpretations of the data and include in their discussion 'contrary occurrences' or 'deviant cases' that might not fit in easily.

The concluding section is where researchers discuss what they learnt in response to their original research question. It is also important to reflect on the strengths and limitations of the study. The researcher is obliged to debate whether or not the questions originally posed when starting out on the journey have been addressed or answered. The findings and implications might be discussed in the context of current policies, practice and research. Everything in the report has to be linked to the original research problem and aim as well as to the context – the setting – where the research took place. The conclusion focuses on essential issues and the implications the findings have for clinical practice. The tale the researcher tells in the research report can never truly present, but might reflect, the social reality of the participants. A number of questions must be answered:

1. Does the research reflect the experience of the participants?

2. Does the research fill a gap in the present knowledge about the area of study?

3. What sense does the writer make of the participant's voice?

4. Does the related literature confirm or challenge ('disconfirm') the findings of the study?

5. Do researchers achieve authenticity in their research?

The story: emic and etic perspectives

Writing descriptions and giving interpretations of the world of the participants are not the only tasks of the researcher. There are many references to 'emic' and 'etic' dimensions (for instance, Harris 1976; Holloway 1997; Darlington and Scott 2002). The emic, or insider's perspective, centres on the ideas of the participants, while the etic dimension leads to the outsider's point of view, that of the researcher. He or she has to go beyond the concepts originating directly in the data collected from the participants – first order concepts – to developing second order concepts (Denzin 1989a), the researcher's own, more abstract and theoretical ideas. This means that the data are not only based on the understanding and accounts of the participants but also transformed by the researcher in the process of analysis and writing. The act of collaboration between the two parties, the researcher and the other participants, develops something new that goes beyond both.

It is unlikely that the researcher completes the study without making some inferences. When researchers relate a story they are at the same time interpreting the stories of the participants. Hence White *et al.* (2003: 287) claim that the challenge lies not only in 'the need to represent the social world that has been researched, but also to re-present it in a way which both remains grounded in the accounts of the participants and explains its subtleties and complexities.' Thus, the most important issue is that of re-presenting, or at least reflecting, the ideas of the participants.

Addressing the audience

The readership of the completed research may comprise health professionals, students or scholars for whom researchers write. Les Todres and I (2004: 88) speak of 'communicative and scientific concerns' in writing. The scientific concern 'cares for' the phenomenon under study and the research participants, while the communicative concern centres on the readers of the research and its eventual purpose. The writer is the mediator who bridges the gap between the participants' perspectives and the reader who tries to understand them. Sometimes the writer appeals to the shared knowledge and education of the professional or scholarly community and uses the first person plural 'we' (the contributors to this book, including myself, also do it occasionally when addressing qualitative researchers). It does make the story more personal and immediate, but, like Alasuutari, I am wary of this. Who is this nebulous 'we'? How do I know that the audience is willing to be involved? In any case in a mixed and varied readership a 'we' does not often exist as each person reads the research differently. On the other hand, I concede that feminist writers attempt to draw those who share their ideas into their writing by using the 'we' more often.

Being context-sensitive

Qualitative research is always situated in context, and in the write-up this has to be shown. The context is the cultural, temporal and physical/geographical setting in which the research occurs. Davies and her colleagues maintain that 'writing is always writing in context and each context (itself constructed) invites particular readings' (Davies *et al.* 2004: 383). Being aware of the context starts at the beginning of the research and does not end until the final account has been written. When collecting data on experience, perspectives and behaviour, we need to have context-intelligence, because contextualization is critical for understanding the reality of the participants.

Writing a piece of qualitative work includes this context so the reader too can grasp the whole picture and does not merely receive a disembodied and context-free text or a description of data that have no connection or link to a storyline. The report presents 'compelling arguments about how things work in a *particular* context' (Mason 2002: 1, her italics). Locality, temporality and culture are reflected in the write-up. Thus the writer sets the scene for a developing an interesting story. I gave some examples in another text (Holloway 1997); a hypothetical example of research with unmarried mothers demonstrates the importance of context: the life of a single mother in the 1940s cannot be compared with that of a single mother in the twenty-first century. Time, culture and history are different and affect the beliefs and assumptions of society and hence the research. Group membership, locality or gender influence interaction, assumptions and experience of participants, and therefore 'thick description' (Geertz 1973) is needed. Denzin (1989b) states that this means contextualization of a study including intentions and meanings. A qualitative research account without contextualization will be lifeless. That's why the criticism of qualitative research as journalistic is inappropriate: *Good* journalists always contextualize and produce a compelling story; as qualitative researchers we can learn from that. However, *good* qualitative research, in addition to generating an interesting story, develops abstract concepts, produces theory and is based on it and thus will never be wholly journalistic. The writer attempts to be imaginative, and fascinate the reader without imagining or inventing the story, truthful to the reality of the participants but not unscientific.

The story of a qualitative research project can only unfold if the writer takes the context into account. Schwandt, however, warns that *context* is a complex term, not merely indicating a physical environment in which people act or conditions against which behaviour can be understood, although this is part of it:

> Context is not simply a background of influences and determinants of meaning, identity, speech and so forth that is detachable from those human actions . . . Rather, context is *produced* in the social practice of asking questions about meaning, identity, speech and so on.
>
> (Schwandt 2001: 37)

Validity or trustworthiness: achieving quality

The terms 'validity' and 'rigour' are most often used in quantitative research. There is no reason, however, why qualitative researchers cannot use these words as long as they realize the different way in which they are understood in qualitative inquiry. To avoid a blurring of boundaries between qualitative and quantitative approaches, other terms have become more common such as trustworthiness and authenticity, credibility, relevance and so on. (I shall not go into detail, nor will I enter the debate as this has been widely discussed elsewhere for instance in Erlandson *et al.* 1993; Hammersley 1998; Murphy *et al.* 1998; Seale 1999, Holloway and Wheeler 2002, and many others). The most commonly used terms are those suggested by Lincoln and Guba (1985) – 'trustworthiness' and 'authenticity'. Whatever term authors select for their study, they must show the truth-value of their research in the write-up, and the account should not contain any internal contradictions (Dahlberg *et al.* 2001).

Writers must be truthful. However, they are not always aware that 'truths are relative, multiple and subject to redefinition' (Charmaz 2004: 983); we do not always recognize it when we see it, but we report the experience and reality of the participants and our own part in the research as accurately as we can. All researchers wish to present a 'valid' and credible piece of research demonstrating rigour and trustworthiness. A piece of research writing that is not trustworthy is unethical, as it does not do justice to the experience of the participants. Writers of qualitative studies are aware that each approach has distinctive criteria for trustworthiness and quality, and Sparkes (2001) states that there is no shared understanding of what is 'good' qualitative research. I would, however, argue that quality in qualitative inquiry is recognized by most experienced qualitative researchers. Many qualitative writers object to the constant preoccupation with the concept of validity (Wolcott 1994; Sparkes 2001; Polkinghorne 2003). It is revealing that most of the authors in this text have discussed, in some form, the notion of validity or its equivalent.

I often find the section on validity boring and difficult, even if the researcher uses alternative terms. It can interrupt the flow of writing and become a turgid legitimization process merely to appease the readers who developed their skills in the quantitative tradition. It is often a form of defence to show that qualitative research is science, just like quantitative research.

Still, scientific writing needs rigour. Quantitative researchers use the term, although qualitative approaches demand this too, for instance Sandelowski (1986) who advises researchers to have rigour. However, in a later article she speaks of 'rigour or rigour mortis', stating that the term is problematic and might imply inflexibility. She sees this rigidity endangering creativity and the search for meaning, because one of the tasks of the researcher is to create 'landscapes of human experience' (Sandelowski 1993: 1). Evidence of rigour is not in itself enough as the essence of qualitative research lies in finding meaning in the data, portraying social life and showing human experience as central in the write-up.

Truth issues are not the only important considerations in qualitative writing. My colleague (Todres 1998: 121) poses the following question: 'What kind of qualitative descriptions of human experience produce a feeling of understanding in the reader? The answer to this question may involve not only issues about truth (validity) but also issues about beauty (aesthetics).' Todres speaks of 'the richness and texture of human experiences'. These need a language that reflects these qualitative dimensions. The significance of aesthetic criteria cannot be overstated. The writing has to do more than engage the readers' intellect; it should also speak to their emotions. The 'good' author invites the reader into the text. Post-modernists, in any case, see the text as local and historical and ever changing through its reading, not as an authoritative account of the 'truth'.

Demonstrating validity

Researchers distinguish between internal and external validity. In qualitative inquiry internal validity – truthfulness and representation of the reality of the participants is most important. Many writers establish this by showing that they have carried out a 'member check' as Lincoln and Guba (1985) suggest. In one of my early research projects I followed the rules, as one is bound to do, and did my member check, that is, I returned to the participants and showed them a summary of their interviews to find out whether I was re-presenting their ideas and their real world. When I gave one of the participants a summary of his interview, he con-gratulated me on capturing his experiences. Only later did I realize that I had given him the interview of one of his colleagues accidentally (not quite ethical but a genuine mistake). I then became aware that the essence of the experience of all participants was very similar, and distinct patterns were found in all their inter-views. This meant that my story would present the social reality of the participants. However, many colleagues argue against the member check and find it proble-matic for a variety of reasons (Bryman 2001). Phenomenologists, in particular, reject the notion of member check as the researcher transforms the data in the process of analysis and writing. Individuals, who have their own unique per-spective, inhabit a social world with others and recognize others' reality to some extent. For the account to have validity, its readers will have grasped not only the essence of the phenomenon but also understood something of the human condi-tion they have in common with the participants – intersubjective understanding.

Thick description – discussed elsewhere in this chapter – is another element in showing internal validity, and this is important as it portrays in a holistic way the reality of the participants. Another way of showing validity is through the accurate and *detailed description of the audit trail* – the record of decision-making during the research process (Lincoln and Guba 1985; Rodgers and Cowles 1993). In a lengthy research study such as a thesis this is not too difficult, but it presents a challenge in a short report or article. Cutcliffe and McKenna (2004), however, see the description of an audit trail as problematic and stress that qualitative research can be valid without being confirmable by an audit trail.

These are only some of the ways in which writers let the readers of their studies know that they have thought about validity. Others are reflexivity, triangulation, peer reviewing and the search for alternative cases. Reflexivity is discussed in the next section of the chapter as it is of major importance in demonstrating validity. I have not detailed all aspects of this large topic, but merely tried to place it in the context of writing up. (There are hundreds of articles and chapters on validity and its elements, including my own chapter in Holloway and Wheeler (2002).)

The search for external validity

In qualitative health research, generalizability is a debated issue within validity. Many feel (for instance Wolcott (1994)) that it is irrelevant as authors often describe specific cases and situations, and their sample is criterion-based, purposive and small. However, generalizability has its uses in the health-care arena so that the research can be shown as valid beyond a single study. Different kinds of qualitative research have different aims in any case. In grounded theory, for instance, researchers can establish external validity through representativeness of concepts, typicality and theory-based generalization where they show that the developed concepts and the theory can be recontextualized into a variety of settings (Strauss and Corbin 1998; Morse and Richards 2002). Phenomenology seeks transfer of meanings and unique variations but not literal generalizability.

Researchers might show where their research fits into the overall inquiry of a particular area, experience and condition, so it is illuminated from many sides to establish its usefulness. This demands a full portrayal of the social reality under study. Mantzoukas (2004: 994) claims: 'The more illustrative, explanatory and sophisticated this portrayal is, the more extended or applicable the acquired knowledge becomes.'

The writer in the tale: reflexivity

Most qualitative texts exhort researchers to be reflective or reflexive. Finlay (2002) declares that the meanings of these words may be open to misconception, and they are often used interchangeably. She suggests that reflection – one might call it 'critical reflection' – takes place after an event or when something has been done, and the researcher reflects on it and thinks about it. It means taking a critical stance towards the research and suggesting ways to improve it or go beyond its limitations as well as thinking about future solutions to the problems encountered. I would suggest that reflection is necessary in all research writing, while reflexivity is a particular characteristic of qualitative research (though it might be used in some form in quantitative research too).

Being reflexive

Reflexivity can be defined as:

> a confessional account of methodology or as examining one's own personal, possibly unconscious, reactions. It can also mean exploring the dynamics of the researcher–researched relationship and how the research is co-constituted.
>
> (Finlay 2002: 536)

Reflexivity is about the interaction of the researcher with the research and the participants as well as reciprocity between the researcher and the process of inquiry. It implies self-awareness, critical evaluation, and self-consciousness of their own role on the part of the researchers. It also needs the recognition of power relationships between themselves and the participants. Reflexivity includes describing and taking account of the unpredictable in the research, unexpected disclosures, expression of deep feelings of participants and of their own emotions during the research. It also involves being self-aware and self-critical about the ethical procedures and issues in the research process (Guillemin and Gillam 2004; see also Freshwater, Chapter 12).

Writers on reflexivity often make explicit, or at least imply, the centrality of the researcher in the research process. I too believe that the researchers' role should be clarified, their assumptions and background uncovered; that is, they should give accounts of their own location and experience as they affect the process, setting and participants of the research. Researchers come to the setting with their own biographies and history. They are themselves participants in the inquiry with their own identities and personal stance; they do not merely retell the experience, feelings and behaviours of those whom they study. Research writing is always an interpretive process, not merely mirroring or describing the views of those involved but also affected directly by the location, perspectives and experience of the researcher. For instance, a doctor or health visitor carrying out research among refugees or people with Aids might ask these questions:

- Do I have assumptions, which might affect my interaction with this group?
- How can I ensure that these don't unduly influence the way I collect or analyze data?
- Can I write about this in a non-judgemental way?

The effect of the researcher's role is by no means always negative. It can also give deeper insight into the phenomenon under study, and thus the subjectivity of the researcher becomes a resource. Indeed, Finlay (2002: 532) suggests that 'through the use of reflexivity, subjectivity in the research can be transformed from a problem to an opportunity'. For instance, the long experience of a health professional with certain conditions from which patients suffer can help develop awareness and expert knowledge of the researcher which determines, or at least affects, the questions which he or she asks the participants.

Researchers account for the ways in which they decided on the research question, data collection and analysis and other parts of the audit trail. Reflexivity is also part of the validation process (see later in this chapter).

Reporting on the relationship with participants

Reflexivity involves not only reporting on or describing the reality of the participants but also shows how the research story came about, how it was constructed and how the researcher's voice complements that of the participants and sometimes even shapes it. The people with whom we do research do react to the researcher as a person and respond to this person (for instance, in Chapter 10, Sharkey and Larsen show how clothing might affect the response of the participants). Thus qualitative researchers identify the reactions of the participants to them as researchers and persons, and their own response to the participants. An example for the latter: one of my colleagues became very upset when interviewing young people with a terminal condition; she found it difficult to finish the interviews.

The writer is both a professional (often with several roles, for instance that of health professional and that of researcher) and also a person with emotions and beliefs; the same is true for the reader. Most importantly, the writer has to recognize that the participants come to the research process with their feelings and thoughts and have their own biographies and histories.

The reflexive 'I'

The use of the 'I', the first person singular in research, shows the researcher's role and place, and demonstrates how he or she as a person is involved in the inquiry in each step of the process. Giving account of themselves and their decisions does not mean a continuous repetition of 'I felt', 'I believe', 'I think', but when discussing their actions, authors uncover their own involvement in the study rather than taking a neutral stance. In any case, a qualitative author does not believe that it is possible to write a wholly neutral and objective account. Authors do not write themselves out of the study but give an account of how the text was produced. Charmaz and Mitchell (1997: 193) shatter 'the myth of silent authorship' and suggest that 'evocative writing' involves the author of the text whose voice can be heard; hearing this voice helps the reader to participate in the research. The use of the 'I' makes the write-up more lively and imaginative if used as a literary device, as well as more credible and real. However, the writer should not use the first person singular too often, otherwise the research sounds like a diary excerpt of a self-centred person and not like a work of science. Also, and more importantly, the 'I' is uncovered in order to amplify the voice of 'the other'.

Finding the participant's 'voice'

I said before that the researcher is important to the research process. This statement is true but also misleading. If researchers have the privilege of entering people's lives, thoughts and feelings, should they not place the participants in the centre of the story? Koch and Harrington (1998) therefore make the case for 'many voiced' qualitative research which is neither self-indulgent nor introspective. In a 'good' text, the author will give the participants – and even the reader – the feeling that their vision of the circumstances and experiences matter. Van Maanen (1988), the ethnographer, speaks of three types of tale that the writer can use: realist, confessional and impressionist. For reasons of space, I shall not discuss all of these here, however, the last is best suited to representing the participant's voice as it centres on the experience, feelings, actions and thoughts of 'the other'. The writer's main task is still storying the participants' lives, not his or her own. In the health arena in particular, by enabling an audience to hear the voices of those who are powerless or vulnerable, the researcher empowers the participants. This is one of the reasons why qualitative researchers don't call those with whom they do research 'subjects'. Even the word 'respondent' does not capture the imagination – though many qualitative researchers use it – nor does it necessarily show that those involved are real people with real lives, not 'objects' to be scrutinized and examined.

It must be remembered here that an impressionistic retelling of the participants' experiences is not enough for a good account – as I have suggested earlier in this chapter. There are other books that do this, such as those of Studs Terkel for instance. Researchers never tell, nor do readers of the research read, the 'pure' story of the participants' lives, and the simplistic notion of 'hearing the voice' does not suffice in an academic piece of writing; indeed, the concept of 'voice' itself is problematic. Atkinson and Silverman (1997) strongly stress the analytical and theoretical elements through which the participants' narrative are transformed into an academic piece of work. (There has been a long and useful debate about this topic in a number of articles including Atkinson (1997), Frank (2000) and Bochner (2001).)

Choosing evidence from the data

The presentation of voice and of the participants' reality is problematic. There is an obligation for the researcher to be mindful of the participants' words and their meaning. Writers select particular parts of the data and show them to the reader in the form of quotes from participants, or excerpts from fieldnotes, to re-present the 'voice' of the participants and to make a distinction between this and their own interpretations. The following is a vivid excerpt from the research of Charmaz that illustrates the feelings of a man who had recently had a heart attack:

> ... you get this invulnerable feeling – this invincible feeling, and all of the sudden the hardest thing to accept is 'Hey you are vulnerable. You can be hurt. You can die.' You know which you never thought of that before, or I never did. So that's still in the back of your mind.
>
> (Charmaz 1997: 40)

In an instant, people who read this grasp the feelings of this 40-year-old man. However, readers do not always recognize that the quotes and excerpts they see are not raw data; the data have already been transformed in the process by the researcher. Even the choice of quotes, quotations and fieldnotes plays a part in the transformation of data into the research story. After all, the writer has a wealth of data from interviews and/or observation and must select some of these while leaving others. In any case, as Coffey (1999: 149) says: '... all writing is edited by those who are putting the pen to paper'. This means that the reader only has access to that which the author chooses to report, never to a wholly complete account of the participants' experience.

Most importantly, however, to represent the social world of the participants adequately, the writer has to be committed to them and not see them as inanimate objects that are either passive or can be manipulated, but as active members of that world who are involved in the construction and re-construction of knowledge.

Ways of writing: style and language

The style of writing in a good qualitative project is personal and lively, and the reader expects a compelling story. Quotations from the participants' talk are part of this tale. Alasuutari (1995) and Frank (2004) both compare writing up research to authoring a detective or mystery story. The readers will be so captured by it that they feel they have to read it to the end to uncover the solution of the research problem. Indeed, many qualitative researchers set the scene to capture the readers' attention and make them curious about what will happen and understand what is at stake. The researchers show 'what is going on' in the setting and why social actors behave in a particular way. Alasuutari (1995) suggests that, even in a piece of scientific work, the writer does not leave spoken language too far behind. Yes, a research report is a piece of scientific writing, but it need not be turgid and incomprehensible. Writing a lively and scholarly account is not easy. Authors sometimes feel that they must state in an introductory paragraph to each chapter what they will write in it and summarize the chapter at the end. In a qualitative study this might disturb the continuity of text and story. Good advice comes from Alasuutari (1995: 191): 'One should aim at a story line that carries the text forward without the need for continuous bridging.' Where bridging is used the writer needs to ensure that it is not artificial, and that chapters or sections flow naturally into each other.

Frank advises researchers to uncover and show incongruities between the expected and the discovered as this produces 'narrative tension'. Authors of the text can also achieve narrative tension by showing that they were surprised by what they found. This might lead to more awareness and insight into people's experiences as well as new theoretical ideas. My own example from the work of a nurse researcher demonstrates some of this: Joy Warren (1995), in her research about the emotional experience of hospital patients expected participants to voice 'fear of dying' as their strongest emotion. Of course, patients did fear death, but their comments centred mostly on 'being embarrassed' as their most overwhelming feeling during the course of their hospital stay. This feeling became part of an interesting and lively discussion.

Another tension is concerned with the structure of the text. An interesting and exciting story is not always well structured. A story that is systematic, complete and ordered may be dry or boring. Of course, the real world is not tightly ordered and systematic, but a piece of academic writing should show that the author has worked within a framework. The author must consider the balance between re-presenting the exciting 'real' world and being mindful of the fact that academic and research work need also be structured. A good narrative alone does not make a research study of high quality. A purely descriptive report that includes statements from the participants and examples from observation is not complete. While Frank gives advice on writing a story, he also stresses the need for theory and the pattern that helps the story hang together. John Diamond's (1998) book on his cancer contains a fascinating, though sad, story; many of the participants in health professionals' research tell a good tale. These narratives are helpful for those who wish to examine an experience of illness, but to become a scholarly text they need to be based on theory or generate it. Readers of the work would expect pattern and theory, and a scholarly text, but the research report does not start out with this; it has to be worked at. Theory is not the only aspect of scholarship, of course. Authors also might have to challenge assumptions and present the 'case' for the findings.

The author's representation also needs immediacy, an 'aha experience' for the reader, a recognition of 'I knew that, I'm sure, but I haven't heard it like this before'. Readers feel this because they share a common humanity with the participants and the researcher and often have similar experiences and feelings. Frank (2004: 432) suggests that readers should 'recognise the problems faced by those being written about as their own problems, and that recognition makes the story compelling'. (Of course, there is never total access to the experiences and feelings of others, as each person inhabits an individual reality as well as sharing a social world.) Often the use of metaphor enriches the writing to help the reader understand the story. In this, again, the research account is like a novel. Throughout the writing process, the story unfolds. Although the authors have an outline given by the experience of the participants, they are still grappling with the findings themselves and try to make sense of what they found.

Conclusion

There is no one single way of writing up research (Woods 1999). Individuals have their own inimitable style and have to write accordingly; their identities can be found in the text. It is not easy to negotiate the fine line between making the story interesting but not sentimental, to have both sense and sensibility, to include both ordinary and scientific language. Arthur Frank's book (1995) is one of the most fascinating accounts of experiences of illness I have read. He achieves an evocative and interesting account without losing out on scholarship. Indeed, he himself suggests (2004: 431) that '... interest becomes a crucial criterion for scholarly writing'. He also stresses the need for commitment (p. 432) '... where there is no commitment, there cannot be any real excitement either, because nothing much is at stake for anyone except fellow specialists'.

Commitment and passion without sentimentality or exaggeration are crucial in writing up qualitative research. Only then can the author convince the reader. An important attribute of a good piece of qualitative research is 'persuasability', a horrible neologism but a simple concept. Each author of a piece of qualitative research has to give a story in which he or she persuades the readers that what they read is authentic and credible. Frank and Wolcott sound convincing when they write about research. I may never be able to write with the same evocative style and excitement as Frank, Eisner or van Manen. I hope, however, that qualitative researchers and readers of this book will find a way to convey the reality of the participants and their own part in the research with vivacity and honesty.

References

Alasuutari, P. (1995) *Qualitative Method and Cultural Studies*. London: Sage.

Atkinson, P.A. (1997) Narrative turn or blind alley? *Qualitative Health Research*, 7 (3): 325–344.

Atkinson, P. and Silverman, D. (1997) Kundera's immortality: the interview society and the invention of the self, *Qualitative Inquiry*, 3 (3): 304–325.

Bochner, A.P. (2001) Narrative's virtues, *Qualitative Inquiry*, 7 (2): 131–157.

Bryman, A. (2001) *Social Research Methods*. Oxford: Oxford University Press.

Charmaz, K. (1997) Identity dilemmas of chronically ill men. In Strauss, A. and Corbin, J. (eds) *Grounded Theory in Practice*. Thousand Oaks: Sage, 35–59.

Charmaz, K. (2003) Grounded Theory. In Smith, J.A. (ed.) *Qualitative Psychology: A Practical Guide to Research Methods*. London: Sage, 81–110.

Charmaz, K. (2004) Premises, principles and practices in qualitative research: revisiting the foundations, *Qualitative Health Research*, 14 (7): 976–993.

Charmaz, K. and Mitchell, R.G. (1997) The myth of silent authorship: self, substance and style in ethnographic writing, *Symbolic Interactionism*, 19 (4): 285–302.

Coffey, A. (1999) *The Ethnographic Self: Fieldwork and the Representation of Identity*. London: Sage.

Cutcliffe, J.R. and McKenna, H.P. (2004) Expert qualitative research and the use of audit trails, *Journal of Advanced Nursing*, 45 (2): 126–135.

Dahlberg, K., Drew, N. and Nyström, M. (2001) *Reflective Life-world Research*. Lund: Studentlitteratur.

Darlington, Y. and Scott, D. (2002) *Qualitative Research: Stories from the Field*. Buckingham: Open University Press.

Davies, B., Browne, J., Gannon, S., Honan, E., Law, C., Mueller-Rockstroh, B. and Bendix Peterson, E. (2004) The ambivalent practices of reflexivity, *Qualitative Inquiry*, 10 (3): 360–389.

Denzin, N.K. (1989a) *The Research Act: A Theoretical Introduction to Sociological Methods*, 3rd edn. New Jersey: Prentice-Hall.

Denzin, N.K. (1989b) *Interpretive Interactionism*. Newbury Park, CA: Sage.

Diamond, J. (1998) *C: Because Cowards Get Cancer Too*. London: Vermilion Press.

Erlandson, D.A., Harris, E.L., Skipper, B.L. and Allen, S.D. (1993) *Doing Naturalistic Inquiry*. Newbury Park: Sage.

Finlay, L. (2002) 'Outing the researcher': The provenance, process and practice of reflexivity, *Qualitative Health Research*, 12 (4): 531–545.

Frank, A.W. (1995) *The Wounded Storyteller: Body, Illness and Ethics*. Chicago: University of Chicago Press.

Frank, A.W. (2000) The standpoint of the storyteller, *Qualitative Health Research*, 10 (3): 354–365.

Frank, A.W. (2004) After methods, the story: From incongruity to truth in qualitative research, *Qualitative Health Research*, 14 (3): 430–440.

Geertz, C. (1973) *The Interpretation of Cultures*. New York: Basic Books.

Guba, E.G. and Lincoln, Y.S. (1989) *Fourth Generation Evaluation*. New York: Sage.

Guillemin, M. and Gillam, L. (2004) Ethics, reflexivity and 'ethically important moments' in research, *Qualitative Inquiry*, 10 (2): 261–280.

Hammersley, M. (1998) *Reading Ethnographic Research: A Critical Guide*, 2nd edn. London: Longman.

Harris, M. (1976) History and significance of the emic/etic distinction, *Annual Review of Anthropology*, 5, 329–350.

Holliday, A. (2002) *Doing and Writing Qualitative Research.* London: Sage.

Holloway, I. (1997) *Basic Concepts in Qualitative Research.* Oxford: Blackwell Science.

Holloway, I. and Wheeler, S. (2002) *Qualitative Research in Nursing*, 2nd edn. Oxford: Blackwell Science.

Koch, T. and Harrington, A. (1998) Reconceptualising rigour: The case for reflexivity, *Journal of Advanced Nursing*, 28: 882–890.

Lewis, C. (2004) Personal communication.

Lincoln, Y.S. and Guba, E.G. (1985) *Naturalistic Inquiry.* Beverly Hills: Sage.

Mantzoukas, S. (2004) Issues of representation within qualitative inquiry, *Qualitative Health Research*, 14 (7): 994–1007.

Mason, J. (2002) *Qualitative Researching*, 2nd edn. London: Sage.

Mattingley, C. (2000) Emergent narratives. In Mattingley, C. and Garro, L.C. (eds) *Narrative and the Cultural Construction of Illness.* Berkeley: University of California Press, 181–211.

Morse, J.M. and Richards, K.L. (2002) *Read me First for a Nurses Guide to Qualitative Methods.* Thousand Oaks: Sage.

Murphy, E., Dingwall, R., Greatbatch, D., Parker, S. and Watson, P. (1998) Qualitative Research Methods in Health Technology Assessment, *Health Technology Assessment*, 2, 16.

Polkinghorne, D. (2003) From presentation at the Conference Qualitative Research in Health and Social Care, Bournemouth University.

Rodgers, B.L. and Cowles, V. (1993) The qualitative audit trail: a complex collection of documentation, *Research in Nursing and Health*, 16: 219–226.

Sandelowski, M. (1986) The problem of rigor in qualitative research. *Advances in Nursing Science*, 8 (3): 27–37.

Sandelowski, M. (1993) Rigor or rigor mortis: the problem of rigor in qualitative research revisited, *Advances in Nursing Science*, 15 (2): 1–8.

Schostak, J.F. (2002) *Understanding, Doing and Conducting Qualitative Research in Education: Framing the Project.* Buckingham: Open University Press.

Schwandt, T.A. (2001) *Dictionary of Qualitative Inquiry.* Thousand Oaks, CA: Sage.

Seale, C. (1999) *The Quality of Qualitative Research.* London: Sage.

Smith, J.A. and Osborn, M. (2003) Interpretative phenomenological analysis. In Smith, J.A. (ed.) *Qualitative Psychology: A Practical Guide to Research Methods.* London: Sage, 51–60.

Sparkes, A. (2001) Myth #94: Qualitative health researchers will agree about validity, *Qualitative Health Research*, 11 (4): 538–552.

Strauss, A. and Corbin, J. (1998) *Basics of Qualitative Research: Techniques and Procedures for Developing Grounded Theory*, 2nd edn. Thousand Oaks: Sage.

Todres, L. (1998) The Qualitative Description of Human Experience: The Aesthetic Dimension, *Qualitative Health Research*, 8 (1): 121–127.

Todres, L. and Holloway, I. (2004) Descriptive phenomenology: life-world as evidence. In Rapport, F. (ed.) *New Qualitative Methodologies in Health and Social Care Research.* London: Routledge, 79–98.

Van Maanen, J. (1988) *Tales of the Field.* London: Sage.

van Manen, M. (2002) *Writing in the Dark: Phenomenological Studies in Interpretive Inquiry.* London, Ontario: Althouse Press.

Warren, J. (1995) The emotional experience of hospital. Unpublished MPhil dissertation, Bournemouth University.

Wetherall, M. (2001) Debates in discourse research. In Wetherall, M., Taylor, S. and Yates, S.J. (eds) *Discourse Theory and Practice*. London: Sage, 380–398.

White, C., Woodfield, K. and Ritchie, J. (2003) Reporting and presenting qualitative data. In Ritchie, J. and Lewis, J. (eds) *Qualitative Research Practice*. London: Sage, 287–320.

Wolcott, H. (1994) *Transforming Qualitative Data: Description, Analysis and Interpretation.* Thousand Oaks, CA: Sage.

Wolcott, H. (2001) *Writing Up Qualitative Research*, 2nd edn. Thousand Oaks, CA: Sage.

Woods, P. (1999) *Successful Writing for Qualitative Researchers*. London: Routledge.

Conclusion: after completion

How to proceed at the end of the research

Most researchers know that there is not much point in carrying out research without disseminating it to a relevant readership and an interested audience; it is of limited use if it gathers dust in a drawer of an agency or the library of a university. Research studies contribute to the knowledge and understanding about a particular phenomenon or a group of people, as well as about of treatment, care and behaviour in clinical or classroom settings. The publication of the research will also help to develop collaboration across the professions and disciplines in the future.

Consequently, communication of findings to appropriate agencies and audiences is a responsibility of the researcher. (A word of warning here: researchers have to be clear about the ownership of the research before publicizing it.) Indeed, academics often start dissemination before the study is complete. For qualitative health researchers the readership or audience generally includes practitioners in the health- and social-care professions, academics and other scholars in the field and, occasionally, the public at large.

The most common way to communicate research results is by presenting them in journal articles. Authors of these generally shape the writing for a specific journal and a particular audience. These journals make different demands on the writer; for instance, the editors of the *British Medical Journal* contain contributions that differ drastically from those in *Social Science and Medicine*. All, however, would expect clarity and high standards. The writing for practitioners would be different from that for scholars, the former would contain an explicit section on implications for practice while the latter would, among other elements, present a theoretical framework.

Oral reports in the form of seminars, presentations at conferences and posters are also common, but they do not usually mirror the depth and width of a research study as well as written work does, though they can be more interesting and useful to the audience. Some researchers present their research in book form – though this happens rarely. All writing and presenting demands not only familiarity with the researcher's own research but also with the literature and research connected to it.

Qualitative research in the health- and social-care field generally develops new questions and demands new answers. Any research study always has limitations and cannot ever be fully finished or include all implications for practice; the latter may only be recognized over time. Also, there is never just one single type of explanation for a phenomenon, for behaviours or feelings, and the researcher is aware of this. Qualitative health research is demanding; it can be challenging and frustrating. Human beings are not wholly predictable as some scientists might have us believe. Nevertheless nothing is more fascinating than obtaining the perspectives of people on their own reality. Gaining insight into their world through observing their behaviour, and grasping the meanings that they give to their experience is interesting and rewarding for the researcher, but it also generates useful knowledge and evidence which assists professionals in practice.

Glossary of main terms used in this text

Many of these terms are used differently in quantitative research or in other contexts. They have been simplified for the purpose of a short glossary.

Action research
A collaborative and cyclical approach to research in which a group of practitioners and/or researchers seek a solution to a problem in practice or to generate change in a setting.

Aide-mémoire (or aide memoir)
A short written note with keywords or points relevant to the research question that the researcher wants to explore.

Assumption
A taken-for-granted belief or assertion which has not necessarily been tested or verified.

Audit trail (or decision trail)
The path of the decision-making processes. The qualitative research report should have a clear audit trail so that trustworthiness or validity of the research can be established.

Authenticity
The extent to which the findings of research represent fairly and accurately the social world of the participants and the phenomenon under study (term used by Lincoln and Guba).

Bias
A distortion in the data collection, analysis or interpretation that prevents neutrality. It means that the subjectivity of the researcher – or the participant – has a strong influence on the research. As subjectivity is seen as one of the resources of the researcher, and the perspectives of the participants are important, this term is not often used in qualitative research.

Bracketing
A suspension of belief and preconceptions.

Category
A cluster of concepts or codes with similar traits.

Code
A name or identifying label given to a specific segment or concept.

Coding
Breaking the data into segments in the process of analysis and assigning a label to them.

Concept
An abstract or generalized idea that describes a phenomenon.

Constant comparison
Qualitative data analysis where the data collected are compared with other incoming data (a term from grounded theory).

Construct
A group of several concepts or categories that has a level of abstraction. The term is often used for a major category that has been developed from collapsing and integrating several smaller categories.

Constructionism (or constructivism)
An approach in social science based on the assumption that human beings construct their social reality, and that the social world cannot exist independently of human beings. In research terms this means that participants and researcher construct meaning together.

Context
The background of culture, location, history and conditions in which the research takes place.

Contextualization
A discussion of the data and findings in relation to the context of the research.

Convenience sample (or opportunistic sample)
A sample chosen because it is easily accessible to the researcher, or the only form of sampling possible, given resource limitations.

Core category
An integrative concept that relates to all other categories developed from the data (from grounded theory).

Credibility
A quality assessment of whether the data convincingly describe the phenomenon which is being researched. The researcher's ability to demonstrate that the study accurately and fairly describes the phenomenon under study.

Criterion
A standard or benchmark by which something is evaluated (plural: criteria).

Critical theory
The critical study of social phenomena and institutions, including their power structures. Its aim is to change society in order to assist marginal and powerless groups to become emancipated.

Data
Information the researcher collects from observations, interviews and other sources (literally 'given things'). Although data is a plural noun, it is often used as though it were singular.

Data analysis
Exploration of the meaning of data through processes of organization, reduction and transformation combined with consulting and linking relevant, related studies in the same field.

Deduction
The procedure of testing a general principle or hypothesis to explain specific phenomena or cases.

Design
The overall plan of the research, including methods and procedures for collecting, analyzing and interpreting data.

Description
A detailed account of the significant phenomenon or phenomena in the research.

Emic perspective
The *insiders'* view of their social world (from anthropology).

Epistemology
An area of philosophy concerned with the nature of human knowledge.

Essence
'The whatness of things' (from Spiegelberg). Essence is what makes something what it is, its most invariant features expressed in linguistic terms.

Ethnography
An approach to research concerned with describing a culture or group and its members' experiences, beliefs, attitudes and behaviours, as well as their location in the culture. It is both process and product: researchers carry out ethnography and write an ethnography.

Ethnomethodology
A branch of sociology that is concerned with social actions and interaction.

Etic perspective
The view of the researcher (or of another outsider to the study) presenting a generalized and theoretically informed perspective.

Evaluation research
The collection of information to explore effectiveness and characteristics of programmes, to improve outcomes.

Feminist research
A stance in research that has as its central concern the lives and voices of women, or is concerned with gender as a variable. The feminist stance might be present in any research approach but is more often associated with qualitative forms of inquiry.

Fieldnotes
A record or description of thoughts, theoretical ideas, observations and quotes from the field.

Fieldwork
Research in the social arena, such as observing, interviewing and other types of work 'in the field'.

Focused interview

An interview in which questions are focused on emerging and relevant issues. In some research approaches, such as grounded theory, interviews become 'progressively more focused'.

Focus group

A group of people often with similar experiences or common traits who are interviewed as a group in order to obtain their thoughts and perceptions about a particular topic, or an exploration of the way in which they talk about these issues within a particular context. Attention to the interaction between research participants is an essential part of this method.

Gatekeepers

People who have the power to allow or restrict access to a setting or people.

Generalizability (also called external validity)

The extent to which the findings of a study apply to other settings or groups in the population. The extent to which a theory grounded in the data can be transferred to similar situations or people (in grounded theory). Qualitative researchers more often use the term 'transferability'.

Grounded theory

An approach to research in which theory is generated from the data through constant comparison.

Hermeneutics

A branch of phenomenology that focuses on the theory and practice of interpretation. In research terms it is interpretation rather than description of a phenomenon.

Hypothesis

An assumption or statement of a relationship between variables which can be tested, verified or falsified.

Immersion

Engagement and involvement in the setting in which the research takes place.

Induction

In qualitative research, an approach to analysis that goes from specific instances of data to general rules or theory.

Informant

A participant in the group or culture under study who provides information for the research (used in ethnography).

Informed consent

A voluntary agreement made by participants after having been informed of the nature and aim of the research.

Interpretivism

An approach to knowledge in the social sciences that focuses on human beings and the way in which they interpret and make sense of their reality.

Intersubjectivity
A process in which human beings share meanings and assumptions with each other. A reciprocity of perspective between people.

Interview (qualitative interview)
A dialogue between the researcher and a research participant with the purpose of eliciting the participants' perspectives or ideas about a phenomenon of interest. (Interviews vary for different research approaches and purposes.)

Interview guide
Questions or keywords which are used flexibly by the interviewer in semi-structured interviews, in order to elicit answers on a particular topic area or research problem.

In vivo code
Labels or names taken from the participants' own words.

Iteration
Continuous movement back and forth between parts of the research text and the whole, between raw data and analyzed data (sometimes called tacking).

Key informant
A member of a culture or group being studied who engages systematically to share his or her knowledge with the researcher. The person generally has long-standing, expert knowledge of its rules, customs and language.

Life-world
People's experience of their lives and environments as they appear naturally and taken for granted in the everyday (from phenomenology).

Member check
A return to the participants with either the transcript, summary of their answers or field-notes from observation to establish whether the description or interpretation truly presents their experience. A member check can be used to establish trustworthiness.

Memoing
Recording in writing a memo or memos.

Memos
Written ideas by the researcher of varying degrees of abstraction when carrying out field-work in the form of notes and records to assist in formulating a theory (term from grounded theory).

Method
Procedures and strategies for collecting, analyzing and interpreting data.

Methodology
The framework of theories and principles on which methods and procedures are based.

Method slurring
An inappropriate mix of methods or approaches.

Narrative
A 'storied representation'. This can be the description of experiences by the participants in a study or the reconstruction of their lives or experiences by the researcher in a research account.

Naturalistic inquiry
Investigation of 'naturally occurring' behaviour and talk. This takes place in a 'natural' setting rather than in a laboratory or artificially created situation. (The term can be misleading as it is often confused with naturalism in quantitative research which approaches social phenomena in the same way as it does natural or physical phenomena.)

Objectivity
A neutral and unbiased stance. Qualitative researchers often maintain that this is impossible to achieve and suggest instead that they need to be clear about the standpoint from which they write and to be reflexive about their approach.

Ontology
A branch of philosophy concerning the nature of being. It is related to assumptions about the nature of reality.

Paradigm
A theoretical perspective or philosophical stance of a community of scholars. This position provides the researcher with a set of beliefs about the world that guide the research.

Participant observation
Observation in which the researcher becomes a participant in the setting that is being researched. There are three types of participant observation on a continuum between complete observer and complete participant.

Phenomenology
A philosophy that focuses on the 'life-world' or 'lived experience' of human beings through their own descriptions. It is also a research approach that explores individuals' lived experiences.

Phenomenon
The main concept, event or occurrence experienced by participants that is being researched or which emerges from the research (plural: phenomena).

Positivism
A paradigm approach to knowledge that aims to find general laws, based on observation and experiment, while applying the methods of the natural sciences. (The term is first used by Comte, the nineteenth-century philosopher.)

Postmodernism
A stance which rejects absolute 'truths' and absolutist frameworks that explain human action or society. The focus is on plurality and diversity rather than a single truth. Postmodernist researchers believe that reality is socially constructed.

Premature closure
Completion of the data collection and analysis before saturation has been achieved.

Progressive focusing
A process that starts with a broad question and becomes more specific and funnelled during the interview or observation process.

Proposition
A hypothesis about categories in research. The researcher develops working hypotheses throughout the research (mainly used in grounded theory and ethnography).

Purposive sample (or purposeful, or criterion-based sample)
A sample of participants selected on the basis of certain criteria relevant to the research.

Reflection
Critical examination of the research process.

Reflexivity
Examining and uncovering the researcher's place in the research process.

Research aim
The intention of the researcher to uncover something about the phenomenon under study in order to answer the research question.

Research question
The statement or problem that is being researched.

Rigour
A standard in research which seeks detail, accuracy, trustworthiness and credibility.

Saturation
A state where no new data of importance to the study emerge and when the elements of all categories are accounted for.

Subjectivity
A personal view influenced by personal background and traits. In qualitative research, subjectivity can be a resource.

Symbolic interactionism
An approach in sociology that focuses on symbols and meaning in interaction. The term was used in the sociology and social psychology of George Herbert Mead.

Tacit knowledge
Implicit knowledge that is shared but not openly articulated and sometimes not even consciously held.

Theoretical sampling
Sampling that proceeds on the basis of emerging, relevant concepts and is guided by developing theory.

Theoretical sensitivity
Awareness and insight of the researcher that assists in detecting meaning in the data (originally from grounded theory but now also used in other approaches).

Theory
A set of interrelated concepts and propositions or a general principle that explains a phenomenon or phenomena, sometimes presented in terms of a model.

Thick description
Dense and conceptual description, including meanings and motivation, that gives a sense and picture of events and actions within the social context. This term is used specifically in ethnography (and discussed by the anthropologist Geertz) but also in other approaches.

Triangulation
The combination of different research methods, data collection approaches, investigators or theoretical perspectives in the study of one phenomenon. This is a way of attempting to ensure validity or credibility.

Trustworthiness
The credibility of the findings in a piece of qualitative research and the extent to which readers can have trust in the research and its findings (term used by Lincoln and Guba).

Validity
The extent to which the researcher's findings reflect the purpose of the study and represent reality and demonstrate integrity and quality. Validity in qualitative research differs from that in quantitative research; qualitative researchers often use the terms 'trustworthiness' and 'authenticity'.

Verification
The testing of a hypothesis through empirical validation. (In Straussian grounded theory it means testing a proposition or a working hypothesis.)

Verstehen
Empathetic and interpretive understanding of the meaning of another person's point of view; grasping the sense of a phenomenon.

Index

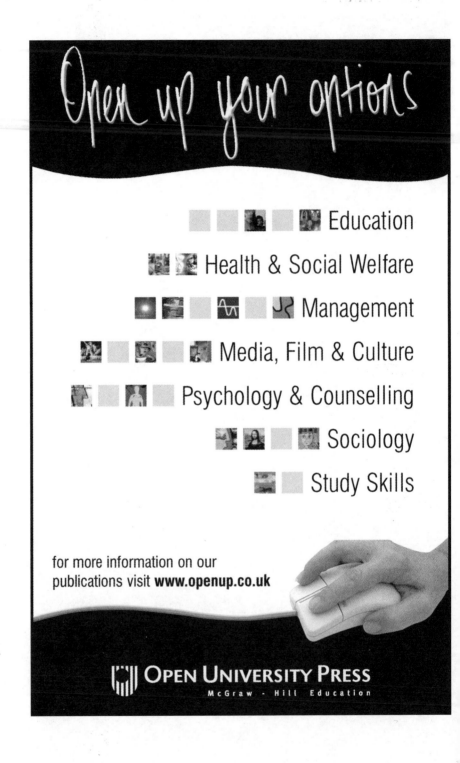